Child and Adolescent Depression

Guest Editors

STUART J. GOLDMAN, MD
FRANCES J. WREN, MD

CHILD AND ADOLESCENT PSYCHIATRIC CLINICS OF NORTH AMERICA

www.childpsych.theclinics.com

Consulting Editor
HARSH K. TRIVEDI, MD

April 2012 • Volume 21 • Number 2

SAUNDERS an imprint of ELSEVIER, Inc.

W.B. SAUNDERS COMPANY
A Division of Elsevier Inc.

Elsevier Inc. • 1600 John F. Kennedy Boulevard • Suite 1800 • Philadelphia, Pennsylvania 19103-2899

http://www.childpsych.theclinics.com

CHILD AND ADOLESCENT PSYCHIATRIC CLINICS OF NORTH AMERICA Volume 21, Number 2
April 2012 ISSN 1056–4993, ISBN-13: 978-1-4557-3840-3

Editor: Joanne Husovski

Child and Adolescent Psychiatric Clinics of North America (ISSN 1056-4993) is published quarterly by Elsevier Inc., 360 Park Avenue South, New York, NY 10010-1710. Months of issue are January, April, July, and October. Business and Editorial Offices: 1600 John F. Kennedy Boulevard, Suite 1800, Philadelphia, PA 19103-2899. Periodicals postage paid at New York, NY and additional mailing offices. Subscription prices are $297.00 per year (US individuals), $453.00 per year (US institutions), $150.00 per year (US students), $343.00 per year (Canadian individuals), $546.00 per year (Canadian institutions), $190.00 per year (Canadian students), $408.00 per year (international individuals), $546.00 per year (international institutions), and $190.00 per year (international students). International air speed delivery is included in all *Clinics* subscription prices. All prices are subject to change without notice. **POSTMASTER:** Send address changes to *Child and Adolescent Psychiatric Clinics of North America,* Elsevier Health Sciences Division, Subscription Customer Service, 3251 Riverport Lane, Maryland Heights, MO 63043. **Customer Service: 1-800-654-2452 (U.S. and Canada); 314-447-8871 (outside U.S. and Canada). Fax: 314-447-8029. E-mail: JournalsCustomerService-usa@ elsevier.com (for print support) or journalsonlinesupport-usa@elsevier.com (for online support).**

Reprints. For copies of 100 or more of articles in this publication, please contact the Commercial Reprints Department, Elsevier Inc., 360 Park Avenue South, New York, New York 10010-1710 Tel.: (212) 633-3812; Fax: (212) 462-1935, e-mail: reprints@elsevier.com.

Child and Adolescent Psychiatric Clinics of North America is covered in *MEDLINE/PubMed (Index Medicus), ISI, SSCI, Research Alert, Social Search, Current Contents,* and *EMBASE/Excerpta Medica.*

Printed and bound by CPI Group (UK) Ltd, Croydon, CR0 4YY
Transferred to Digital Print 2012

Contributors

CONSULTING EDITOR

HARSH K. TRIVEDI, MD
Associate Professor of Psychiatry, Vanderbilt University School of Medicine; and Executive Medical Director, and Chief of Staff, Vanderbilt Psychiatric Hospital, Nashville, Tennessee

CONSULTING EDITOR EMERITUS

ANDRÉS MARTIN, MD, MPH

FOUNDING CONSULTING EDITOR

MELVIN LEWIS, MBBS, FRCPSYCH, DCH

GUEST EDITORS

STUART J. GOLDMAN, MD
Associate Professor of Psychiatry, Harvard Medical School; Director of the Mood Disorders Clinic, Children's Hospital Boston, Boston, Massachusetts

FRANCES J. WREN, MD, MB, MRCPsych
Adjunct Clinical Associate Professor, Department of Psychiatry and Behavioral Sciences, Stanford University School of Medicine, Stanford, California

AUTHORS

JOAN R. ASARNOW, PhD
Professor of Psychiatry and Biobehavioral Sciences, UCLA Semel Institute for Neuroscience and Human Behavior, Los Angeles, California

TARA M. AUGENSTEIN, BA
Research Assistant, Department of Psychiatry, Children's Hospital Boston, Boston, Massachusetts

WILLIAM R. BEARDSLEE, MD
Director, Baer Prevention Initiatives; Chairman Emeritus, Department of Psychiatry, Children's Hospital; Gardner/Monks Professor of Child Psychiatry, Harvard Medical School; Judge Baker Children's Center, Boston, Massachusetts

BORIS BIRMAHER, MD
Professor of Psychiatry, Endowed Chair in Early Onset Bipolar Disease, Western Psychiatric Institute and Clinic, University of Pittsburgh Medical Center, Pittsburgh, Pennsylvania

KATHRYN DINGMAN BOGER, PhD
Clinical Instructor in Psychiatry, McLean Hospital, Belmont; Harvard Medical School, Boston, Massachusetts

DAVID A. BRENT, MD
Western Psychiatric Institute and Clinic, Department of Psychiatry, University of Pittsburgh School of Medicine, Pittsburgh, Pennsylvania

GREG CLARKE, PhD
Kaiser Permanente Center for Health Research, Portland, Oregon

EUGENE J. D'ANGELO, PhD
Chief, Division of Psychology, Department of Psychiatry; Director, Outpatient Psychiatry Service, Department of Psychiatry; Children's Hospital Boston; Associate Professor of Psychology, Department of Psychiatry, Harvard Medical School, Boston, Massachusetts

JANE MESCHAN FOY, MD
Professor, Department of Pediatrics, Wake Forest University School of Medicine, Winston-Salem, North Carolina

TRACY R.G. GLADSTONE, PhD
Department of Psychiatry, Children's Hospital; Judge Baker Children's Center, Boston; Wellesley Centers for Women, Wellesley College, Wellesley, Massachusetts

STUART J. GOLDMAN, MD
Associate Professor of Psychiatry, Harvard Medical School, Director of the Mood Disorders Clinic, Children's Hospital Boston, Boston, Massachusetts

ALLISON G. HARVEY, PhD
Department of Psychology, University of California, Berkeley, Berkeley, California

PATRICIA I. IBEZIAKO, MD
Assistant Professor in Psychiatry, Harvard Medical School; Psychiatry Consult Service, Children's Hospital Boston, Boston, Massachusetts

ROBERT Li KITTS, MD
Clinical Instructor of Psychiatry, Harvard Medical School; Attending Psychiatrist, Children's Hospital Boston, Boston, Massachusetts

MARIA KOVACS, PhD
Distinguished Professor of Psychiatry, Department of Psychiatry, University of Pittsburgh School of Medicine, Pittsburgh, Pennsylvania

NESTOR L. LOPEZ-DURAN, PhD
Assistant Professor, Department of Psychology, University of Michigan, Ann Arbor, Michigan

FADI T. MAALOUF, MD
Assistant Professor of Psychiatry, Department of Psychiatry, American University of Beirut Medical Center, Beirut, Lebanon; Adjunct Assistant Professor of Psychiatry, University of Pittsburgh School of Medicine, Pittsburgh, Pennsylvania

ERIN E. O'CONNOR, BA
Judge Baker Children's Center, Boston, Massachusetts

UMA RAO, MD
Center for Molecular and Behavioral Neuroscience, Department of Psychiatry and Behavioral Sciences, Meharry Medical College; Department of Psychiatry, Vanderbilt University School of Medicine, Nashville, Tennessee

DARA SAKOLSKY, MD, PhD
Instructor of Psychiatry, Western Psychiatric Institute and Clinic, University of Pittsburgh Medical Center, Pittsburgh, Pennsylvania

MARTHA C. TOMPSON, PhD
Associate Professor, Department of Psychology, Boston University, Boston, Massachusetts

JOHN M. WEIR, PhD, MPH
Center for Molecular and Behavioral Neuroscience, Meharry Medical College, Nashville, Tennessee

FRANCES J. WREN, MD, MB, MRCPsych
Adjunct Clinical Associate Professor, Department of Psychiatry and Behavioral Sciences, Stanford University School of Medicine, Stanford, California

ARTHURINE ZAKAMA
Vanderbilt University, Nashville, Tennessee

Contents

> Definitions, understanding, and treatment of childhood depressive disorders are changing. The last 40 years have seen a move from questioning whether depression even existed in younger children to evidence-based descriptive models. The field is now moving toward developmentally informed multifactorial models that more accurately reflect the complexity, heterogeneity, and dimensionality of depressive disorders. Knowledge about genetic, temperamental, and developmental risks has increased. Inability to self-regulate seems to be common in depressive and related disorders. Positive modulation can be promoted through experiences, psychotherapies, and, possibly, medications. The authors provide an overview of childhood depressive disorders with emphasis on the developmental/etiologic underpinnings.

> This article discusses recent findings on the neurobiology of pediatric depression as well as the interplay between genetic and environmental factors in determining the risk for the disorder. Utilizing data from both animal and human studies, the authors focus on the evolving understanding of the developmental neurobiology of emotional regulation, cognitive function and social behavior as it applies to the risk and clinical course of depression. Treatment implications and directions for future research are also discussed.

> This article focuses on discussing risks for depression onset and the role of environmental factors in promoting resilience in children and adolescents. The authors review the current literature on specific (eg, family history of depression) and nonspecific (eg, poverty, stressful life events) risk factors for youth depression to underscore the need for prevention efforts promoting resiliency in this population.

article begins with the authors' definition of the elements that should comprise such an intervention. A succinct summary of this contextual emotion regulation therapy is then provided, including its explanatory paradigm of depression, followed by an exposition of how it addresses the various definitional criteria of a developmentally informed intervention. The article concludes with a brief overview of the challenges of implementing a developmentally sensitive psychotherapy for depressed children and adolescents.

Treatment models for youth depression that emphasize interpersonal functioning, particularly family relationships, may be particularly promising. This article first reviews the current state of knowledge on the efficacy of psychosocial treatments for depression in youth, with an emphasis on family involvement in treatment. It then discusses developmental factors that may impact the applicability and structure of family-focused treatment models for preadolescent and adolescent youth. Finally, two family-based treatment models that are currently being evaluated in randomized clinical trials are described: one focusing on preadolescent depressed youth and the other on adolescents who have made a recent suicide attempt.

Psychological and pharmacologic treatments for youth depression yield post-acute response and remission rates that are modest at best. Improving these outcomes is an important long-term goal. The authors examine the possibility that a youth cognitive behavioral therapy *insomnia* intervention may be an adjunct to traditional depression-focused treatment with the aim of improving depression outcomes. This "indirect route" to improving youth depression treatment outcomes is based on research indicating that the risk of depression is increased by primary insomnia and that sleep problems interfere with depression treatment success and on emerging *adult* depression randomized controlled trial results. The authors describe the protocol they developed.

SECTION III: DISSEMINATING DEVELOPMENTALLY INFORMED INTERVENTIONS FOR CHILD AND ADOLESCENT DEPRESSION

This article outlines the importance of primary health care in addressing the public health challenge presented by pediatric depressive disorders. The current realities of depression management in primary care

are discussed. The models emerging from intervention research and the barriers to their implementation in practice are then reviewed. Drawing on this background, recent new standards for primary care management of pediatric depressive disorders are discussed, along with resources that have been developed to support their achievement.

Robert Li Kitts and Stuart J. Goldman

This article is intended to assist educators in the medical field in promoting competency among medical students and trainees on the key issues in child and adolescent depression, including approach, understanding, and management. Using clinical vignettes, up-to-date research, and expert opinion and referencing accessible guidelines, resources, and tools, the authors' goal is to create information that is engaging and useful. It is designed to reach a broad audience with emphasis on trainees who are early in their career path (eg, medical students or interns) and/or who are going into primary care.

CHILD AND ADOLESCENT PSYCHIATRIC CLINICS

FORTHCOMING ISSUES

Anxiety Disorders
Moira A. Rynn, MD, Hilary Vidair, PhD,
and Jennifer U. Blackford, PhD,
Guest Editors

Psychopharmacology
Harsh K. Trivedi, MD, and
Kiki Chang, MD, *Guest Editors*

Psychodynamic Psychotherapy
Rachel Ritvo, MD, and
Shirley Papilsky, MD,
Guest Editors

RECENT ISSUES

January 2012
Evidence-Based School Psychiatry
Jeffrey Q. Bostic, MD, EdD, and
Alexa L. Bagnell, MD, FRCPC,
Guest Editors

October 2011
**Gender Variant Childern and
Transgender Adolescents**
Richard R. Pleak, MD, *Guest Editor*

July 2011
Forensic Psychiatry
William Bernet, MD, and
Bradley W. Freeman, MD, *Guest Editors*

RELATED INTEREST

Psychiatric Clinics of North America, March 2012
Depression
David L. Mintz, MD, *Guest Editors*
http://www.psych.theclinics.com/

NOW AVAILABLE FOR YOUR iPhone and iPad

Preface

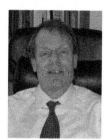

Stuart J. Goldman, MD   Frances J. Wren, MD
Guest Editors

The childhood depressive disorders, in aggregate, affect approximately 15% of all children and adolescents by the age of 18. The toll on individuals and families is immense. As a field we are evolving from a static, linear descriptive concept of the depressive disorders to a broader developmentally informed, transactional model of understanding. Our knowledge of biological vulnerability, expressed through genetic, temperamental, and developmental risk, and its transactions with the environment is ever-expanding. Recent work on emotional regulation gives a powerful new lens through which to view the evolution across childhood and adolescence of the lived experience and clinical presentation of depression. We have a richer picture of the depressed child, and the child at risk for depression, in interaction with family and the wider world. We know more about the development and the developmental psycho-pathology of coping strategies. These advances give provocative clues to the actual processes whereby well-established risk and protective factors might interact to produce, sustain, or curtail a depressive syndrome. This in turn opens the door to treatment and prevention approaches that are truly developmentally informed. It is through this complex, rapidly evolving set of developmentally informed lenses that we present the articles in this monograph.

This presentation emphasizes a developmentally informed approach and is organized into three sections. The first, Development and Depression, presents four topics, beginning with a developmentally informed overview of the depressive disorders. Then, the next two topics cover the biological and experiential underpinnings of depression, followed by a developmentally informed approach to assessment.

The second section, Developmentally Informed Interventions for Child and Adolescent Depression, begins with an overview of interventions. It then presents a more detailed review of the pharmacological interventions and continues on to three novel intervention frameworks. The first is a novel, evidence-based approach to school-age children, *Contextual Emotional Regulation Therapy*, that integrates cutting-edge developmentally informed approaches to regulation and is delivered

Child Adolesc Psychiatric Clin N Am 21 (2012) xiii–xiv
doi:10.1016/j.chc.2012.03.001
1056-4993/12/$ – see front matter

childpsych.theclinics.com

through collaboration with parents. The second appreciates the systemic, family-based nature of the depressive disorders and discusses two promising, developmentally informed family interventions with depressed youth. The third expands the complex biological reverberations of the depressive disorders into the realm of sleep and offers novel approaches to treatment of this biological disruption as an adjunctive intervention for Depressive Disorders.

The third, final section recognizes that no treatment or preventive strategy can be effective unless it is available to children and families. Given the very modest number of child and adolescent mental health specialists, any effective strategy to make it more available must incorporate primary health care. In addition, there must be effective education directed toward professionals and students, at all levels, within the health care field. The first of the last two topics addresses these challenges by looking at depression in primary care and at recent advances in tools and concepts to support primary care clinicians. The final topic offers a case-based template as a model for educating health care professionals about childhood depression.

Stuart J. Goldman, MD
Harvard Medical School, Children's Hospital Boston
Boston, MA 02115, USA

Frances J. Wren, MD
Department of Psychiatry and Behavioral Sciences
Stanford University School of Medicine
Stanford, CA 94305, USA

E-mail addresses:
Stuart.goldman@childrens.harvard.edu (S.J. Goldman)
fwren@standford.edu (F.J. Wren)

Erratum

Reference Omission

The author of: Goldstein, TR (2009). Suicidality in Pediatric Bipolar Disorder. Child and Adolescent Psychiatric Clinics of North America, 18:339-352 wishes to recognize that page 346 (Safety Planning) contains material drawn from the following source:

Brent, D., Brown, G., Curry, J., Goldstein, T., Hughes, J., Kennard, B., Poling, K., Schlossberg, M., Stanley, B., Wells, K. (Version 7, September, 2008). Cognitive Behavioral Therapy for Adolescent Suicide Attempters (CBTASA) Manual. Unpublished manuscript.

Child Adolesc Psychiatric Clin N Am 21 (2012) xv
doi:10.1016/j.chc.2012.01.009

childpsych.theclinics.com

1056-4993/12/$ – see front matter © 2012 Elsevier Inc. All rights reserved.

Developmental Epidemiology of Depressive Disorders

Stuart Goldman, MD[a,b],*

KEYWORDS

- Depressive disorders • Children
- Developmental epidemiology • Evidence-based

Definitions, understanding, and treatment of childhood depressive disorders are dramatically changing. The last 40 years have seen a move from questioning whether depression even existed in younger children to the evidence-based descriptive models framed by the first through fourth, and soon fifth, editions of the *Diagnostic and Statistical Manual of Mental Disorders* (*DSM*). The field is now moving toward developmentally informed, multifactorial models that more accurately reflect the complexity, heterogeneity, and dimensionality of the syndromes called depressive disorders. Knowledge of biological vulnerability, expressed through genetic, temperamental, and developmental risk, and its interactions with the environment have grown logarithmically. Complex transactional models for depression must continue to be developed, and earlier linear models are far too limited. In a simple but overarching way, it is now recognized that an underlying or acquired inability to self-regulate is a common cornerstone for depressive and related disorders (anxiety, oppositional, substance abuse, and so forth) and that self-regulation is a multidetermined skill that can be modulated or learned. Positive modulation can be promoted developmentally through everyday experiences or through specific psychotherapies, and possibly medications. In many ways the brain, like the rest of the body, is an experience- or practice-dependent organ. Good practice (experience and subsequent learning) promotes emotional regulation, and poor practice promotes the dysregulation that, in interaction with genetic vulnerability, may lead to depression and anxiety as well as a myriad of other difficulties. Seen through this lens, understanding and promoting the brain's developmental "experience" at self-regulation becomes a critical frame for patients, parents, clinicians, and researchers.

The authors have nothing to disclose.
[a] Harvard Medical School, USA
[b] Mood Disorders Clinic, Children's Hospital Boston, USA
* Corresponding author.
E-mail address: Stuart.goldman@childrens.harvard.edu

Child Adolesc Psychiatric Clin N Am 21 (2012) 217–235
doi:10.1016/j.chc.2011.12.002
1056-4993/12/$ – see front matter © 2012 Elsevier Inc. All rights reserved.

childpsych.theclinics.com

Increasingly, treatment as well as diagnosis have been grounded in evidence-based observation, a vital shift in the field. The current diagnostic schema (*Diagnostic and Statistical Manual of Mental Disorders, Fourth Edition, Text Revision, DSM-IVTR*) classifies depressive disorders by their severity (both symptoms and dysfunction) and the presence or absence of mania. To enhance interrater reliability it treats the depressive disorders as discrete categories. However, this approach has not been without acknowledged compromises.[1] It falls far short of appreciating that patients, development, and depression all exist on a continuum that occurs in a specific context and that understanding, diagnosis, and subsequent interventions must too.[1] Striking the balance between the individual case and the class or category is an unresolved challenge.[1] In this article the authors provide an overview of childhood depressive disorders with particular emphasis on their developmental/etiologic underpinnings. This overview sets the stage for the more detailed developmentally informed wide-ranging articles to follow.

CLASSIFYING DEPRESSION—WHAT'S IN A NAME?

The study of any disease or disorder begins with reliably and validly being able to name the disorder. For all the depressive disorders, especially in the pediatric population, this identification has been problematic. Most would agree that the hallmark of depressive disorders, across all ages, is persistent and impairing dysphoria, anhedonia, or mania. However, without clear causes or biological markers, the diagnosis becomes phenomenologically based on symptoms known to be continuously distributed within the population,[2] inherently making depressed patients a heterogeneous group.[2] Using cutoff score approaches, as in *DSM -IVTR*, one can reliably identify "patients," but the resultant group heterogeneity severely limits the ability to understand, define, treat, and predict outcomes for all depressed patients.[2] This difficulty becomes even more limiting for children and adolescents because *DSM-IVTR*, with rare exceptions, uses only adult-derived criteria to define the child and adolescent depressive disorders, minimizing the known developmental variations between children, adolescents, and adults. However, because there is no current alternative, one must rely on the *DSM*-based classification system. The *DSM* classification begins with the presence or absence of mania and goes on to categorize mood disorders into mania/hypomania *absent* the set of unipolar disorders; in other words, major depressive episode or dysthymia and the mania/hypomania *present* set of bipolar disorders. As in each *DSM* diagnosis, the symptoms must cause dysfunction and are not primarily due to other causes. Following is a closer look at the present criteria.

Criteria for Major Depressive Episode

DSM-acknowledged developmental considerations are bolded.

A. Five (or more) of the following symptoms have been present during the same 2-week period and represent a change from previous functioning; at least one of the symptoms is either (1) depressed mood or (2) loss of interest or pleasure.
   1. Depressed mood most of the day, nearly every day, as indicated by either subjective report (eg, feels sad or empty) or observation made by others (eg, seems tearful). **Note: in children and adolescents, can be irritable mood.**
   2. Markedly diminished interest or pleasure in all, or almost all, activities most of the day, nearly every day (as indicated by either subjective account or observation made by others).

3. Significant weight loss when not dieting or weight gain (eg, a change of more than 5% of body weight in a month), or decrease or increase in appetite nearly every day. **Note: in children, consider failure to make expected weight gains.**
4. Insomnia or hypersomnia nearly every day.
5. Psychomotor agitation or retardation nearly every day (observable by others, not merely subjective feelings of restlessness or being slowed down).
6. Fatigue or loss of energy nearly every day.
7. Feelings of worthlessness or excessive or inappropriate guilt (which may be delusional) nearly every day (not merely self-reproach or guilt about being sick).
8. Diminished ability to think or concentrate, or indecisiveness, nearly every day (either by subjective account or as observed by others).
9. Recurrent thoughts of death (not just fear of dying), recurrent suicidal ideation without a specific plan, or a suicide attempt or a specific plan for committing suicide.

B. The symptoms do not meet criteria for a mixed episode.
C. The symptoms cause clinically significant distress or impairment in social, occupational, or other important areas of functioning.

Criteria for Dysthymic Disorder

Changes for children and adolescents are bolded.

A. Depressed mood for most of the day, for more days than not, as indicated either by subjective account or observation by others, for at least 2 years. **Note: in children and adolescents, mood can be irritable and duration must be at least 1 year.**
B. Presence, while depressed, of two (or more) of the following:
   1. Poor appetite or overeating.
   2. Insomnia or hypersomnia.
   3. Low energy or fatigue.
   4. Low self-esteem.
   5. Poor concentration or difficulty making decisions.
   6. Feelings of hopelessness.

Criteria for Mania

Note: there are no *DSM* developmental considerations.

A. A distinct period of abnormally and persistently elevated, expansive, or irritable mood, lasting at least 1 week (or hospitalization). Hypomania symptoms are the same but lasting at least 4 days.
B. During the mood disturbance three (four if the mood is only irritable) or more of the following have persisted or have been present to a significant degree:
   1. Inflated self-esteem or grandiosity.
   2. Decreased need for sleep (but feels rested).
   3. More talkative or pressure to keep talking.
   4. Flight of ideas.
   5. Distractibility.
   6. Increase in goal-directed activity (socially, work, or sexually).
   7. Excessive involvement in pleasurable activities that have a high potential for adverse consequences.

From a developmental framework many of these criteria are reasonably applicable, with modest developmental consideration, to adolescent patients, particularly the older ones. However, earlier in childhood many of the criteria (excessive guilt, indecisiveness, worthlessness, thoughts of suicide, among others) have varying to minimal developmental applicability. Additionally, when other "developmentally adapted criteria" (for instance, marked irritability) are seen as being a depressive or manic equivalent in children, the results have complicated and further muddied already challenging waters.[3] **Table 1** represents a composite of the variability in depressive symptoms across the developmental span when using today's symptom criteria.

From the table (see **Table 1**), one sees in children that the depressive disorders are appreciably more symptomatically variable and that this variability (both within age group and when compared with adults) decreases with chronological age. Additionally, for younger children, many of the symptoms may be observed rather than self-reported. However, somewhat paradoxically, whereas depressed teens look increasingly like adults, they still do not respond to clinical interventions like adults, based on the outcomes of a myriad of antidepressant studies. This disparity has resulted in the lack of US Food and Drug Administration (FDA) approval for all but a few of the antidepressants approved for adult usage. Although it is clear that age/development moderates depressive symptomology, it is unclear as to the extent and the details of how age/development mediates symptom presentation. This uncertainty and the biological differences between children, adolescents, and adults clearly are arenas for future exploration.

For bipolar disorders and diagnosing mania, the field has been muddled even more. Whereas it is almost unquestioned that juvenile bipolar disorder was underdiagnosed in the more distant past, the ultimately unsubstantiated "developmental" adaptations[4] had broadened the diagnosis, (particularly of bipolar II and not otherwise specified, or NOS) well beyond a meaningful category.[5] As a field, we are now just recovering.[5] Whereas this has been an evolving story, at least for the present, based on *DSM*, developmental considerations take the form of how the core symptoms are developmentally expressed (moderated by age), rather than that there are different core symptoms expressed at different ages (mediated by age). In other words, the core symptoms of mania: rapid thoughts, decreased sleep, grandiosity, and increased, often inappropriate, goal-directed activity (including hyper-sexuality) all are seen as critical but take on an age-adjusted form. So grandiosity may present as, "I am smarter than my teacher," rather than, "I am going to make a million dollars in the next year." Hypersexuality may present as inappropriate, poorly modulated behaviors or interests, like peering under the desks rather than actual overt sexual acts. Of course, in all cases additional etiologic and developmental considerations should be taken into account.

Naming the disorder becomes even more complex and perhaps even less meaningful when one considers additional factors beyond the lack of developmental modification:

First, the vast majority of children and adolescents with a depressive disorder have a comorbid disorder or disorders[6] (anxiety, attention-deficit/hyperactivity disorder, substance abuse, or other) seen in both the identified patient and the family.

Second, whereas certain childhood disorders (depression, anxiety, oppositional defiant disorder) do seem to predict an increased risk of depression across the lifespan, they also predict increases in anxiety, behavioral disorders, and substance abuse disorders.

Issues of continuity and heterotypic and homotypic predictions of risk remain to be sorted out. For example Reinherz and colleagues[7] found that childhood anxiety cluster symptoms predict depression in 18- to 26-year-olds, and in a recent

Table 1
Presentation of depression symptoms by age group

Symptom	Preschool	School Age	Adolescent	Adult
Dysphoria	+++ but more time/activity variability, can be challenging to elicit	+++ more persistent than in younger children, but still variable	+++ can present as isolation	+++
Anhedonia	+++ but varies in time—seems to not have much fun	+++ varies but less so over time—seems to lack or reports lack of fun	+++ may also present as boredom	+++
Irritability	+++	+++	+++	++
Acting Out	+++	+++	+++	+
Decreased Energy	+	++	+++	+++
Sleep Disturbance	+/−	+/−	+++	+++
Weight Loss/Appetite Change	+	+	++	+++
Other Somatic Complaints	+++	+++	++	+
Delusions	Very rare	Very rare	+	++ but increases with age

+++ common, ++ less frequent, + infrequent, +/− variably present longitudinal study, Copeland and colleagues[8] found that it was only comorbid anxiety and behavioral disorders that accounted for the link between adolescent depression and adult depressive disorders; adolescent depression did not. This was further substantiated by Kendler and colleagues'[9] finding of shared (anxiety and depression) genetic risk in a Swedish twin study. At the clinical level, depressive and anxiety-based disorders generally respond to the same pharmacologic interventions (selective serotonin reuptake inhibitors, SSRIs), further suggesting a common biological diathesis or set of diatheses and resultant physiology. So, when multiple sources of evidence are taken together, we seem to be identifying patients who at their core have a neurobiologic diathesis for what Andrews and colleagues[10] have called emotional cluster disorders and others have labeled neuroticism.[11] In other words, the depressive disorders are one of a set of disorders embedded in a core inability to emotionally self-regulate, and this inability takes on several interrelated forms or sets of symptoms that may lead to separate or interrelated diagnoses.

Despite these limitations, current nomenclature is vital in that it serves as scaffold and springboard that allow us to study and care for patients. Our current nomenclature offers comfort for patients, families, and clinicians by providing a "name." However, it is also clear that the aforementioned concerns, among others, make it imperative that clinicians and researchers recognize that current nomenclature only provides a clinical and scientific way station on the road to greater understanding.[1] This and subsequent articles of necessity rely on the structure of the current nosology but also strive to go beyond. They describe the leading efforts at moving from the current, static, limited yet reliable, phenomenological frameworks to the dynamic, developmental, and complex individualized processes that offer a far better fit to the growing body of clinical and research evidence and have the potential to ultimately result in improved clinical interventions.

VULNERABLE CHILDREN

Identifying vulnerable children offers insight into understanding, preventing, diagnosing, and treating depressive disorders. Current models of vulnerability are almost universally grounded in a gene by environment (G×E) pathway, but specific, valid, and reproducible findings have been elusive.[12] Complicating matters further is that biological and experiential factors sort into those that present nonspecific general risk (learning disabilities, poverty, family dysfunction) and those that may be more specific to the depressive disorders (prior or family history of depression, low positive affectivity). (For further details see article by Beardslee and colleagues elsewhere in this issue.) In any case, fundamental identification of vulnerability needs to start with the biological underpinnings, and biological risk has been well-established. Genetic studies have repeatedly demonstrated the heritability of depressive disorders. Monozygotic twin studies have found concordance rates of 40% to 65%.[13] In families, both bottom-up (children to parents) and top-down (parents to children) studies have found that there is a 2- to 4-fold[14] bidirectional increase in unipolar depression among first-degree relatives. However, increased rates of anxiety, behavioral, and substance abuse disorders may also be seen. Genetic factors in pediatric bipolar disorders are more complex to ascertain, but the data seem to be at least as compelling, with both bottom-up and top-down studies finding significant increases in rates (3 to 6 times)[15] and monozygotic twin concordance rates in the up-to-60% range.[15]

The exact nature of what makes up biological vulnerability is less clear. Transporter genes, the hypothalamic-pituitary-adrenal (HPA) axis, affective and vagal tone, cerebral variations (in both form and development), as well as cognitive style all seem transactionally interrelated and have been implicated as components of biological vulnerability. (See article by Singh and Gotlib elsewhere in this issue.) Additionally, with the marked increase in depression seen at age 13 (especially for girls),[16] pubertal hormonal factors, along with the marked neurophysiologic/neurocognitive changes of adolescence, also must be accounted for. If the current trends continue, it seems that depressive disorders are the end product of multiple processes that are both highly complex and heterogeneous. However, because these factors all seem to mediate the broad category called the ability to self-regulate, reliable epigenetic measures, particularly those effecting self-regulation, may evolve that allow better identification and estimation of risk.

Reflective of this mediation, Kovacs and Lopez-Duran[17] have found that children at risk for depression have less positive affectivity, less mood repair (the appropriate attenuation of sad, dysphoric affect), and evidence of impaired functioning in the three intertwined physiologic systems noted previously (HPA, cerebral, vagal). This combination may make both for greater reactivity to environmental factors and also impair affective repair, resulting in a feed-forward process that makes their affective state even more highly dysregulated. Similarly, Luby and colleagues[18] found that vulnerable preschoolers are less able to attenuate their dysphoria and demonstrate less positive and more negative behaviors.

Environmental factors are also highly important, and twin studies have shown that environmental[9] factors are at least as powerful as genes in determining depressive disorders. The range of known adverse experiences that increase depressive risk is extensive, broadly predicting multiple adverse outcomes including depression.[19,20] These risk factors include poverty, stressful life events, parental psychopathology (depression, substance abuse, and criminality), as well as low family cohesion.[19,20] More direct familial maltreatment of children in the form of abuse, neglect, and harsh parenting has also been implicated, as has maltreatment by peers (bullying). Losses of all types including bereavement and medical illness also increase rates of depression.[19,20] Physiologically, all of these stressors certainly impact the HPA axis; however, why some go on to develop disorders and others do not is under investigation.

Current efforts at unpacking the nature of both depression-specific and general environmental risk have examined risk factors stratified in multiple manners. Among the more productive has been examination of the specific risk factors stratified by the age of depression onset (childhood, adolescence, young adulthood) and proximity (recency) to adverse events.[21] In contrast to earlier studies, the investigators found that childhood onset and young adult onset depression shared common risk factors that were best explained by a recency-based (proximity in time) approach to predicating risk. In contrast, adolescent onset depression seemed to follow a somewhat separate risk model, perhaps accounted for by increases in pubertal hormones[16] or biopsychosocial and cognitive interactions,[22] or the rapid neurologic remodelling characteristic of this age. (For more details see the article by Singh and Gotlib elsewhere in this issue.) An important exception to the recency model of risk was that childhood-occurring poverty, loss, or violence predicted future depression[21] across all ages as well as predicting a range of other difficulties.

Cognitive vulnerability emerges transactionally from biological and experiential factors. The development of cognitive vulnerability has been variously defined as depressive attributional style,[23] negative cognitive schemata, and as a negatively biased processing of information.[24] Studies of children and adolescents have linked preexisting cognitive vulnerabilities as factors that lead to increases in depression as well as products of being depressed.[24] Directly altering attributions, schema, and biased processing are the targets of cognitive behavioral therapy (CBT), the most evidence-based psychotherapy.

These biological, experiential, and cognitive factors seem almost to conspire transactionally in a feed-forward manner toward depression. Young children having as few as two depressive symptoms for a week are highly likely to have a depressive episode as they get older.[17] From a distance, and somewhat simply put, the following equation seems to capture the likelihood of a depressive outcome: (negative affectivity-positive affectivity) $\times$ environment = depression. That is, the biologically at-risk with high negative affectivity and low positive affectivity need only a minimal environmental multiplier to become depressed, whereas the biologically less vulnerable (low negative, high positive affectivity) need major environmental multipliers. Given the challenges of reliably identifying genetic risk,[12] using affectivity as an epigenetic marker may ultimately be more productive.

MAKING THE DIAGNOSIS—AN OVERVIEW

In the current schema, the diagnosis of each of the depressive disorders is a descriptive one, with *DSM* as the gold standard. This gold standard has been unpacked and then repackaged in multiple instruments (for more details see the article by D'Angelo and Augenstein elsewhere in this issue) including structured interviews (K-SADS, DISC) and questionnaires (CDI, HAM-D). *DSM*-based criteria also serve as the standard for making the diagnosis by carefully elicited clinical history from both the parents/guardians and the child, coupled with the child interview/ mental status examination. Most clinicians and some studies use both approaches, but because almost all current diagnostic approaches and validation studies derive from the same *DSM*-based original source, they do not provide true convergent validity.

This tautologic dilemma becomes the first main dilemma in making a diagnosis, because all of the gold standards can be no more valid than the original *DSM*-derived criteria that they are based on.

Muddying the diagnostic waters even further and becoming the second major diagnostic dilemma is that with some of the unipolar depressive disorders, and even more so with the bipolar disorders (particularly those other than bipolar I), nonvalidated modifications or extensions of *DSM* criteria were promoted. In the most dramatic instance this promotion led to a tidal wave of bipolar diagnoses and bipolar treatments, none of which had been validated. This trend added a major layer of uncertainty in diagnosis and treatment to an already questionable foundation. Fortunately, this surge seems to be waning.[3]

The third problem is that developmentally and clinically, children are much more embedded in a family context. There are compelling data (see article by Tompson and Asarnow elsewhere in this issue) that family context is vital toward understanding, preventing (see article by Beardslee and colleagues elsewhere in this issue), and treating depressed children (see article by Kovacs and Lopez-Duran and Tompson and Asarnow elsewhere in this issue), particularly preadolescents. Current diagnostic tools almost universally fail to recognize the importance of context as a both a mediator and moderator for depressive disorders.

Finally, clinicians must be mindful that many disorders mimic or have overlapping symptoms with the depressive disorders; these include bereavement or adjustment disorders, oppositional defiant disorder, pervasive developmental disorder, and substance abuse, as well as a myriad of medical disorders including hypothyroidism, infections, some cancers, and autoimmune diseases. Careful clinical consideration and exclusion of these disorders should be part of any best-practice approach.

Although we remain constrained by our current schema, as noted earlier, exciting efforts at capturing a truer essence of the depressive and other disorders are under way.[10]

EPIDEMIOLOGY

All discussions on prevalence are innately constrained by the diagnostic limitations described previously. It is thought that lifetime rates of depression in adults are about 20%, with an annual rate approaching 10%, and that the vast majority of these begin in childhood. In adults, women are approximately twice as likely (25%) as men (10% to 15%) to suffer from depression, according to the *DSM*. Societal costs for adults are estimated in the tens of billions of dollars (30-plus), and this estimate is without the additional costs of pediatric depression. Adolescent rates of unipolar depression seem relatively comparable to those for adults. It is estimated that by the end of adolescence, upwards of 20%[6] will have a depressive episode (major depression or dysthymia), with girls twice as likely as boys to be affected. Annual rates of adolescent depression are estimated in the 4% to 9%[6] range, pooling both the dysthymic and major depressive disorders. For the majority of these adolescents, symptoms that are quite consistent with adult depression are present.

Rates of the bipolar disorders in adolescents and children are less clear but are presumed to be lower than in the adult population and are estimated in aggregate to be approximately 1% to 2%.[15] It is estimated that over 20% of youths presenting with unipolar depression will have a future bipolar episode/disorder,[25] with earlier onset depression presenting a greater risk.[25] Expert consensus is that the cardinal symptoms of mania (as described previously) must be present to meaningfully make the diagnosis.[26]

In prepubertal children, ascertaining the prevalence rates of depression is more challenging. However, with the appropriate developmental diagnostic accommodations[27] there is compelling support for lower but reliably diagnosable rates as early as in the preschool population. Although symptoms in the younger age groups are appreciably more varied, the core symptoms of anhedonia (with its lowered positive affectivity) and dysphoria remain the most reliable cornerstones.[27] The estimates of combined major depression and dysthymia in the prepubertal group are in the 1% to 2.5% range, with boys and girls having comparable rates.[6]

In the prepubertal population the epidemiology of bipolar disorders has been clouded by controversy, as noted previously. Most clinicians believe, with good reason, that bipolar disorders in the prepubertal population are far rarer than in adolescents, for whom bipolar disorder is rarer than in adults. Applying a developmentally adjusted set of criteria based on the actual manic or hypomanic criteria is now the standard of practice.[26] However, additionally, there is a clear population of highly dysregulated, challenging school-aged children that fits poorly into current nomenclature, does not grow up to have adult bipolar disorder, and has been described by Leibenluft[3] to have "severe mood dysregulation."[3] Clearly, these children have a mood-disordered dimensional problem, but they have been poorly served when forced into the bipolar category.[3]

Further supporting the idea of dimensionality in this prepubertal population is that anxiety disorders are a more prevalent set of problems than depressive disorders, with annual rates (6% to 8%)[28] that approximate later those of depression in adolescents. The potential that developmentally, the majority of children at risk for clinically significant dysregulation manifest it as anxiety in childhood and as depression in adolescents represents another important avenue to be explored.[28]

This broader conceptual frame of emotional dysregulation vulnerability is further supported by the high comorbidity seen in the major depressive disorders. Forty percent to 80% of children with major depressive disorders have a comorbid diagnosis, including anxiety disorders (30% to 80%), disruptive disorders (10% to 80%) and substance disorders (20% to 30%).[15,29] Clearly, there is much work to be done.

INTERVENTION

The ideal intervention is primary prevention, and clear progress in early primary intervention has been demonstrated.[30] (For further details see article by Beardslee and colleagues elsewhere in this issue.) Whereas depression for most children is a readily treatable disorder, the roots of and ongoing impact of all the depressive disorders are almost invariably complex and multidetermined. Quality care then demands that a detailed, multidimensional, systemic assessment of the biological, experiential, familial, social, and educational contributors should be part of any comprehensive assessment and intervention plan.[31] Once comprehensively assessed, care should be based on the best evidence-based practice and then individualized to address each factor as it presents in the specific child and family. Problematically, here is often where causative considerations, clinical practice, and research diverge. Causes are almost invariably multidimensional, and research trials are almost always, for many good reasons, monodimensional. Narrowing their focus, researchers may, in their pursuit of good science, inadvertently provide a disservice to patients and practitioners by not developing and studying the real-world integrated care that is needed. However, in all cases there is support for psychoeducation (**Appendix 1**), environmental and family support, and ongoing careful screening for existent or emergent comorbid disorders (anxiety, substance abuse, and so forth) or risky behaviors (suicide, self-injury) as part of every care plan.[31] Additionally, given the recurrent nature of depressive disorders, a plan that includes acute, maintenance, and monitoring components should be the default clinical plan and should be extended with regular meetings for at least 6 to 12 months after remission.[31] For many patients, longer term, less frequent monitoring (eg, monthly, quarterly) is recommended.[31]

In the mildest of depression, psychoeducation and environmental support may suffice. In more serious cases of unipolar depression (see article by Brent elsewhere in this issue), randomized clinical trials (RCTs) have demonstrated that approximately 60% of teens respond to CBT,[32] interpersonal psychotherapy,[33] or medication[32]; however, the size of the response is often modest. Whereas CBT is the most extensively studied and documented intervention, the effect size for CBT is clearly modest (0.36).[34] Furthermore, in a large study of teen depression (Treatment of Adolescents With Depression Study, or TADS), CBT was not superior to pill placebo and was inferior to fluoxetine in the first 12 weeks.[32] However, in the same study, rates of response to medication, CBT, and combined medication/CBT merged at 9 months,[32] and over the longer term, adding CBT had a positive impact on both secondary prevention and suicidality.[35,36] Although CBT has been adapted to preadolescents, the data are far less compelling.

Family-based interventions (see article by Tompson and Asarnow elsewhere in this issue) have the advantage of addressing the critical context that all children exist in and are not dependent on yet-to-be-developed cognitive skills (see article by Tompson and Asarnow elsewhere in this issue). Family-based intervention has increasingly been demonstrated over the last decade as an efficacious intervention in all children[37] and uniquely with younger children.[38]

RCT support exists for the use of certain SSRIs in adolescents and older children. (See article by Emslie elsewhere in this issue.) However, only fluoxetine (age 8) and escitalopram (age 12) have current FDA approval. The response rates have been approximately 60% (50% respond to placebo) with the number needed to treat in the range of 5% to 10.[39,40] The high pill placebo response rates (upwards of 45 to 50%[40]) have made demonstrating efficacy more challenging, and many attribute the modest effect size of SSRIs to high placebo response rate as well as potentially to other developmental factors. Venlafaxine has also been RCT-supported but does not have FDA approval for use by adolescents and older children.[41] To date, RCT support does not exist for use of SSRIs in the prepubertal population for depression except for fluoxetine. Despite this lack of support and perhaps encouraged by both the RCT and subsequent FDA support of SSRIs in prepubertal anxiety disorders, many practitioners have cautiously prescribed SSRIs for this population off-label, but without FDA support.

Whereas there are relatively few RCT studies of combined (pharmacologic and psychotherapeutic; see TADS[32]) intervention, practitioners most often recommend combination therapy for all of the moderate, severe, or refractory unipolar depressive disorders, particularly in adolescents. Further study is needed to better define optimal care indications and combinations. Ideally, these studies would include head-to-head comparisons; unfortunately, such comparison is rarely undertaken.

For bipolar disorders, multidimensional care is the standard of practice, and the care plan should include all of the general interventions noted previously. RCT studies of CBT and other psychotherapies have shown some support for use as a helpful adjunct,[15,26] (eg, in helping with adherence) but have not shown an adequate primary effect.[15,26] RCT and subsequent FDA support exists for lithium, valproate, and the majority of the novel neuroleptics (except ziprasidone) in adolescents, but there is no support to date in prepubertal populations. Whereas some clinical and case reports support this off-label extension to a younger population, many have expressed concern that an inappropriately low diagnostic threshold for this practice has led to overuse.

COURSE AND PROGNOSIS

The biological and experiential diathesis that makes one vulnerable to depressive disorders also seems to makes one vulnerable to reoccurrences and increases the risk of related disorders. These related disorders include anxiety (30%–80%), disruptive behaviors (10%–80%), and substance abuse (20%–30%). These interrelationships are seen both top-down and bottom-up for both individuals and families. The natural history in most patients of unipolar depressive disorders is that they remit over time and then reoccur. Almost all systematic follow-up in children has been limited to adolescents. For adolescents with major depression, the average untreated duration is 6 to 8 months,[42] and for those with dysthymia, 3.5 years.[43] Both conditions reoccur more often (up to 70% of the time) than not over the course of the next 5 years.[44] With treatment, about 60% of the depressive disorders at least partially respond within 3 to 4 months, and over time about 15% to 20% more respond.[32] This rate puts the aggregate response rate at over 80%.[32] However, looking more closely, the timing of these delayed responders bumps up against spontaneous remission (at 6 to 8 months), making the sorting out of later treatment responders from spontaneous (natural) remitters challenging. In one study, Treatment of Resistant Depression in Adolescents (TORDIA), that looked at SSRI treatment-resistant patients, 61% of nonresponders gained remission with successive treatments by 72 weeks.[45] Again, differentiating true responders from spontaneous remitters is challenging. Prognostically, in the TORDIA study, the investigators found that those who had more severe symptoms, failure to remit or long delays to fully remit, and comorbid disorders (including substance abuse) and already had a reoccurrence were individually at greatest risk for ongoing functional difficulties and future recurrences, albeit with some possible moderation by environment.[45]

For those with bipolar I disorder, the course and prognosis is more ominous. Whereas the percentage of those eventually recovering is comparable (70% to over 80%),[46] the time to recovery is far longer, with a median time of 78 weeks.[46] Additionally, the postrecovery course is compounded by significant, subsyndromic recurrent symptoms[47] and general functional impairment,[46] as well as common (60% to 70%) full syndromic recurrence in relatively short periods of time (10 to 12 months).[15] The juvenile form of bipolar I is truly a challenging disorder for children, families, and their care providers. Given the controversies and absence of reliable diagnostic data on children with bipolar II or NOS, course and prognosis cannot be reliably ascertained. However, for children who meet formal bipolar II or NOS diagnoses or those who approximate them dimensionally based on their level of dysfunction, there are clear reasons for concern, and ongoing, multidimensional interventions are indicated.

Given the chronic, intermittent, and often pervasive dysfunction associated with the depressive disorders, efforts at prevention are critical. Although some primary prevention efforts have demonstrated efficacy,[48,49] demonstrating secondary and tertiary prevention is still in the early stages.

SUICIDE

Children and adolescents with any of the depressive disorders are at risk for attempted or completed suicide, and approximately 70% of youths who complete suicide have a depression diagnosis.[50] Increased risk is undoubtedly driven by pervasive dysphoria/anhedonia, common known causes (trauma, loss), and comorbid risk factors (such as substance abuse), as well as the associated cognitive distortions (hopelessness and helplessness that are developmentally dependent) seen in depressive disorders.[51] Risk in the pediatric population is stratified by age and by diagnosis as it is in the general population, although detailed studies, particularly in younger patients, need to be carried out. In aggregate, suicide attempts by age 18 run from about 20% in major depression to 44% of bipolar I or II patients.[52] Fortunately, completed suicide rates remain in the vicinity of 1 in 10,000 for all adolescents, although completed suicides are statistically more common in the mood-disordered population. Identifying those adolescents most at risk is crucial, and struggling nonremitting depressed adolescent patients with substance abuse or prior history of attempts, including so-called nonsuicidal self-injury,[53] should be clinically flagged.

CONTROVERSIES

Depressive disorders that have been at the center of several controversies in the last decade have made the study and care of this patient population more complex. The "epidemic" of bipolar disorder noted in the professional literature from the mid- to late 1990s onward and in the lay literature over the last 5 to 10 years dramatically muddied the clinical waters. Whereas the disorder was likely underdiagnosed in earlier times, the broadening of the term to functionally include almost any child with serious disruptive behavior rendered the term highly controversial.[26] Far more critically, such reports led many parents to believe that their child had a lifelong, recurrent, often disabling illness and to well-documented overprescription, generally off-label, of powerful, complex, expensive, and often not benign medications. Eventually, longitudinal, systematic study was used to counter the epidemic (with new diagnostic[3] or even dimensional frames[10] being studied. However, despite these evolving patterns, the downstream ramifications continue still, albeit with some anecdotal evidence of slowing.

The bipolar epidemic also was one of the major sources of the pharmacy and polypharmacy pandemic seen today in the treatment of depressive disorders. This epidemic has resulted in the all-too-common treatment of subsyndromic or dysthymic irritability or negativity with powerful and often side effect–laden "mood stabilizers," all without a clear evidence base.[26,31] Additionally, whereas a significant portion of both bipolar and unipolar depressions may be refractory, there are no RCTs that clearly support the efficacy of polypharmacy for either unipolar or bipolar depression. Balance between the clinical need to treat according to the evidence base and doing no harm has at times been lost, spawning many controversial and some harmful clinical interventions. Although treating mood disorders can present notable challenges and clinicians are often pressed to do something, practitioners must rely on an evolving evidence base, doing no harm in the process.[26,31]

The relationship between SSRIs for depression and suicidality frames that last controversy. In 2003, based on an "evidence base,"[54] the FDA put a black box warning on what eventually evolved to all SSRIs and other antidepressants in the under-25 population. In the next year prescription rates dropped, and in parallel adolescent suicide rates went up for the first time in a decade.[54] Careful follow-up studies did demonstrate a two-fold increase in reported adverse suicide events, but all of these were in ideation or attempts; there has been no increase in suicide completions.[40] Importantly, a clinical study found that 12 times more depressed adolescents show a clinical response than an increase in suicidality.[40] Unfortunately, suicide rates have yet to return to pre–black box levels. Caution and careful monitoring should be part of every practitioner's care, with medications being judiciously used only as indicated as part of a comprehensive plan. With the exception of patients in a stable maintenance phase, medication alone is rarely good care.[26,31]

FUTURE DIRECTIONS

Our conceptualization of the complex nature of depressive disorders, although still limited, has grown much more rapidly than our ability to prevent, cure, or even minimize their impact. Far more complex and transactional models are being developed to help us understand the heterogeneous causes and presentation of depressive disorders. Ongoing efforts at refining both common and uniquely individualized elements of depressive disorders are also under way. How does depression evolve with development? What are the meta factors underlying depression and the other emotional dysregulatory disorders? What are the common underlying vulnerabilities to the cooccurring disorders, and what are the factors that determine the possible various outcomes? Can we use this evolving knowledge to refine our efforts at prevention? When prevention fails, can we then develop multidimensional integrated treatments that address the actual and specific way depression evolves in individuals and the systems around them? In the biological realm can we evolve clear, individual, and family-based pharmacogenomics to guide care? These concerns all bump up against the real limitations that define depression as a series of discrete disorders versus the clearly dimensional nature that risk, presentation, comorbidity, treatment, and prognosis present, all making an evolving diagnostic nomenclature almost inevitable.

These and other questions will serve as the foundation for future efforts, some of which are described in other articles in this issue. For clinicians, the question will always be, "How do we first understand and then apply evidence-based, best practice knowledge to the care of patients and their families in our office?" Shedding light on this complex question is a major focus of this issue.

APPENDIX 1
Psychoeducation in care plan for depression in children and adolescents

Introduction

- Depression is a complex disorder that is the end result of many factors that include stress, emotions, and biology. Whereas all depression has certain common features, each person's situation is unique. We are going to review with you those areas that are most often common to all depression, and then we will speak particularly about your or your child's depression. We will answer any questions that you may have as we go along.

Biology

- Depression is a biological illness that may include a variety of types of trouble with the brain's chemical messengers. We know that these changes can occur because of stress and that this stress can be emotional, environmental, or physical. There is a strong link between brain biology and the way we experience the world. Thus, serious depression is more than just being sad; most people generally cannot just "get over it" right away. We will help by addressing all the stresses (emotional, environmental, and biological) that we can, regardless of their source.
- Depression has a genetic underpinning in many people, which means that it runs in certain families and that it can at times be associated with other illness including anxiety, behavioral problems, and substance abuse disorders.
- There are two basic types of depression: one that only has symptoms on the down side (unipolar) and one that includes both ups and downs (bipolar).
- Depression may start in response to a serious or not-so-serious (to the outside observer) event or circumstance, but then it seems to be self-sustaining. We do know that for many people it is a product of stresses over time and that this stress and the subsequent depression can make people feel bad about themselves. This feeling is the source of the low self-esteem that is generally part of the depression.
- Depression is more common in adolescents and adults than in children and more common in women than men. Estimates are that about 1 in 5 teenagers will have a significant episode (far more girls than boys), and lifetime estimates are that up to about 1 in every 4 women and 1 in every 6 men will be affected.
- Depression is a recurrent illness. Most people will have more than one episode in their lifetime, and once you have been depressed, your vulnerability throughout life is increased.
- Most important, depression is a *highly treatable illness*. We will help tailor a treatment program for you and your family to help you get well. We will also identify ways in which you can minimize the likelihood of future episodes or manage them more easily should they reoccur.

Presentation

- Depression may have different types of onset but most often includes some type of unpleasant mood. This may be one of sadness, irritability, or anger, which can appear as hopelessness, severe boredom, or decreased self-esteem.

- There are less common disturbances of mood in patients with bipolar disorder that may present as a mixture of depression symptoms and increased energy, sleeplessness, being driven, and poorly controlled behaviors compounded by poor judgment.
- These difficulties may be episodic or present around-the-clock, but there is some continuity from day to day, and they must last for days or even weeks to be diagnosed as bipolar.
- Pediatric bipolar illness is uncommon, and most children with disruptive behaviors do not have bipolar disorder.
- Mood disturbances are almost always accompanied by symptoms of decreased performance at home and school and by social isolation. In addition, there may be physical symptoms with impairment in sleep, energy and appetite, and concentration. In some cases people may feel so bad that they become self-destructive.

Cognition

- Depression alters the way people think about the world and themselves.
- Negative thoughts and pessimism characterize depressed thinking. Depressed thinking means that people almost always see the world and themselves as a series of "half-empty glasses," rather than coming to an accurate perception of things as they are.
- Depressed thinking makes people believe that they are to blame for negative events.
- Depressed thinking makes people feel that they are powerless to change for the better.
- Depressed thinking makes people "forget" the positive events.
- Depressed thinking generally changes with intervention, and when it does, the depressed mood changes as well.

Impact on Family

- Children and adolescents exist in the context of a family.
- Families want the best for their children.
- Caregivers and children are not to blame for the illness.
- Depression, like any serious illness, disrupts family functioning.
- Family therapy or support will be helpful for the family and their child and often can make a big difference.
- Having an opportunity to tell "their family story" will help in managing the illness and in family functioning as a system.

Treatment

- Depression is a highly treatable disease that is best approached multimodally However, not every approach is right for every patient, and we will collaboratively, with their help, design an individual treatment plan.
- Individual work with the child will focus on identifying and resolving faulty, depressed thinking; interpersonal binds; an inability to soothe himself or herself or problem-solve; and any other problems as they emerge.
- Family therapy collaboration and support is vital to the child's progress.
- For some younger (school-aged) children, family therapy may be the primary intervention.

- Medication is quite safe when appropriately monitored and can be very helpful for more severe depression or more modest depression that fails to respond to psychotherapy.
- We use medication interventions to target specific symptoms that we will track. If a medication is not clearly helpful, we will not continue your child on that medication; however, if the depression remains, we may try additional medications or combinations of medications to help address the problem.

Prognosis

- The majority of depressions will resolve over time on their own; however, we can dramatically shorten the time course and lessen the child's suffering.
- About two-thirds of patients respond to psychotherapy.
- About two-thirds of patients who need medication respond to medication.
- The vast majority of patients will dramatically improve with intervention.
- However, most depression has a tendency to reoccur.
- Preventative efforts and follow-up will be part of the ongoing care to lessen the long-term impact of the depressive disorder.

The patient and family are then given a chance to review this information, and any questions are addressed.

REFERENCES

1. Hyman SE. The diagnosis of mental disorders: the problem of reification. Annu Rev Clin Psychol 2010;6:155–79.
2. Vitiello B. Prevention and treatment of child and adolescent depression: challenges and opportunities. Epidemiol Psychiatr Sci 2011;20:37–43.
3. Leibenluft E. Severe mood dysregulation, irritability, and the diagnostic boundaries of bipolar disorder in youths. Am J Psychiatry 2011;168:129–42.
4. Wozniak J, Biederman J, Kiely K, et al. Mania-like symptoms suggestive of childhood-onset bipolar disorder in clinically referred children. J Am Acad Child Adolesc Psychiatry 1995;34:867–76.
5. Carlson GA, Glovinsky I. The concept of bipolar disorder in children: a history of the bipolar controversy. Child Adolesc Psychiatr Clin N Am 2009;18:257–71, vii.
6. Costello EJ, Mustillo S, Erkanli A, et al. Prevalence and development of psychiatric disorders in childhood and adolescence. Arch Gen Psychiatry 2003;60:837–44.
7. Reinherz HZ, Paradis AD, Giaconia RM, et al. Childhood and adolescent predictors of major depression in the transition to adulthood. Am J Psychiatry 2003;160:2141–7.
8. Copeland WE, Shanahan L, Costello EJ, et al. Childhood and adolescent psychiatric disorders as predictors of young adult disorders. Arch Gen Psychiatry 2009;66:764–72.
9. Kendler KS, Gardner CO, Gatz M, et al. The sources of co-morbidity between major depression and generalized anxiety disorder in a Swedish national twin sample. Psychol Med 2007;37:453–62.
10. Andrews G, Goldberg DP, Krueger RF, et al. Exploring the feasibility of a meta-structure for DSM-V and ICD-11: could it improve utility and validity? Psychol Med 2009;39:1993–2000.
11. Ormel J, Stewart R, Sanderman R. Personality as modifier of the life change-distress relationship. A longitudinal modelling approach. Soc Psychiatry Psychiatr Epidemiol 1989;24:187–95.
12. Brzustowicz L, Freedman R. Digging more deeply for genetic effects in psychiatric illness. Am J Psychiatry 2011;168:1017–20.

13. Todd RD, Botteron KN. Family, genetic, and imaging studies of early-onset depression. Child Adolesc Psychiatr Clin N Am 2001;10:375–90.
14. Weissman MM, Wickramaratne P, Nomura Y, et al. Families at high and low risk for depression: a 3-generation study. Arch Gen Psychiatry 2005;62:29–36.
15. Pavuluri MN, Birmaher B, Naylor MW. Pediatric bipolar disorder: a review of the past 10 years. J Am Acad Child Adolesc Psychiatry 2005;44:846–71.
16. Angold A. Adolescent depression, cortisol and DHEA. Psychol Med 2003;33:573–81.
17. Kovacs M, Lopez-Duran N. Prodromal symptoms and atypical affectivity as predictors of major depression in juveniles: implications for prevention. J Child Psychol Psychiatry 2010;51:472–96.
18. Luby JL, Sullivan J, Belden A, et al. An observational analysis of behavior in depressed preschoolers: further validation of early-onset depression. J Am Acad Child Adolesc Psychiatry 2006;45:203–12.
19. Gilman SE, Kawachi I, Fitzmaurice GM, et al. Socio-economic status, family disruption and residential stability in childhood: relation to onset, recurrence and remission of major depression. Psychol Med 2003;33:1341–55.
20. Jaffee SR, Moffitt TE, Caspi A, et al. Differences in early childhood risk factors for juvenile-onset and adult-onset depression. Arch Gen Psychiatry 2002;59:215–22.
21. Shanahan L, Copeland WE, Costello EJ, et al. Child-, adolescent- and young adult-onset depressions: differential risk factors in development? Psychol Med 2011: 41:2265–74.
22. Ge X, Conger RD, Elder GH Jr. Pubertal transition, stressful life events, and the emergence of gender differences in adolescent depressive symptoms. Dev Psychol 2001;37:404–17.
23. Asarnow JR, Bates S. Depression in child psychiatric inpatients: cognitive and attributional patterns. J Abnorm Child Psychol 1988;16:601–15.
24. Kendall PC, Stark KD, Adam T. Cognitive deficit or cognitive distortion in childhood depression. J Abnorm Child Psychol 1990;18:255–70.
25. Geller B, Fox LW, Clark KA. Rate and predictors of prepubertal bipolarity during follow-up of 6- to 12-year-old depressed children. J Am Acad Child Adolesc Psychiatry 1994;33:461–8.
26. McClellan J, Kowatch R, Findling RL. Practice parameter for the assessment and treatment of children and adolescents with bipolar disorder. J Am Acad Child Adolesc Psychiatry 2007;46:107–25.
27. Luby JL, Heffelfinger A, Koenig-McNaught AL, et al. The Preschool Feelings Checklist: a brief and sensitive screening measure for depression in young children. J Am Acad Child Adolesc Psychiatry 2004;43:708–17.
28. Axelson DA, Birmaher B. Relation between anxiety and depressive disorders in childhood and adolescence. Depress Anxiety 2001;14:67–78.
29. Angold A, Costello EJ. Depressive comorbidity in children and adolescents: empirical, theoretical, and methodological issues. Am J Psychiatry 1993;150:1779–91.
30. Horowitz JL, Garber J, Ciesla JA, et al. Prevention of depressive symptoms in adolescents: a randomized trial of cognitive-behavioral and interpersonal prevention programs. J Consult Clin Psychol 2007;75:693–706.
31. Birmaher B, Brent D, Bernet W, et al. Practice parameter for the assessment and treatment of children and adolescents with depressive disorders. J Am Acad Child Adolesc Psychiatry 2007;46:1503–26.
32. Kennard B, Silva S, Vitiello B, et al. Remission and residual symptoms after short-term treatment in the Treatment of Adolescents with Depression Study (TADS). J Am Acad Child Adolesc Psychiatry 2006;45:1404–11.

33. Klomek AB, Mufson L. Interpersonal psychotherapy for depressed adolescents. Child Adolesc Psychiatr Clin N Am 2006;15:959–75, ix.

34. Weisz JR, McCarty CA, Valeri SM. Effects of psychotherapy for depression in children and adolescents: a meta-analysis. Psychol Bull 2006;132:132–49.

35. Kennard BD, Silva SG, Tonev S, et al. Remission and recovery in the Treatment for Adolescents with Depression Study (TADS): acute and long-term outcomes. J Am Acad Child Adolesc Psychiatry 2009;48:186–95.

36. Emslie G, Kratochvil C, Vitiello B, et al. Treatment for Adolescents with Depression Study (TADS): safety results. J Am Acad Child Adolesc Psychiatry 2006;45:1440–55.

37. Asarnow JR, Scott C, Mintz J. A combined cognitive-behavioral family education intervention for depression in children: a treatment development study. Cognit Ther Res 2002;26:221–9.

38. Tompson MC, Pierre CB, McNeil Haber F, et al. Family-focused treatment for childhood-onset depressive disorders: results of an open trial. Clin Child Psychol Psychiatry 2007;12:403–20.

39. Bridge JA, Birmaher B, Iyengar S, et al. Placebo response in randomized controlled trials of antidepressants for pediatric major depressive disorder. Am J Psychiatry 2009;166:42–9.

40. Bridge JA, Iyengar S, Salary CB, et al. Clinical response and risk for reported suicidal ideation and suicide attempts in pediatric antidepressant treatment: a meta-analysis of randomized controlled trials. JAMA 2007;297:1683–96.

41. Emslie GJ, Findling RL, Yeung PP, et al. Venlafaxine ER for the treatment of pediatric subjects with depression: results of two placebo-controlled trials. J Am Acad Child Adolesc Psychiatry 2007;46:479–88.

42. Kovacs M. Presentation and course of major depressive disorder during childhood and later years of the life span. J Am Acad Child Adolesc Psychiatry 1996;35:705–15.

43. Kovacs M, Obrosky S, Gatsonis C, et al. First-episode major depressive and dysthymic disorder in childhood: clinical and sociodemographic factors in recovery. J Am Acad Child Adolesc Psychiatry 1997;36:777–84.

44. Kovacs M, Feinberg TL, Crouse-Novak MA, et al. Depressive disorders in childhood. Arch Gen Psychiatry 1984;41:643–9.

45. Vitiello B, Emslie G, Clarke G, et al. Long-term outcome of adolescent depression initially resistant to selective serotonin reuptake inhibitor treatment: a follow-up study of the TORDIA sample. J Clin Psychiatry 2010;72:388–96.

46. Birmaher B, Axelson D. Course and outcome of bipolar spectrum disorder in children and adolescents: a review of the existing literature. Dev Psychopathol 2006;18:1023–35.

47. DelBello MP, Hanseman D, Adler CM, et al. Twelve-month outcome of adolescents with bipolar disorder following first hospitalization for a manic or mixed episode. Am J Psychiatry 2007;164:582–90.

48. Beardslee WR, Gladstone TR. Prevention of childhood depression: recent findings and future prospects. Biol Psychiatry 2001;49:1101–10.

49. Beardslee WR, Gladstone TR, Wright EJ, et al. A family-based approach to the prevention of depressive symptoms in children at risk: evidence of parental and child change. Pediatrics 2003;112:e119–31.

50. Shaffer D, Gould MS, Fisher P, et al. Psychiatric diagnosis in child and adolescent suicide. Arch Gen Psychiatry 1996;53:339–48.

51. Brent DA, Perper JA, Goldstein CE, et al. Risk factors for adolescent suicide. A comparison of adolescent suicide victims with suicidal inpatients. Arch Gen Psychiatry 1988;45:581–8.

52. Strober M, Schmidt-Lackner S, Freeman R, et al. Recovery and relapse in adolescents with bipolar affective illness: a five-year naturalistic, prospective follow-up. J Am Acad Child Adolesc Psychiatry 1995;34:724–31.
53. Wilkinson P, Kelvin R, Roberts C, et al. Clinical and psychosocial predictors of suicide attempts and nonsuicidal self-injury in the Adolescent Depression Antidepressants and Psychotherapy Trial (ADAPT). Am J Psychiatry 2011;168:495–501.
54. Pfeffer CR. The FDA pediatric advisories and changes in diagnosis and treatment of pediatric depression. Am J Psychiatry 2007;164:843–6.

Developmental Risk I: Depression and the Developing Brain

John M. Weir, PhD, MPH[a], Arthurine Zakama[b], Uma Rao, MD[a,b,c],*

KEYWORDS

- Adolescent • Depression • Brain • Development
- Neurobiology

In the past three decades, public health recognition of depression in children and adolescents has increased significantly. The prevalence of pediatric depression is on the rise,[1–4] and depression during this developmental period is associated with significant impairment in multiple social domains.[5–8] Further, there is evidence that early depressive episodes persist or recur into adult life along with ongoing psychosocial difficulties.[8,9] A growing body of research has been identifying the neurobiological and psychological correlates.[8,10,11] In addition, recent studies have begun to identify specific genetic and experiential risk factors.[12–15] The aim of this article is to describe recent findings on the neurobiology of pediatric depression as well as the interplay between genetic and environmental factors in determining the risk for the disorder. In particular, utilizing data from both animal and human studies, the authors focus on the evolving understanding of the developmental neurobiology of emotional regulation, cognitive function, and social behavior as it applies to the risk and clinical course of depression. Treatment implications and directions for future research are also discussed.

This work was supported, in part, by the following grants from the National Institutes of Health (DA17805, MH68391, RR003032 and RR026140) and from the Endowed Chair in Brain and Behavior Research at Meharry Medical College.
The authors have no financial conflicts to disclose.
[a] Center for Molecular and Behavioral Neuroscience, Meharry Medical College, 1005 Dr D.B. Todd Jr Boulevard, Nashville, TN 37208, USA
[b] Vanderbilt University, 2201 West End Avenue, Nashville, TN 37235, USA
[c] Department of Psychiatry and Behavioral Sciences, Meharry Medical College, 1005 Dr D.B. Todd Jr Boulevard, Nashville, TN 37208, USA
* Corresponding author. Center for Molecular and Behavioral Neuroscience, Meharry Medical College, 1005 Dr D.B. Todd Jr Boulevard, Nashville, TN 37208.
E-mail address: urao@mmc.edu.

Child Adolesc Psychiatric Clin N Am 21 (2012) 237–259
doi:10.1016/j.chc.2012.01.004
1056-4993/12/$ – see front matter © 2012 Elsevier Inc. All rights reserved.
childpsych.theclinics.com

DEVELOPMENTAL INFLUENCES ON THE VULNERABILTY TO DEPRESSION

The risk for depression increases markedly during the transition from childhood to adolescence.[1] Adolescence is a crucial developmental stage marked by a confluence of physical, biological, psychological, and social challenges.[16–19] There are significant physical maturational changes (eg, the onset of puberty), social–cognitive advances (eg, ability for more abstract thinking and generalizations across situations and time), interpersonal transitions (eg, changes in social roles in family and peer relationships), and social–contextual changes (eg, school transitions). Although these maturational transitions offer tremendous opportunities for youth, because the developing brain regions underlying emotional, cognitive, and behavioral systems mature at different rates, and because these systems are under the control of both common and independent biological processes, this developmental period also is marked by heightened vulnerability.[16,18,20–22] The normative developmental transitions associated with adolescence might serve as sensitive periods for the activation of specific processes involved in the onset, persistence, and recurrence of depressive episodes.[23–25]

THE DEVELOPMENTAL NEUROBIOLOGY OF ADOLESCENCE

Adolescence is perhaps the greatest time of neural change and maturation since infancy.[26,27] Simultaneously, this period of brain maturation is marked by improvements in the ability to understand social and emotional cues, as well as an increase in the responsiveness to and importance of peer and other interpersonal relationships.[28–31] Also, there is a gradual increase in the capacity for cognitive control and executive function, including abstract thought, organization, decision making and planning, and response-inhibition.[16,30,32,33] Until recently, there was limited research on the neurobiological changes that accompany the emotional and cognitive changes that occur during adolescence. The application of magnetic resonance imaging (MRI) techniques has enabled researchers to examine the specific areas and circuits within the brain that are involved in the development of emotional and cognitive abilities.[31,34–36]

Although there is a minimal increase in brain size after early school-age years, remodeling of gray and white matter occurs throughout adolescence and into early adulthood.[34,37] In the gray matter, these changes are nonlinear and region specific. The gray matter changes take the form of increased myelination of different cortical connections or synaptic pruning or both, with a net reduction in volume.[26,37–40] There is a simultaneous linear increase in white matter density associated with increases in the diameter and myelination of the axons forming the fiber tracts alongside increased neural size and proliferation of glia.[27,39–42]

Myelination increases the speed of neural transmission.[27,43] Synaptic pruning is the process by which excess connections (synapses) between neurons are removed. Synapse elimination is believed to reduce the immature pattern of processing.[44] The elimination of this immature pattern of processing is adaptive in that in its immature state it requires greater metabolic activity and the recruitment of a wider array of structures.[44] In addition, pruning appears to increase the efficiency of cognitive processing through the creation of dedicated neural networks.[36] For instance, synaptic overproduction followed by selective pruning allows for maximum efficiency in associative memory functions.[45,46] Disturbances in these developmental patterns can adversely affect behavioral, emotional, and cognitive control.[21,22]

Neural Circuits

Prominent developmental transformations are seen in prefrontal cortex (PFC) and limbic brain regions of adolescents across a variety of species.[16,18] The previously described emotional and cognitive processes and social behavior (ie, self-regulation) appear to depend on the maturation of PFC and limbic system interconnectivity.[47-51] The limbic system consists of diverse neural structures, including the cingulate cortex, amygdala, and hippocampus, and it regulates emotional experience and motivational learning.[48,49,51-55] Further, maturation of connections between the PFC, basal ganglia, and cerebellum also appear to be crucial for the development of higher cognitive functions.[56]

The PFC mediates the highest cognitive capacities, including reasoning, planning, and behavioral control.[57,58] This relatively large and complex associative brain region has been shown to develop along with other higher-order association regions as children mature from adolescence into adulthood.[26,58] Structural neuroimaging studies using growth mapping techniques suggest that the prefrontal cortex matures more slowly than other regions of the brain,[26,59] and that its development parallels the improvements in cognitive control and behavioral inhibition that emerge during the adolescent transition into adulthood.[60] Frontal lobe maturation, particularly thinning of the cortical gray matter, has been associated with better performance on verbal memory tests in children aged 7–16 years,[61] and PFC volume in healthy adolescents has been associated with greater ability to inhibit behavioral responses.[62] Changes in white matter microstructure have been studied by means of diffusion tensor imaging (DTI) technology. These studies indicated that anisotropy, a measure that reflects myelin-related restriction of water diffusion across axons, was significantly lower in the frontal white matter in children than in adults, suggesting less myelination.[63,64]

Functional MRI (fMRI) studies indicate that core regions of the neural circuitry underlying cognitive control are on-line early in development.[32] However, age-related changes in localized processes across the brain, and in establishing long-range connections that support top-down (cortical–subcortical) modulation of behavior and more effective neural processing for optimal mature executive function, have been demonstrated.[32,65-70] With respect to affect regulation, adolescents seem to show a greater magnitude of amygdala activation in response to facial expressions of emotion compared to children and adults.[71-73] The exaggerated amygdala activation in response to emotional cues in adolescents might be related to their intense and variable emotional responses.[74-76] In contrast to the exaggerated amygdala responses to emotional cues, preliminary evidence indicates that the PFC is under-recruited in adolescents compared to adults.[73,77]

Although some neuroscientists describe cognition and emotion as separable processes implemented by different regions of the brain, such as the amygdala for emotion and the PFC for cognition, functional interactions between the amygdala and PFC mediate emotional influences on cognitive processes and vice versa. These mental processes are inextricably linked and represented in dynamic neural networks composed of interconnected prefrontal and limbic brain structures.[48,49,51] During adolescence, social relationships take on a new importance and adolescents become adept at reading social and emotional cues and modulating their affective responses.[28,78] Evidence suggests that children have difficulty managing interference from competing distractions, and the level of difficulty seems to correlate with the immaturity of posterior and frontal association cortices.[70] As children mature, they show an increased ability to attend to incoming information and control their behavior in a goal-directed manner.[60,68,77,79] This development seems to emerge in conjunction with a progressive "frontalization" of functional activity associated with inhibitory processing.[32,66,70]

Neurotransmitter Systems

In addition to connective and structural changes in the central nervous system, adolescents undergo dramatic alterations in virtually all neurotransmitter systems, including innervation patterns, neurotransmitter levels, and signaling mechanisms.[18,80,81] Developmental studies have shown that neurotransmitter systems generally follow a trajectory of overproduction and pruning, such that changes in expression typically peak during late childhood/early adolescence and are then reduced to reach adult levels. This pattern of overproduction and regressive elimination are believed to fine-tune the brain for efficiency but it also represents a state of vulnerability to exogenous influences.[18,22,80]

Cholinergic neurons projecting from the basal forebrain innervate the cerebral cortex during critical periods of neural development.[82] Acetylcholine stimulation may help to promote a favorable environment for neuronal maturation and the refinement of cortical connectivity. Acetylcholine also is likely to play a critical role in neural plasticity. Nicotinic acetylcholine receptors (nAChRs) appear early during development and are expressed throughout the nervous system. They not only exist on neuronal cell bodies and dendrites but also are located on axon terminals and are involved in multiple neurotransmitter release, including acetylcholine, dopamine, 5-hydroxytryptamine (5-HT), γ-aminobutyric acid (GABA), glutamate, and norepinephrine.[83] Muscarinic receptors gradually appear in the postnatal cortex and may be more dependent on the presence of nAChRs.[84] The cholinergic receptors are expressed at high levels in the developing cortex but then decline progressively to a significant extent during adolescence, with the cholinergic innervation of the PFC reaching mature levels.[18] The timing of cholinergic cortical innervation is of primary importance for the normal development of cognitive functions as nAChRs are involved in attention, learning, and memory.[85]

The mesostriatal and mesocorticolimbic dopamine pathways are involved in processing natural rewards and reward-directed behavior.[86,87] The mesostriatal–mesocorticolimbic dopamine system includes reciprocal dopamine projections from the ventral tegmental area in the midbrain into the ventral striatum, the limbic structures (amygdala in particular), and the orbitofrontal cortex.[88] The temporal relationships among exposure to rewards, dopamine neuronal firing activity, and extracellular dopamine concentrations suggest that ventral striatal dopamine release is involved in forming associations between salient contextual stimuli and internal rewarding events.[86,89]

Adolescence is associated with substantial development of the dopaminergic system. There is an increase in dopaminergic input to the PFC indexed by an increase in the density of dopaminergic fibers and transporters,[18] which is partially offset by developmental decline in dopamine synthesis and turnover after early adolescence.[80] Dopamine receptors are overproduced in early adolescence, followed by pruning that is more evident in subcortical than prefrontal regions.[18,90] The net effect of increased dopaminergic projection to the PFC, which shows less pronounced receptor pruning, is a shift in the relative balance between subcortical and cortical dopaminergic systems, with dominance of the mesocortical dopaminergic system. The development of the dopamine system during adolescence is likely to have an influence on the pruning of PFC neurons.[18] Dopaminergic input to the PFC, then, likely contributes to the coupling of salient cortico–cortical connections, and concomitantly to the pruning of connections that do not have significant salience, thereby influencing the important adolescent neurodevelopmental process of prefrontal pruning and myelination.[24]

Serotonin (5-HT) is involved in neural plasticity, a process through which modification of the functional properties of neurons and their networks occurs based on experience.[91] It has been hypothesized that neural plasticity occurs through a reversal of neuronal maturation that reinstates neuronal functions lost during development.[92] Such a dynamic process may involve a number of mechanisms, including neurite outgrowth, synaptogenesis, neurogenesis, and cell survival during brain development and even in adulthood.[91] There is evidence of significant 5-HT synaptic pruning in the basal forebrain around puberty in rats,[93] and 5-HT1A receptor binding appears to decrease most dramatically in humans during adolescence.[94]

Serotonin inhibits and opposes dopamine activity, particularly in relation to dopamine's role in aggressive and impulsive behaviors.[95–97] By puberty, dopamine input to the PFC is up to three times greater than serotonin input,[98] and PFC concentrations of dopamine precursor are much greater than those of 5-HT precursor in pubertal rhesus monkeys.[99] The relative imbalance in the dopamine–serotonin activity during adolescence might explain the enhanced sensitivity to appetitive (rewarding) situations, resulting in a higher prevalence of risky behaviors.[18,100,101]

Maturational changes during adolescence also have been detected in glutaminergic and GABAergic systems. The behavioral effects of agonists for a specific glutamate receptor, the N-methyl-D-aspartate (NMDA) receptor, appear to peak late in the preadolescent period in rats,[102] and this coincides with greater NMDA agonist sensitivity.[103] Glutaminergic inputs to the PFC appear to decrease during adolescence.[18] GABA opposes the modulating excitatory effects of glutamate.[104] GABA receptors achieve maturity in adolescence,[105] and GABAergic input to the PFC appears to decrease strongly through adolescence in humans.[18]

In summary, there are significant developmental changes in the neural circuits involved in emotional and cognitive regulation from childhood through adolescence. The following sections discuss how these maturational changes might be associated with increased vulnerability to depression during adolescence.

THE DEVELOPMENTAL NEUROBIOLOGY OF DEPRESSIVE DISORDER: THEORETICAL MODELS

Utilizing developmental, integrative, and neuroscience frameworks, several theoretical models have been proposed for the increased vulnerability to depression during adolescence. Some of these models are described.

The Social Information Processing Model

Nelson and colleagues[106] have proposed that developmental changes in social behavior during adolescence correlate with the maturation of a brain system referred to as the social information processing network. This network consists of three specific nodes: the detection node, the affective node, and the cognitive–regulatory node. They hypothesized that these nodes develop along different trajectories, such that the development of the affective node, approximately equivalent to the subcortical limbic system, outpaces maturation of the cortically based cognitive–regulatory node. The mismatch is proposed to create a vulnerability in which strong emotional responses to social stimuli are not tempered by the yet-to-mature regulatory mechanisms.

The Triadic Model

Ernst and Korelitz[21] put forth a triadic model comprising three primary systems: the affective system (which includes the amygdala), the reward system (which includes the ventral striatum), and the cognitive/response inhibition system (which includes the PFC). Each system/node has its own developmental trajectory, which creates a state of flux during adolescence. Final behavioral outcomes are likely to depend on the dominant node of a given stage or could result from a weakened node that fails to perform regulatory functions. In its simplified form, the triadic model explains exaggerated reactivity to a number of emotional stimuli,[74–76] changes in reward sensitivity,[107,108] and the significant lag in cortical control and cognitive development.

The Dysregulated Positive Affect Model

A third model, proposed by Forbes and Dahl,[109] focuses on the relationship between adolescent depression and the development of the reward system. They conceptualized depression as a reduction in positive affectivity (a factor that indexes active engagement with the environment). The approach system is a motivational system whose function is the pursuit of reward, and it is posited to include brain structures (eg, the nucleus accumbens) that mediate processing of reward information. From this view, depression is associated with deficits in the approach system. They posited a link between the development of neural systems underlying reward processing, which may become vulnerable to dysregulation as a consequence of remodeling during adolescence, and a predisposition to depression, particularly in vulnerable youth with a temperamental characteristic of low positive affect.

Integration of the Theoretical Models

An integration of the various models suggests that the increased vulnerability to depression and other psychiatric disorders during adolescence may be due to an imbalance between the relative structural and functional maturity of brain systems critical to emotional and incentive-based behavior (subcortical regions such as the amygdala and ventral striatum) compared to brain systems mediating cognitive and impulse control (eg, PFC), suggesting that the PFC exerts less regulatory control over subcortical regions relative to adults.[16,20,21,101,106]

This framework provides a heuristic model for explaining the neurodevelopmental basis for the affective and behavioral changes observed in adolescence. By demonstrating how the development of regulatory mechanisms lag behind development of affective brain systems, the model seems particularly appropriate for explaining the increased rates of dysregulated behaviors, especially antisocial behaviors, that emerge during adolescence but decline during adulthood when regulatory brain systems have reached adult levels of maturity.[110,111] However, it is not able to explain the increased rates of depression that start in adolescence but persist through adulthood,[9] by which time, presumably, the regulatory mechanisms whose delayed development putatively gave rise to affective dysregulation have matured.[26,40] The theory also appears to hold that affective and motivational systems are composed primarily of subcortical structures, whereas the regulatory systems are cortical. Recently, the concept that affect and affective regulation (or affect and cognition) can even be said to exist as separable processes has been questioned.[112–115]

In contrast to the models described in the preceding text that implicated the delayed development of the PFC compared to limbic areas as being responsible for the increased vulnerability to depression in adolescence, Davey and colleagues[24] proposed that the maturation of the PFC itself might be responsible for the development and maintenance of depression. According to this model, there is a cost to the ability of the PFC to make decisions in complex social environments that take into account the consequences of decisions into the future, resulting in a heightened vulnerability to depression when anticipated future rewards are not attained.

As described earlier, there is substantial remodeling and maturation of the dopaminergic reward system and PFC during adolescence, which coincides with the adolescent entering the complex world of adult peer and romantic relationships, in which the rewards that can be obtained (such as group affiliation, romantic love, social status) are abstract and temporally distant from the proximal context. Development of the PFC makes it possible to pursue such complex and distal rewards, which are, however, tenuous and more readily frustrated than the more immediate rewards. Davey and colleagues[24] hypothesized that when these distant rewards are unattainable, they suppress the reward system. When such suppression is extensive and occurs for an extended period of time, it manifests as depressive disorder.

The functional significance of the dopaminergic system's more extensive integration with PFC during adolescence is that the nature of the represented rewards becomes more sophisticated. The net result is the ability of adolescents to be motivated by, and to respond to, rewards that are more distal and complex.[86,89] Serotonin interacts with the dopaminergic system to further shape reward function,[116,117] possibly by reducing impulsive over-responding to proximal affective stimuli in favor of maintaining affective engagement with the long-term goals.[96,118]

Davey and colleagues[24] proposed that the initial episodes of clinical depression during adolescence often result from the frustration, or omission, of a highly anticipated social reward(s). Abstract social rewards have a greater salience and are associated with an active state of arousal.[119,120] When an anticipated reward is omitted, it has the effect of transiently suppressing the neural reward system.[86] Omission of rewards that are extended in their representation into the more distant future will cause a correspondingly prolonged suppression of the reward system, resulting in depression.

THE DEVELOPMENTAL NEUROBIOLOGY OF DEPRESSIVE DISORDER: EMPIRICAL DATA
Structural Brain Changes

Hippocampus
The hippocampus has been a focal area of research in both animal and human studies because depression is recognized as a stress-sensitive illness and the hippocampus is highly sensitive to stress, particularly during the early developmental period.[121–124] The hippocampus also is involved in mood regulation and cognitive function.[125] In animal models, extreme or chronic psychosocial stress was associated with dendritic atrophy of hippocampal pyramidal neurons and impaired neurogenesis in the dentate gyrus.[126–128] In a recent investigation, adult female cynomolgus macaques that exhibited spontaneously occurring depressive behavior manifested reduced volume compared with nondepressed controls specifically in the anterior portion of the hippocampus.[129] This finding is notable in that this region of the hippocampus has been implicated in emotional functioning. In a developmental study, subjecting infant monkeys to early-life stress led to reductions in glucocorticoid and mineralocorticoid receptors in the hippocampus during adolescence (compared to nonstressed controls[130]).

Human studies, including both pediatric and adult patients, also reported a reduction in hippocampal volume in association with depression.[121,131] In a recent study, reduced hippocampal volume was observed in healthy adolescents at high familial risk for depression, particularly in those who experienced high levels of adversity in childhood.[132] Among youth who experienced high levels of adversity, reduced hippocampal volume partly accounted for the increased vulnerability to depression during longitudinal follow-up.[132] In another investigation, adult patients with depression showed a greater decline in gray matter density of the hippocampus than controls after 3 years, particularly those who failed to remit from the index depressive episode.[133] Although morphologic changes in the hippocampus have been associated with depression, not all studies replicated these findings. The variability in findings might be attributed to sample size, developmental stage of the sample, number of depressive episodes, duration of illness, family history of depression, history of early-life adversity, comorbid symptoms, and methodology of the morphometric analysis.[131,134]

Amygdala

The amygdala is of importance to depression research due to its posited role in stress responses, as well as emotional and mood processes. In human adult studies, there was significant variability in amygdala changes associated with depression.[135] The variability across studies was accounted for by medication status such that studies that included only medicated individuals showed increased amygdala volume, whereas studies with only unmedicated persons showed a decrease in amygdala volume.[135] In a pediatric sample of medication-naïve patients with depression, an increased ratio of the amygdala to hippocampal volume was observed compared to age-matched and gender-matched controls, but this difference was accounted for by the severity of associated anxiety symptoms.[136] In a separate investigation, depressed youngsters had significant reductions of left and right amygdala volumes compared with healthy subjects. No significant correlations were found between amygdala volumes and depressive symptom severity, age at onset of illness, or illness duration.

Frontal lobes

In adult human studies, depressed patients showed large volume reductions in frontal regions, especially in the anterior cingulate and orbitofrontal cortex, and subgenual region of the PFC.[137,138] Gender, medication status, stage of illness, and family history appear to affect the nature of the findings in a region-specific manner. In a study of pediatric patients, those with nonfamilial depression had significantly increased left PFC volume compared to patients with familial depression as well as with healthy controls.[139] Left PFC volume correlated with severity of depression in familial but not in nonfamilial patients with depression.[139] Taken together, decreased left PFC volume in familial depression in youth and adults might result from degeneration of the left PFC,[139–141] whereas larger left PFC volume in pediatric patients with nonfamilial depression might be due to developmental alterations in PFC maturation.

Striatum

Several studies in depressed adults reported gray matter deficits in the striatum, especially in the caudate nucleus.[137,142] Reduced caudate volume also was observed in adolescents with depression.[143]

Summary of structural brain changes

Morphometric changes have been observed in a number of brain regions in association with depressive disorder, particularly those involving corticostriatal and corticolimbic networks, in adults.[144,145] Limited studies in pediatric samples showed similar patterns.[146,147] Several DTI studies reported reduced white matter integrity (fractional anisotropy) in adult patients with depression, particularly in the frontal and temporal regions.[148–151] Microstructural white matter abnormalities also were detected during the first episode of depression in young adult patients[152] as well as in depressed adolescents.[153] In a pilot study, we reported alterations in white matter tracts in healthy adolescents at high familial risk for depression, suggesting that it might be a vulnerability marker for depression.[154] Postmortem studies in animals and adult humans revealed alterations in glial cells in these networks.[155–157] Glial cells not only protect neurons through the production of myelin, but they are also dynamic partners participating in brain metabolism and communication between neurons.[157]

Functional Brain Changes

Consistent with structural brain changes associated with depressive disorder, functional imaging (fMRI) studies in adults also implicated impaired corticostriatal and corticolimbic circuits.[51,144,158,159] Most of this research has focused on resting state data[160,161] or the processing of negative or positive emotional stimuli.[161,162] A summary of these data indicates that patients with depression show increased neural activity in response to negative cues and diminished neural activity in response to positive stimuli in emotion-related brain circuits (eg, amygdala and ventral striatum). Some of these abnormalities in the processing of emotional information persist after symptom remission and they have also been found in healthy individuals who are at heightened risk for the development of mood disorders. Reports based on limited data in pediatric populations also indicated similar deficits in these neural networks, although the direction of change (ie, increased vs decreased response) was not consistent across pediatric studies or in comparison with adult data.[147,163–168]

Biochemical studies utilizing magnetic resonance spectroscopy (MRS) reported alterations in N-acetyl aspartate, glutamate/glutamine/GABA, creatinine/phosphocreatinine, choline, and myoinositol concentrations in specific regions of the corticostriatal and corticolimbic networks in adult patients with depression.[161,169–171] A modest amount of research in pediatric samples is consistent with the findings in adults, suggesting developmental continuities.[147,171–173]

In summary, data from functional neuroimaging studies in youngsters and adults indicate alterations in corticolimbic and corticostriatal circuits, similar to structural brain changes.

Summary of Neuroimaging Findings in Pediatric Depression

Although a growing body of research in pediatric depression has identified structural and functional brain changes, it has raised more questions than answers. This is, in great part, due to the modest sample sizes with cross-sectional designs. For instance, it is not clear how the maturational changes across child, adolescent, and adult development relate to the vulnerability and maintenance of depression. More information is needed on which neural changes are specific to depression and how family history, severity of illness, symptom patterns, and comorbid conditions influence the findings.[131] Also, it is not known whether the neural changes are preexisting and increase vulnerability to the disorder or if they are a consequence of the illness.[132,154,166] Further, it is not known with any certainty if the observed brain changes are temporary, statelike conditions that resolve without any sequalae, are temporary but still place an individual on a delayed trajectory toward normal development, or whether any disruption to the normal maturational process during this period permanently and deleteriously affects the neurobiological systems. The last of these possibilities may well be the most likely explanation based on data regarding the increased risk for recurrent depressive episodes.[174,175] The effect of disease course on the neurobiological substrate also has not been studied.[133] The utility of these neural markers in the diagnosis, treatment, and prognosis of the disorder should be established, as well as neurobiological changes in response to treatment.[176,177] In the final section of this article, future research directions are discussed that address these issues.

INDIVIDUAL DIFFERENCES IN DEVELOPMENT AND VULNERABILITY TO DEPRESSION

Although adolescence is associated with dramatic maturational changes in multiple domains and this developmental period is marked by vulnerability to depression, it is important to recognize that the behavioral and neurobiological responses are highly subject to individual differences and only a small subset develops the disorder. Such individual differences may take the form of heritable characteristics such as stable personality traits, differences in neurotransmitter profiles and biologically governed changes in hormones, or other effects of puberty. Environmental factors (eg, the social context, such as one's social status among peers) also make a contribution to individual differences. Depression itself has a significant heritable component,[178] but stress interacts with the genetic diathesis to determine the clinical manifestation of the disorder.[179–181] In the following section, the moderating influence of genetic and environmental factors on the relationship between neurobiological markers and vulnerability to depressive illness is described.

Gene–Environment Interactions in Determining the Risk for Depression

Research indicates that genetic factors account for anywhere between 24% and 58% of the variance in depression.[178] The relative contribution of genetics to depression vulnerability seems to vary with age. Some studies reported that the genetic influence on depression appears to increase with age, such that depression in adolescents appears to be influenced more by genes than is depression in children.[182,183] Contrary to this finding, other investigators found that the influence of genes decreases as children grow into adolescence.[184,185] The genetic risk also may be moderated by gender. Eley and Stevenson[186] found that genetic factors made a greater contribution to depression in boys but not girls. Silberg and colleagues[187] reported the opposite finding, with genes playing a greater role in girls as they matured into adolescence, but not with boys. Clearly, more research is needed before any meaningful conclusions can be made with regard to the relationships among genetic factors, development, gender, and depression vulnerability.

A growing body of research has indicated that the genetic vulnerability is modified by adverse environmental conditions, particularly during early development, to increase the risk for depression.[179,188] For instance, in a longitudinal study of a birth cohort, Caspi and colleagues[189] found that individuals with the short allele of the serotonin transporter gene-linked polymorphic region (5-HTTLPR) were at elevated risk for developing a depressive episode in adult life only if they experienced severe maltreatment in childhood. On the other hand, another investigation showed the presence of positive social support to be protective against depression in children with 5-HTTLPR short allele and a prior maltreatment history.[190] However, not all studies found a relationship between 5-HTTLPR polymorphism in determining the risk for depression.[191] In addition to methodologic differences across studies, factors such as stress sensitivity might determine the contribution of environmental factors on vulnerability to depression. For instance, Wichers and colleagues[181] found that greater stress sensitivity required less environmental influence for the clinical manifestation of depression.

Another candidate gene that has received significant attention in depression research is the corticotropin-releasing hormone type 1 receptor (*CRHR1*) because it mediates the hormonal responses to stress.[179,192] In a large community study of adults, a single nucleoside polymorphism (rs110402) of the *CRHR1* gene moderated the effects of childhood abuse on depressive symptoms in adult life in men only; women with childhood maltreatment were at elevated risk for depressive symptoms regardless of the genetic alleles.[192] In addition, the presence of the rare allele (the *A* allele in the case of rs110402) was protective against depression in men who had been exposed to childhood abuse.

Genetic variants of the Val66Met polymorphism of brain-derived neurotrophic factor (BDNF) gene also have been studies in relation to gene–environment interactions on depression risk.[193] In such studies, childhood adversity seems to have a greater impact on depressive symptoms in Met allele carriers of the *BDNF* gene than in the Val/Val group. *BDNF* is important for neural plasticity.[194] In animal models, depressive states were associated with reduced *BDNF* levels in the brain, and central administration of *BDNF* has been shown to reverse such depressive states. In an investigation of children with and without maltreatment, a three-way interaction was observed among *BDNF* genotype, 5-HTTLPR, and maltreatment history in predicting depression.[195] Children with the Met allele of the *BDNF* gene and two short alleles of 5-HTTLPR had the highest depression scores, but the vulnerability associated with these two genotypes was evident only in maltreated children. However, social support was protective against depression in the vulnerable group.

Taken together, these data support gene–environment interactions in the etiology of depression across the lifespan.

Genetic and Environmental Influences on Neurobiological Responses and Vulnerability to Depression

There is a growing interest in understanding genetic influences on the variability in brain structure and function.[196–198] For example, genetic variants of the 5-HTTLPR and *BDNF* polymorphisms were associated with amygdala, hippocampal, and prefrontal volumes.[196,198,199] Moreover, individuals carrying the 5HTTLPR short (risk) allele or *BDNF* Met allele had smaller hippocampal or amygdala volumes, or both, when they had a history of childhood maltreatment compared with those who had only one risk factor (environmental or genetic). Independent of genetic risk, childhood stress predicted additional hippocampal white matter alterations.[196,199] Although depressed patients had reduced PFC volume, individuals carrying the non-risk (long) allele and who also experienced high levels of childhood stress had larger PFC volumes, suggesting a protective effect.[199] Structural brain changes due to stress represent part of the mechanism by which the illness risk and outcome might be genetically mediated.

Genetic factors also influence neurobiological responses. In a meta-analysis, there was an association between the magnitude of amygdala activation in response to emotional cues and 5-HTTLPR.[197] To our knowledge, there are no data on the gene–environment interactions in brain responses in relation to depressive disorder. In the study described in the preceding text, the *A* allele of *CRHR1* gene was associated with a less robust hormonal response in men, possibly serving as a potential mediator of protection against depression.[192]

Summary of Findings on the Associations Among Genes, Neurobiology, Environment, and Depression

Genetic polymorphisms modulate brain structure and function. The structural and functional brain changes might serve as intermediate phenotypes in determining the risk for depressive illness. Environmental insults can further exacerbate the neurobiological alterations in at-risk individuals and magnify the risk for the disorder. In a similar vein, enriched/supportive environment can ameliorate the risk in genetically vulnerable persons. A better understanding of the gene–environment interactions, and the mechanisms (eg, neurobiological changes) through which risk and resilience for the disorder occur, will be helpful in developing more specific and effective preventive and treatment interventions.

Treatment Implications for Depression

Although there is still much to learn in terms of understanding the neurobiology of depressive illness across the lifespan in general and pediatric depression in particular, the available data offer potential options for intervention. Given that depression is associated with reduced hippocampal volume and possibly other structural brain changes, interventions that can potentially reverse these changes could be helpful. Potential therapies such as antidepressant agents, electroconvulsive therapy, and exercise that have been shown to promote neurogenesis ought to be considered.[200–202] Lithium has been found to reverse the glial cell changes.[203] Anti-glucocorticoid agents and CRH antagonists can be helpful in reducing the toxic effects of hypercortisolemia.[204] Psychotherapeutic interventions also can induce brain changes.[205]

FUTURE DIRECTIONS FOR RESEARCH

Perhaps the most obvious implication from the current article is the need for more prospective longitudinal research in youngsters. Investigators should identify clear structure/function hypotheses that utilize, but go beyond, the current diagnostic system to translate findings from clinical neuroscience research into a new classification system based on pathophysiology and etiological processes.[206] Such models also may be able to explain the high rates of comorbidity between depression and other psychiatric conditions. Studies of depressed children and adolescents have a number of advantages compared with studies of adults; confounding factors such as repeated episodes, long duration of illness, multiple medications, and co-occurring medical problems are minimized. It is also important to include high-risk youth who have not yet developed a depressive episode to identify premorbid factors. Another focus of future research should center on evaluating the stability of biological abnormalities. Given that adolescence is a high-risk period for the onset of depression, in a relatively short follow-up period, it is possible to identify both preexisting and "scar" markers of the illness.

It is important to obtain functional neuroimaging measures before and after pharmacologic or behavioral interventions. Results from such studies will shed light on the mechanisms through which treatments work and may provide new intervention targets for drug development.[207,208] In addition to identifying potential mediators of different treatments, it is important for neuroimaging studies to identify baseline predictors of treatment outcome (ie, the moderators). The identification of mediators and moderators of treatment would help move the field toward more "personalized" care.[209] Exciting times lie ahead in our efforts to tackle the mechanisms involved in pediatric depression and its treatment response.

REFERENCES

1. Kessler RC, Avenevoli S, Ries Merikangas K. Mood disorders in children and adolescents: an epidemiologic perspective. Biol Psychiatry 2001;49(12):1002–14.
2. Kovacs M, Gatsonis C. Secular trends in age at onset of major depressive disorder in a clinical sample of children. J Psychiatr Res 1994;28(3):319–29.
3. Lewinsohn PM, Hops H, Roberts RE, et al. Adolescent psychopathology: I. Prevalence and incidence of depression and other DSM-III-R disorders in high school students. J Abnorm Psychol 1993;102(1):133–44.
4. Ryan ND, Williamson DE, Iyengar S, et al. A secular increase in child and adolescent onset affective disorder. J Am Acad Child Adolesc Psychiatry 1992;31(4):600–5.
5. Puig-Antich J, Lukens E, Davies M, et al. Psychosocial functioning in prepubertal major depressive disorders. I. Interpersonal relationships during the depressive episode. Arch Gen Psychiatry 1985;42(5):500–7.
6. Puig-Antich J, Lukens E, Davies M, et al. Psychosocial functioning in prepubertal major depressive disorders. II. Interpersonal relationships after sustained recovery from affective episode. Arch Gen Psychiatry 1985;42(5):511–7.
7. Puig-Antich J, Kaufman J, Ryan ND, et al. The psychosocial functioning and family environment of depressed adolescents. J Am Acad Child Adolesc Psychiatry 1993; 32(2):244–53.
8. Rao U, Chen LA. Characteristics, correlates, and outcomes of childhood and adolescent depressive disorders. Dialogues Clin Neurosci 2009;11(1):45–62.
9. Rao U. Links between depression and substance abuse in adolescents: neurobiological mechanisms. Am J Prev Med Dec 2006;31(6 Suppl 1):S161–74.
10. Hankin BL, Oppenheimer C, Jenness J, et al. Developmental origins of cognitive vulnerabilities to depression: review of processes contributing to stability and change across time. J Clin Psychol 2009;65(12):1327–38.
11. Zalsman G, Oquendo MA, Greenhill L, et al. Neurobiology of depression in children and adolescents. Child Adolesc Psychiatr Clin North Am 2006;15(4):843–68, vii–viii.
12. Franic S, Middeldorp CM, Dolan CV, et al. Childhood and adolescent anxiety and depression: beyond heritability. J Am Acad Child Adolesc Psychiatry 2010;49(8): 820–9.
13. Rice F. The genetics of depression in childhood and adolescence. Curr Psychiatry Rep. 2009;11(2):167–73.
14. Rutter M. Gene-environment interplay. Depress Anxiety 2010;27(1):1–4.
15. Schlossberg K, Massler A, Zalsman G. Environmental risk factors for psychopathology. Isr J Psychiatry Relat Sci 2010;47(2):139–43.
16. Somerville LH, Jones RM, Casey BJ. A time of change: behavioral and neural correlates of adolescent sensitivity to appetitive and aversive environmental cues. Brain Cogn 2010;72(1):124–33.
17. Sisk CL, Foster DL. The neural basis of puberty and adolescence. Nat Neurosci 2004;7(10):1040–7.
18. Spear L. Neurobehavioral changes in adolescence. Curr Dir Psychol Sci 2000;9(4): 111–4.
19. Blakemore SJ, Burnett S, Dahl RE. The role of puberty in the developing adolescent brain. Human Brain Mapp 2010;31(6):926–33.
20. Brenhouse HC, Andersen SL. Developmental trajectories during adolescence in males and females: a cross-species understanding of underlying brain changes. Neurosci Biobehav Rev 2011;35(8):1687–703.
21. Ernst M, Korelitz KE. Cerebral maturation in adolescence: behavioral vulnerability. L'Encephale 2009;35(Suppl 6):S182–9.

22. Paus T, Keshavan M, Giedd JN. Why do many psychiatric disorders emerge during adolescence? Nat Rev Neurosci 2008;9(12):947–57.

23. Andersen SL, Teicher MH. Stress, sensitive periods and maturational events in adolescent depression. Trends Neurosci 2008;31(4):183–91.

24. Davey CG, Yucel M, Allen NB. The emergence of depression in adolescence: development of the prefrontal cortex and the representation of reward. Neurosci Biobehav Rev 2008;32(1):1–19.

25. Rudolph KD, Hammen C, Daley SE. Mood disorders. In: Wolfe DA, Mash EJ, editors. Behavioral and emotional disorders in adolescents: nature, assessment, and treatment. New York: Guilford Press; 2006. p. 300–42.

26. Gogtay N, Giedd JN, Lusk L, et al. Dynamic mapping of human cortical development during childhood through early adulthood. Proc Natl Acad Sci USA 2004;101(21): 8174–9.

27. Paus T. Growth of white matter in the adolescent brain: myelin or axon? Brain Cogn 2010;72(1):26–35.

28. Herba C, Phillips M. Annotation: development of facial expression recognition from childhood to adolescence: behavioural and neurological perspectives. J Child Psychol Psychiatry Allied Disciplines 2004;45(7):1185–98.

29. Rosso IM, Young AD, Femia LA, et al. Cognitive and emotional components of frontal lobe functioning in childhood and adolescence. Ann NY Acad Sci 2004; 1021:355–62.

30. Yurgelun-Todd D. Emotional and cognitive changes during adolescence. Curr Opin Neurobiol 2007;17(2):251–7.

31. Burnett S, Sebastian C, Cohen Kadosh K, et al. The social brain in adolescence: evidence from functional magnetic resonance imaging and behavioural studies. Neurosci Biobehav Rev 2011;35(8):1654–64.

32. Luna B, Padmanabhan A, O'Hearn K. What has fMRI told us about the development of cognitive control through adolescence? Brain Cogn 2010;72(1):101–13.

33. Paus T. Mapping brain maturation and cognitive development during adolescence. Trends Cogn Sci 2005;9(2):60–8.

34. Durston S, Hulshoff Pol HE, Casey BJ, et al. Anatomical MRI of the developing human brain: what have we learned? J Am Acad Child Adolesc Psychiatry 2001; 40(9):1012–20.

35. Chugani HT. Biological basis of emotions: brain systems and brain development. Pediatrics 1998;102(5 Suppl E):1225–9.

36. Luna B, Sweeney JA. The emergence of collaborative brain function: FMRI studies of the development of response inhibition. Ann NY Acad Sci 2004;1021:296–309.

37. Wilke M, Krageloh-Mann I, Holland SK. Global and local development of gray and white matter volume in normal children and adolescents. Exp Brain Res Exp Hirnforsch Exp Cerebrale 2007;178(3):296–307.

38. Sowell ER, Thompson PM, Holmes CJ, et al. In vivo evidence for post-adolescent brain maturation in frontal and striatal regions. Nat Neurosci 1999;2(10):859–61.

39. Giorgio A, Watkins KE, Chadwick M, et al. Longitudinal changes in grey and white matter during adolescence. NeuroImage 2010;49(1):94–103.

40. Giedd JN, Blumenthal J, Jeffries NO, et al. Brain development during childhood and adolescence: a longitudinal MRI study. Nat Neurosci 1999;2(10):861–3.

41. Schmithorst VJ, Yuan W. White matter development during adolescence as shown by diffusion MRI. Brain Cogn 2010;72(1):16–25.

42. Asato MR, Terwilliger R, Woo J, et al. White matter development in adolescence: a DTI study. Cereb Cortex 2010;20(9):2122–31.

43. Yurgelun-Todd DA, Killgore WD, Young AD. Sex differences in cerebral tissue volume and cognitive performance during adolescence. Psychol Rep 2002;91(3 Pt 1):743–57.
44. Durston S, Casey BJ. What have we learned about cognitive development from neuroimaging? Neuropsychologia 2006;44(11):2149–57.
45. Chechik G, Meilijson I, Ruppin E. Synaptic pruning in development: a computational account. Neural Comput. 1998;10(7):1759–77.
46. Mimura K, Kimoto T, Okada M. Synapse efficiency diverges due to synaptic pruning following overgrowth. Phys Rev E 2003;68(3 Pt 1):031910.
47. Disner SG, Beevers CG, Haigh EA, et al. Neural mechanisms of the cognitive model of depression. Nat Rev Neurosci 2011;12(8):467–77.
48. Heatherton TF, Wagner DD. Cognitive neuroscience of self-regulation failure. Trends Cogn Sci 2011;15(3):132–9.
49. Price JL, Drevets WC. Neurocircuitry of mood disorders. Neuropsychopharmacology 2010;35(1):192–216.
50. Liston C, Watts R, Tottenham N, et al. Frontostriatal microstructure modulates efficient recruitment of cognitive control. Cereb Cortex 2006;16(4):553–60.
51. Mayberg HS. Modulating dysfunctional limbic-cortical circuits in depression: towards development of brain-based algorithms for diagnosis and optimised treatment. Br Med Bull 2003;65:193–207.
52. Bellani M, Baiano M, Brambilla P. Brain anatomy of major depression II. Focus on amygdala. Epidemiol Psychiatr Sci 2011;20(1):33–6.
53. Hamani C, Mayberg H, Stone S, et al. The subcallosal cingulate gyrus in the context of major depression. Biol Psychiatry 2011;69(4):301–8.
54. Hariri AR, Bookheimer SY, Mazziotta JC. Modulating emotional responses: effects of a neocortical network on the limbic system. NeuroReport 2000;11(1):43–8.
55. Rogers MA, Bradshaw JL, Pantelis C, et al. Frontostriatal deficits in unipolar major depression. Brain Res Bull 1998;47(4):297–310.
56. Heyder K, Suchan B, Daum I. Cortico-subcortical contributions to executive control. Acta Psychol [Amst]. 2004;115(2-3):271–89.
57. Baxter MG. Introduction to the special section on "translational models of prefrontal cortical function." Behav Neurosci 2011;125(3):279–81.
58. Fuster JM. Frontal lobe and cognitive development. J Neurocytol 2002;31(3–5): 373–85.
59. Sowell ER, Thompson PM, Leonard CM, et al. Longitudinal mapping of cortical thickness and brain growth in normal children. J Neurosci 2004;24(38):8223–31.
60. Casey BJ, Tottenham N, Liston C, et al. Imaging the developing brain: what have we learned about cognitive development? Trends Cogn Sci 2005;9(3):104–10.
61. Sowell ER, Thompson PM, Rex D, et al. Mapping sulcal pattern asymmetry and local cortical surface gray matter distribution in vivo: maturation in perisylvian cortices. Cereb Cortex 2002;12(1):17–26.
62. Casey BJ, Castellanos FX, Giedd JN, et al. Implication of right frontostriatal circuitry in response inhibition and attention-deficit/hyperactivity disorder. J Am Acad Child Adolesc Psychiatry 1997;36(3):374–83.
63. Lebel C, Walker L, Leemans A, et al. Microstructural maturation of the human brain from childhood to adulthood. NeuroImage 2008;40(3):1044–55.
64. Klingberg T, Vaidya CJ, Gabrieli JD, et al. Myelination and organization of the frontal white matter in children: a diffusion tensor MRI study. NeuroReport 1999;10(13): 2817–21.

65. Casey BJ, Cohen JD, Jezzard P, et al. Activation of prefrontal cortex in children during a nonspatial working memory task with functional MRI. NeuroImage 1995; 2(3):221–9.

66. Rubia K, Overmeyer S, Taylor E, et al. Functional frontalisation with age: mapping neurodevelopmental trajectories with fMRI. Neurosci Biobehav Rev 2000;24(1): 13–9.

67. Schlaggar BL, Brown TT, Lugar HM, et al. Functional neuroanatomical differences between adults and school-age children in the processing of single words. Science 2002;296(5572):1476–9.

68. Tamm L, Menon V, Reiss AL. Maturation of brain function associated with response inhibition. J Am Acad Child Adolesc Psychiatry 2002;41(10):1231–8.

69. Gaillard WD, Hertz-Pannier L, Mott SH, et al. Functional anatomy of cognitive development: fMRI of verbal fluency in children and adults. Neurology 2000;54(1): 180–5.

70. Durston S, Davidson MC, Tottenham N, et al. A shift from diffuse to focal cortical activity with development. Dev Sci 2006;9(1):1–8.

71. Somerville LH, Fani N, McClure-Tone EB. Behavioral and neural representation of emotional facial expressions across the lifespan. Dev Neuropsychol 2011;36(4): 408–28.

72. Guyer AE, Monk CS, McClure-Tone EB, et al. A developmental examination of amygdala response to facial expressions. J Cogn Neurosci 2008;20(9):1565–82.

73. Hare TA, Tottenham N, Galvan A, et al. Biological substrates of emotional reactivity and regulation in adolescence during an emotional go-nogo task. Biol Psychiatry 2008;63(10):927–34.

74. Arnett JJ. Adolescent storm and stress, reconsidered. Am Psychol 1999;54(5): 317–26.

75. Buchanan CM, Eccles JS, Becker JB. Are adolescents the victims of raging hormones: evidence for activational effects of hormones on moods and behavior at adolescence. Psychol Bull 1992;111(1):62–107.

76. Larson RW, Moneta G, Richards MH, et al. Continuity, stability, and change in daily emotional experience across adolescence. Child Dev 2002;73(4):1151–65.

77. Monk CS, McClure EB, Nelson EE, et al. Adolescent immaturity in attention-related brain engagement to emotional facial expressions. NeuroImage 2003;20(1):420–8.

78. Baird AA, Gruber SA, Fein DA, et al. Functional magnetic resonance imaging of facial affect recognition in children and adolescents. J Am Acad Child Adolesc Psychiatry 1999;38(2):195–9.

79. Luna B, Garver KE, Urban TA, et al. Maturation of cognitive processes from late childhood to adulthood. Child Dev 2004;75(5):1357–72.

80. Andersen SL. Trajectories of brain development: point of vulnerability or window of opportunity? Neurosci Biobehav Rev 2003;27(1-2):3–18.

81. Daws LC, Gould GG. Ontogeny and regulation of the serotonin transporter: providing insights into human disorders. Pharmacol Ther 2011;131(1):61–79.

82. Bruel-Jungerman E, Lucassen PJ, Francis F. Cholinergic influences on cortical development and adult neurogenesis. Behav Brain Res 2011;221(2):379–88.

83. Dani JA. Overview of nicotinic receptors and their roles in the central nervous system. Biol Psychiatry 2001;49(3):166–74.

84. Aubert I, Cecyre D, Gauthier S, et al. Comparative ontogenic profile of cholinergic markers, including nicotinic and muscarinic receptors, in the rat brain. J Comp Neurol 1996;369(1):31–55.

85. Berger-Sweeney J. The cholinergic basal forebrain system during development and its influence on cognitive processes: important questions and potential answers. Neurosci Biobehav Rev 2003;27(4):401–11.

86. Schultz W. Dopamine signals for reward value and risk: basic and recent data. Behav Brain Funct 2010;6:24.

87. Berridge KC, Robinson TE. Parsing reward. Trends Neurosci 2003;26(9):507–13.

88. Ongur D, Price JL. The organization of networks within the orbital and medial prefrontal cortex of rats, monkeys and humans. Cereb Cortex 2000;10(3):206–19.

89. Spanagel R, Weiss F. The dopamine hypothesis of reward: past and current status. Trends Neurosci 1999;22(11):521–7.

90. Andersen SL, Thompson AT, Rutstein M, et al. Dopamine receptor pruning in prefrontal cortex during the periadolescent period in rats. Synapse 2000;37(2):167–9.

91. Mattson MP, Maudsley S, Martin B. BDNF and 5-HT: a dynamic duo in age-related neuronal plasticity and neurodegenerative disorders. Trends Neurosci 2004;27(10):589–94.

92. Kobayashi K, Ikeda Y, Sakai A, et al. Reversal of hippocampal neuronal maturation by serotonergic antidepressants. Proc Natl Acad Sci USA 2010;107(18):8434–9.

93. Dinopoulos A, Dori I, Parnavelas JG. The serotonin innervation of the basal forebrain shows a transient phase during development. Brain Res Dev Brain Research 1997;99(1):38–52.

94. Dillon KA, Gross-Isseroff R, Israeli M, et al. Autoradiographic analysis of serotonin 5-HT1A receptor binding in the human brain postmortem: effects of age and alcohol. Brain Res 1991;554(1-2):56–64.

95. Goveas JS, Csernansky JG, Coccaro EF. Platelet serotonin content correlates inversely with life history of aggression in personality-disordered subjects. Psychiatry Res 2004;126(1):23–32.

96. Katz LD. Dopamine and serotonin: integrating current affective engagement with longer-term goals. Behav Brain Sci 1999;22(3):527.

97. van der Vegt BJ, Lieuwes N, Cremers TI, et al. Cerebrospinal fluid monoamine and metabolite concentrations and aggression in rats. Hormones Behav 2003;44(3):199–208.

98. Lambe EK, Krimer LS, Goldman-Rakic PS. Differential postnatal development of catecholamine and serotonin inputs to identified neurons in prefrontal cortex of rhesus monkey. J Neurosci 2000;20(23):8780–7.

99. Goldman-Rakic PS, Brown RM. Postnatal development of monoamine content and synthesis in the cerebral cortex of rhesus monkeys. Brain Res 1982;256(3):339–49.

100. Zeeb FD, Robbins TW, Winstanley CA. Serotonergic and dopaminergic modulation of gambling behavior as assessed using a novel rat gambling task. Neuropsychopharmacology 2009;34(10):2329–43.

101. Steinberg L, Albert D, Cauffman E, et al. Age differences in sensation seeking and impulsivity as indexed by behavior and self-report: evidence for a dual systems model. Dev Psychol 2008;44(6):1764–78.

102. Frantz KJ, Van Hartesveldt C. The locomotor effects of quinpirole in rats depend on age and gender. Pharmacol Biochem Behav 1999;64(4):821–6.

103. Subramaniam S, McGonigle P. Regional profile of developmental changes in the sensitivity of the N-methyl-D-aspartate receptor to polyamines. J Neurochem 1994;62(4):1408–15.

104. Johnson BA. Recent advances in the development of treatments for alcohol and cocaine dependence: focus on topiramate and other modulators of GABA or glutamate function. CNS Drugs 2005;19(10):873–96.

105. Nurse S, Lacaille JC. Late maturation of GABA(B) synaptic transmission in area CA1 of the rat hippocampus. Neuropharmacology 1999;38(11):1733–42.

106. Nelson EE, Leibenluft E, McClure EB, et al. The social re-orientation of adolescence: a neuroscience perspective on the process and its relation to psychopathology. Psychol Med 2005;35(2):163–74.

107. Ernst M, Paulus MP. Neurobiology of decision making: a selective review from a neurocognitive and clinical perspective. Biol Psychiatry 2005;58(8):597–604.

108. Galvan A, Hare TA, Parra CE, et al. Earlier development of the accumbens relative to orbitofrontal cortex might underlie risk-taking behavior in adolescents. J Neurosci 2006;26(25):6885–92.

109. Forbes EE, Dahl RE. Neural systems of positive affect: relevance to understanding child and adolescent depression? Dev Psychopathol 2005;17(3):827–50.

110. Moffitt TE. Adolescence-limited and life-course-persistent antisocial behavior: a developmental taxonomy. Psychol Rev 1993;100(4):674–701.

111. Rutter M, Kim-Cohen J, Maughan B. Continuities and discontinuities in psychopathology between childhood and adult life. J Child Psychol Psychiatry Allied Disciplines 2006;47(3-4):276–95.

112. Campos JJ, Frankel CB, Camras L. On the nature of emotion regulation. Child Dev 2004;75(2):377–94.

113. Phillips ML, Drevets WC, Rauch SL, et al. Neurobiology of emotion perception I: The neural basis of normal emotion perception. Biol Psychiatry 2003;54(5):504–14.

114. Salzman CD, Fusi S. Emotion, cognition, and mental state representation in amygdala and prefrontal cortex. Annu Rev Neurosci 2010;33:173–202.

115. Wager TD, Davidson ML, Hughes BL, et al. Prefrontal-subcortical pathways mediating successful emotion regulation. Neuron 2008;59(6):1037–50.

116. Benloucif S, Galloway MP. Facilitation of dopamine release in vivo by serotonin agonists: studies with microdialysis. Eur J Pharmacol 1991;200(1):1–8.

117. Di Mascio M, Di Giovanni G, Di Matteo V, et al. Selective serotonin reuptake inhibitors reduce the spontaneous activity of dopaminergic neurons in the ventral tegmental area. Brain Res Bull 1998;46(6):547–54.

118. Spoont MR. Modulatory role of serotonin in neural information processing: implications for human psychopathology. Psychol Bull 1992;112(2):330–50.

119. Panksepp J. Affective neuroscience of the emotional BrainMind: evolutionary perspectives and implications for understanding depression. Dialogues Clin Neurosci 2010;12(4):533–45.

120. Bechara A, Damasio AR. The somatic marker hypothesis: a neural theory of economic decision. Games Econ Behav 2005;52:336–72.

121. MacQueen G, Frodl T. The hippocampus in major depression: evidence for the convergence of the bench and bedside in psychiatric research? Mol Psychiatry 2011;16(3):252–64.

122. Sapolsky RM. Stress and plasticity in the limbic system. Neurochem Res 2003; 28(11):1735–42.

123. Spinelli S, Chefer S, Suomi SJ, et al. Early-life stress induces long-term morphologic changes in primate brain. Arch Gen Psychiatry 2009;66(6):658–65.

124. McEwen BS. Stress and hippocampal plasticity. Annu Rev Neurosci 1999;22: 105–22.

125. Campbell S, Macqueen G. The role of the hippocampus in the pathophysiology of major depression. J Psychiatry Neurosci JPN 2004;29(6):417–26.

126. Samuels BA, Hen R. Neurogenesis and affective disorders. Eur J Neurosci 2011; 33(6):1152–9.

127. Thomas RM, Hotsenpiller G, Peterson DA. Acute psychosocial stress reduces cell survival in adult hippocampal neurogenesis without altering proliferation. J Neurosci 2007;27(11):2734–43.

128. Fuchs E, Flugge G. Chronic social stress: effects on limbic brain structures. Physiol Behav 2003;79(3):417–27.

129. Willard SL, Friedman DP, Henkel CK, et al. Anterior hippocampal volume is reduced in behaviorally depressed female cynomolgus macaques. Psychoneuroendocrinology 2009;34(10):1469–75.

130. Arabadzisz D, Diaz-Heijtz R, Knuesel I, et al. Primate early life stress leads to long-term mild hippocampal decreases in corticosteroid receptor expression. Biol Psychiatry 2010;67(11):1106–9.

131. McKinnon MC, Yucel K, Nazarov A, et al. A meta-analysis examining clinical predictors of hippocampal volume in patients with major depressive disorder. J Psychiatry Neurosci JPN 2009;34(1):41–54.

132. Rao U, Chen LA, Bidesi AS, et al. Hippocampal changes associated with early-life adversity and vulnerability to depression. Biol Psychiatry 2010;67(4):357–64.

133. Frodl TS, Koutsouleris N, Bottlender R, et al. Depression-related variation in brain morphology over 3 years: effects of stress? Arch Gen Psychiatry 2008;65(10): 1156–65.

134. Campbell S, Marriott M, Nahmias C, et al. Lower hippocampal volume in patients suffering from depression: a meta-analysis. Am J Psychiatry 2004;161(4):598–607.

135. Hamilton JP, Siemer M, Gotlib IH. Amygdala volume in major depressive disorder: a meta-analysis of magnetic resonance imaging studies. Mol Psychiatry 2008;13(11): 993–1000.

136. MacMillan S, Szeszko PR, Moore GJ, et al. Increased amygdala: hippocampal volume ratios associated with severity of anxiety in pediatric major depression. J Child Adolesc Psychopharmacol 2003;13(1):65–73.

137. Koolschijn PC, van Haren NE, Lensvelt-Mulders GJ, et al. Brain volume abnormalities in major depressive disorder: a meta-analysis of magnetic resonance imaging studies. Hum Brain Mapp 2009;30(11):3719–35.

138. Lorenzetti V, Allen NB, Fornito A, et al. Structural brain abnormalities in major depressive disorder: a selective review of recent MRI studies. J Affect Disord 2009;117(1-2):1–17.

139. Nolan CL, Moore GJ, Madden R, et al. Prefrontal cortical volume in childhood-onset major depression: preliminary findings. Arch Gen Psychiatry 2002;59(2):173–9.

140. Botteron KN, Raichle ME, Drevets WC, et al. Volumetric reduction in left subgenual prefrontal cortex in early onset depression. Biol Psychiatry 2002;51(4):342–4.

141. Drevets WC. Neuroimaging studies of mood disorders. Biol Psychiatry 2000;48(8): 813–29.

142. Kim MJ, Hamilton JP, Gotlib IH. Reduced caudate gray matter volume in women with major depressive disorder. Psychiatry Res 2008;164(2):114–22.

143. Shad MU, Muddasani S, Rao U. Grey matter differences between healthy and depressed adolescents: a voxel-based morphometry study. Journal of Child and Adolescent Psychopharmacology, in press.

144. Drevets WC, Price JL, Furey ML. Brain structural and functional abnormalities in mood disorders: implications for neurocircuitry models of depression. Brain Struct Funct 2008;213(1-2):93–118.

145. Peng J, Liu J, Nie B, et al. Cerebral and cerebellar gray matter reduction in first-episode patients with major depressive disorder: a voxel-based morphometry study. Eur J Radiol 2011;80(2):395–99.

146. Pine DS. Brain development and the onset of mood disorders. Semin Clin Neuro-psychiatry 2002;7(4):223–33.

147. Rosenberg DR, Macmaster FP, Mirza Y, et al. Reduced anterior cingulate glutamate in pediatric major depression: a magnetic resonance spectroscopy study. Biol Psychiatry 2005;58(9):700–4.

148. Kieseppa T, Eerola M, Mantyla R, et al. Major depressive disorder and white matter abnormalities: a diffusion tensor imaging study with tract-based spatial statistics. J Affect Disord 2010;120(1–3):240–4.

149. Maller JJ, Thomson RH, Lewis PM, et al. Traumatic brain injury, major depression, and diffusion tensor imaging: making connections. Brain Res Rev 2010; 64(1):213–40.

150. Sexton CE, Mackay CE, Ebmeier KP. A systematic review of diffusion tensor imaging studies in affective disorders. Biol Psychiatry 2009;66(9):814–23.

151. Shimony JS, Sheline YI, D'Angelo G, et al. Diffuse microstructural abnormalities of normal-appearing white matter in late life depression: a diffusion tensor imaging study. Biol Psychiatry 2009;66(3):245–52.

152. Ma N, Li L, Shu N, et al. White matter abnormalities in first-episode, treatment-naive young adults with major depressive disorder. Am J Psychiatry 2007;164(5):823–6.

153. Cullen KR, Klimes-Dougan B, Muetzel R, et al. Altered white matter microstructure in adolescents with major depression: a preliminary study. J Am Acad Child Adolesc Psychiatry 2010;49(2):173–83,e171.

154. Huang H, Fan X, Williamson DE, et al. White matter changes in healthy adolescents at familial risk for unipolar depression: a diffusion tensor imaging study. Neuropsychopharmacology 2011;36(3):684–91.

155. Hamidi M, Drevets WC, Price JL. Glial reduction in amygdala in major depressive disorder is due to oligodendrocytes. Biol Psychiatry 2004;55(6):563–9.

156. Leventopoulos M, Ruedi-Bettschen D, Knuesel I, et al Long-term effects of early life deprivation on brain glia in Fischer rats. Brain Res 2007;1142:119–26.

157. Rajkowska G, Miguel-Hidalgo JJ. Gliogenesis and glial pathology in depression. CNS Neurol Disord Drug Targets 2007;6(3):219–33.

158. Pizzagalli DA, Holmes AJ, Dillon DG, et al. Reduced caudate and nucleus accumbens response to rewards in unmedicated individuals with major depressive disorder. Am J Psychiatry 2009;166(6):702–10.

159. Rigucci S, Serafini G, Pompili M, et al. Anatomical and functional correlates in major depressive disorder: the contribution of neuroimaging studies. World J Biol Psychiatry 2010;11(2 Pt 2):165–80.

160. Greicius MD, Flores BH, Menon V, et al. Resting-state functional connectivity in major depression: abnormally increased contributions from subgenual cingulate cortex and thalamus. Biol Psychiatry 2007;62(5):429–37.

161. Hasler G, Northoff G. Discovering imaging endophenotypes for major depression. Mol Psychiatry 2011;16(6):604–19.

162. Leppanen JM. Emotional information processing in mood disorders: a review of behavioral and neuroimaging findings. Curr Opin Psychiatry 2006;19(1):34–9.

163. Davey CG, Allen NB, Harrison BJ, et al. Increased amygdala response to positive social feedback in young people with major depressive disorder. Biol Psychiatry 2011;69(8):734–41.

164. Forbes EE, Christopher May J, Siegle GJ, et al. Reward-related decision-making in pediatric major depressive disorder: an fMRI study. J Child Psychol Psychiatry Allied Disciplines 2006;47(10):1031–40.

165. Forbes EE, Hariri AR, Martin SL, et al. Altered striatal activation predicting real-world positive affect in adolescent major depressive disorder. Am J Psychiatry 2009; 166(1):64–73.

166. Gotlib IH, Hamilton JP, Cooney RE, et al Neural processing of reward and loss in girls at risk for major depression. Arch Gen Psychiatry 2010;67(4):380–7.

167. Roberson-Nay R, McClure EB, Monk CS, et al. Increased amygdala activity during successful memory encoding in adolescent major depressive disorder: an FMRI study. Biol Psychiatry 2006;60(9):966–73.

168. Shad MU, Bidesi AP, Chen LA, et al. Neurobiology of decision making in depressed adolescents: a functional magnetic resonance imaging study. J Am Acad Child Adolesc Psychiatry 2011;50(6):612–21,e612.

169. Konarski JZ, McIntyre RS, Soczynska JK, et al. Neuroimaging approaches in mood disorders: technique and clinical implications. Ann Clin Psychiatry 2007; 19(4):265–77.

170. Milne A, MacQueen GM, Yucel K, et al. Hippocampal metabolic abnormalities at first onset and with recurrent episodes of a major depressive disorder: a proton magnetic resonance spectroscopy study. NeuroImage 2009;47(1):36–41.

171. Yildiz-Yesiloglu A, Ankerst DP. Review of 1H magnetic resonance spectroscopy findings in major depressive disorder: a meta-analysis. Psychiatry Res 2006;147(1): 1–25.

172. Kondo DG, Hellem TL, Sung YH, et al. Review: magnetic resonance spectroscopy studies of pediatric major depressive disorder. Depress Res Treat 2011;2011: 650450.

173. Olvera RL, Caetano SC, Stanley JA, et al. Reduced medial prefrontal N-acetyl-aspartate levels in pediatric major depressive disorder: a multi-voxel in vivo(1)H spectroscopy study. Psychiatry Res 2010;184(2):71–6.

174. Kessler RC, Walters EE. Epidemiology of DSM-III-R major depression and minor depression among adolescents and young adults in the National Comorbidity Survey. Depress Anxiety 1998;7(1):3–14.

175. Birmaher B, Arbelaez C, Brent D. Course and outcome of child and adolescent major depressive disorder. Child Adolesc Psychiatr Clin North Am 2002;11(3):619–37, x.

176. Gerber AJ, Peterson BS. Applied brain imaging. J Am Acad Child Adolesc Psychiatry 2008;47(3):239.

177. Pavuluri MN, Sweeney JA. Integrating functional brain neuroimaging and developmental cognitive neuroscience in child psychiatry research. J Am Acad Child Adolesc Psychiatry 2008;47(11):1273–88.

178. Uhl GR, Grow RW. The burden of complex genetics in brain disorders. Arch Gen Psychiatry 2004;61(3):223–9.

179. Nugent NR, Tyrka AR, Carpenter LL, et al. Gene-environment interactions: early life stress and risk for depressive and anxiety disorders. Psychopharmacology 2011; 214(1):175–96.

180. Silberg JL, Maes H, Eaves LJ. Genetic and environmental influences on the transmission of parental depression to children's depression and conduct disturbance: an extended Children of Twins study. J Child Psychol Psychiatry Allied Disciplines 2010;51(6):734–44.

181. Wichers M, Geschwind N, Jacobs N, et al. Transition from stress sensitivity to a depressive state: longitudinal twin study. Br J Psychiatry 2009;195(6):498–503.

182. Rice F, Harold GT, Thapar A. Assessing the effects of age, sex and shared environment on the genetic aetiology of depression in childhood and adolescence. J Child Psychol Psychiatry Allied Disciplines 2002;43(8):1039–51.

183. Scourfield J, Rice F, Thapar A, et al. Depressive symptoms in children and adolescents: changing aetiological influences with development. J Child Psychol Psychiatry Allied Disciplines 2003;44(7):968–76.

184. Gjone H, Stevenson J, Sundet JM, et al. Changes in heritability across increasing levels of behavior problems in young twins. Behav Genet 1996;26(4):419–26.

185. O'Connor TG, Neiderhiser JM, Reiss D, et al. Genetic contributions to continuity, change, and co-occurrence of antisocial and depressive symptoms in adolescence. J Child Psychol Psychiatry Allied Disciplines 1998;39(3):323–36.

186. Eley TC, Stevenson J. Exploring the covariation between anxiety and depression symptoms: a genetic analysis of the effects of age and sex. J Child Psychol Psychiatry Allied Disciplines 1999;40(8):1273–82.

187. Silberg J, Pickles A, Rutter M, et al. The influence of genetic factors and life stress on depression among adolescent girls. Arch Gen Psychiatry 1999;56(3):225–32.

188. Karg K, Burmeister M, Shedden K, et al. The serotonin transporter promoter variant (5-HTTLPR), stress, and depression meta-analysis revisited: evidence of genetic moderation. Arch Gen Psychiatry 2011;68(5):444–54.

189. Caspi A, Sugden K, Moffitt TE, et al. Influence of life stress on depression: moderation by a polymorphism in the 5-HTT gene. Science 2003;301(5631):386–9.

190. Kaufman J, Yang BZ, Douglas-Palumberi H, et al. Social supports and serotonin transporter gene moderate depression in maltreated children. Proc Natl Acad Sci USA 2004;101(49):17316–21.

191. Risch N, Herrell R, Lehner T, et al. Interaction between the serotonin transporter gene (5-HTTLPR), stressful life events, and risk of depression: a meta-analysis. JAMA 2009;301(23):2462–71.

192. Heim C, Bradley B, Mletzko TC, et al. Effect of childhood trauma on adult depression and neuroendocrine function: sex-specific moderation by CRH receptor 1 gene. Front Behav Neurosci 2009;3:41.

193. Aguilera M, Arias B, Wichers M, et al. Early adversity and 5-HTT/BDNF genes: new evidence of gene-environment interactions on depressive symptoms in a general population. Psychol Med 2009;39(9):1425–32.

194. Castren E, Rantamaki T. Role of brain-derived neurotrophic factor in the aetiology of depression: implications for pharmacological treatment. CNS Drugs 2010;24(1):1–7.

195. Kaufman J, Yang BZ, Douglas-Palumberi H, et al. Brain-derived neurotrophic factor-5-HTTLPR gene interactions and environmental modifiers of depression in children. Biol Psychiatry 2006;59(8):673–80.

196. Gatt JM, Nemeroff CB, Dobson-Stone C, et al. Interactions between BDNF Val66Met polymorphism and early life stress predict brain and arousal pathways to syndromal depression and anxiety. Mol Psychiatry 2009;14(7):681–95.

197. Munafo MR, Brown SM, Hariri AR. Serotonin transporter (5-HTTLPR) genotype and amygdala activation: a meta-analysis. Biol Psychiatry 2008;63(9):852–7.

198. Frodl T, Moller HJ, Meisenzahl E. Neuroimaging genetics: new perspectives in research on major depression? Acta Psychiatr Scand 2008;118(5):363–72.

199. Frodl T, Reinhold E, Koutsouleris N, et al. Childhood stress, serotonin transporter gene and brain structures in major depression. Neuropsychopharmacology 2010;35(6):1383–90.

200. Duman RS, Monteggia LM. A neurotrophic model for stress-related mood disorders. Biol Psychiatry 2006;59(12):1116–27.

201. Griffin EW, Mulally S, Foley C, et al. Aerobic exercise improves hippocampal function and increases BDNF in the serum of young adult males. Physiol Behav 2011;104(5):934–41.

202. Lucassen PJ, Meerlo P, Naylor AS, et al. Regulation of adult neurogenesis by stress, sleep disruption, exercise and inflammation: implications for depression and antidepressant action. Eur Neuropsychopharmacol 2010;20(1):1–17.

203. Bowley MP, Drevets WC, Ongur D, et al. Low glial numbers in the amygdala in major depressive disorder. Biol Psychiatry 2002;52(5):404–12.

204. Holsboer F, Ising M. Central CRH system in depression and anxiety — evidence from clinical studies with CRH1 receptor antagonists. Eur J Pharmacol 2008;583(2-3): 350–7.

205. Linden DE. Brain imaging and psychotherapy: methodological considerations and practical implications. Eur Arch Psychiatry Clin Neurosci 2008;258(Suppl 5):71–5.

206. Regier DA, Narrow WE, First MB, et al. The APA classification of mental disorders: future perspectives. Psychopathology 2002;35(2-3):166–70.

207. Leibenluft E. Skating to where the puck will be: the importance of neuroimaging literacy in child psychiatry. J Am Acad Child Adolesc Psychiatry 2008;47(11): 1213–6.

208. Mason GF, Krystal JH. MR spectroscopy: its potential role for drug development for the treatment of psychiatric diseases. NMR Biomed 2006;19(6):690–701.

209. Kraemer HC, Wilson GT, Fairburn CG, et al. Mediators and moderators of treatment effects in randomized clinical trials. Arch Gen Psychiatry 2002;59(10):877–83.

Developmental Risk of Depression: Experience Matters

William R. Beardslee, MD[a,b,*], Tracy R.G. Gladstone, PhD[a,b,c],
Erin E. O'Connor, BA[b]

KEYWORDS

- Depression • Risk • Resiliency • Youth • Prevention

Key Abbreviations: DEVELOPMENTAL RISK OF DEPRESSION	
ACE	Adverse childhood experiences
CNS	Central nervous system
CWS	Coping With Stress course
HPA	Hypothalamic–pituitary–adrenal
MDD	Major depressive disorder
NCS	National Comorbidity Survey
PRP	Penn Resiliency Program
SES	Socioeconomic status
subACC	Subgenual region of the anterior cingulate cortex

Youth depression is a problem of major proportions, with 1-year prevalence rates of about 2% in childhood, and ranging from 4% to 7% in adolescence.[1] According to the National Comorbidity Survey (NCS),[2] the lifetime prevalence of major depressive disorder (MDD) in adolescents aged 15 to 18 years is 14%, and an estimated 20% of adolescents will have had a depressive disorder by the time they are 18 years old.[3,4] Although depression is a treatable disorder, most depressed youth do not receive treatment for depressive symptoms or disorder,[5] and even though successful treatments for youth depression have been explored, such as antidepressants, cognitive behavioral interventions, and interpersonal psychotherapy, such treatments have been found effective for only about 50% to 60% of cases under controlled research conditions.[6] Overall, although treatment for youth depression is important

William R. Beardslee and Tracy R.G. Gladstone have received funding from the Sidney R. Baer, Jr. Foundation. Erin O'Connor has nothing to disclose.
[a] Department of Psychiatry, Children's Hospital, 300 Longwood Avenue, Boston, MA 02115, USA
[b] Judge Baker Children's Center, 53 Parker Hill Avenue, Boston, MA 02120, USA
[c] Wellesley Centers for Women, Wellesley College, 106 Central Street, Wellesley, MA 02484, USA
* Corresponding author. Children's Hospital Boston, 21 Autumn Street, Suite 130.2, Boston, MA 02215.
E-mail address: william.beardslee@childrens.harvard.edu

and can be beneficial, many who receive treatment for depression do not respond, have residual symptoms, or experience relapses of disorder.[7–10]

Similar to adult depression, adolescent depression frequently is persistent and recurring.[3,4,11] Twelve percent of children will relapse within 1 year, 40% will relapse within 2 years, and 75% will experience a second episode within 5 years.[12,13] Adolescent depression is associated with negative long-term functional and psychiatric outcomes, including impairment in school, work, interpersonal relationships, and substance abuse.[14–20] Of particular note is the association between adolescent depression and suicidal behavior. Suicide is the third leading cause of death in adolescents.[21] Over a 1-year period, 13.8% of adolescents in the United States reported seriously considering suicide, 10.9% had made suicidal plans, and 6.3% reported making a suicide attempt.[22] Moreover, up to 70% of youth who completed suicide had multiple comorbid psychiatric disorders, with the risk of suicide completion increasing as the degree of comorbidity increased.[23,24] Depression is the most common mental disorder associated with suicide.[25–27] For example, in the review paper by Gould and colleagues,[28] 49% to 64% of adolescent suicide victims were found to have a corresponding depressive disorder.

Given the prevalence of youth depression and the limitations of current treatment options, it follows that efforts to prevent the onset of youth depression are warranted. Prevention approaches have the potential to reach a large number of youth and may be more acceptable than seeking treatment for many youth. This is in part because prevention can be rendered in nonclinic settings that are more acceptable to youth, such as schools, and also because receiving prevention services does not require identifying oneself as ill. Efficacious preventive efforts are developed from the understanding of risk and protective factors for youth depression. That is, understanding risks for depression onset, and the role of environmental factors in promoting resilience in children and adolescents, identifies targets for programs that focus on youth depression. In this article, we focus on discussing risks for depression onset and the role of environmental factors in promoting resilience in children and adolescents.

RISKS FOR DEPRESSION

Risks for depression can be grouped into two classes:

1. Those specific for depression, such as having a depressed parent
2. Those nonspecific risk factors that affect a wide range of psychiatric outcomes including depression (eg, poverty, child abuse).

It should be noted that it is a constellation of adversities that leads to poorer outcomes, as multiple risk factors have more impact than does any single risk factor.[29–32]

Specific Risk Factors

Specific risk factors are those factors that have been associated with increased risk for youth depression in empirical investigations. Specific risk factors for adolescent depression include[33,34]:

- A family history of depression
- Prior experience of depression
- A negative cognitive style
- Bereavement.

Family history of depression
In the case of youth depression, one of the strongest factors for the development of depression is having a parent with a depressive illness.[35,36] Depression is remarkably common among parents.[33] According to an Institute of Medicine report, at least 15 million children are living with a depressed parent. In addition, because many parents who recover from an episode of depression continue to experience subclinical levels of depressive symptomatology, many children are repeatedly exposed to depression, and to associated disruptions in parenting.[37]

Disorders of offspring of depressed parents Offspring of depressed parents are at a two- to fourfold increased risk of developing depressive disorders, and more than half of the parents bringing their depressed adolescents for services themselves have current mood disorders.[35] Research in the past 20 years suggests that children who grow up with depressed parents have more internalizing disorders such as depression and anxiety, more externalizing disorders such as conduct disorder and attention deficit disorder,[38] more cognitive delays and academic difficulties, and more social difficulties.[35] Thus, many depression prevention efforts in youth have targeted either those with symptoms or those whose parents have depression.

Over the past 12 years, data have accumulated on several longitudinal samples of depressed parents and their offspring[39–42] Weissman and colleagues have followed a sample of the offspring of depressed and nondepressed parents (n = 47) over the course of 20 years, such that all of the offspring are now adults and have their own children.[40] At the last assessment, rates of diagnoses of depressive disorders, as well anxiety and substance use disorders, were threefold in the now adult offspring compared to the comparison group.[43] Moreover, the authors found that offspring were at the greatest risk for depression between the ages of 15 and 20.[43]

Genetic influences on depression Recently, much more work has been done in the area of genetics and what specifically confers risk of depression from parent to child. Overall, this research suggests that various kinds of family history of depression contribute to an increased risk for depression in the face of stressful life events. Specific genes have been identified as key in the transmission of depression from parent to child, such as the presence of two short alleles in 5-HTTLPR polymorphism in context of chronic stress (girls),[44] the gene *BDNF*,[45] and homozygous carriers of the *T* allele (MTHFR allele). Unfortunately, a number of recent meta-analyses of the 5-HTTLPR polymorphism have failed to replicate many of these findings.[46,47] The lack of replication points to an overarching problem plaguing these genetic studies. Often, these studies look at one specific or "candidate" gene and its role in the presentation of various diseases and disorders. However, disorders rarely result from the expression of a single gene.

Genetic-environmental influences on depression The unique genetic influences of *individual* genes may be modest, but when coupled with environmental influences, the contribution of heritable factors provides us with invaluable information about which individuals are most at risk. The gene–environment interaction is especially potent when it comes to determining outcomes of those who are at risk for depression. Applying this model to the heritability of depression, a child who inherits a certain genetic makeup from a depressed parent has the raw materials for developing depressive symptoms, but only when certain environmental effects come into play does the combination of gene and environment create the finished product, namely a depressive disorder. The impact of the environment on the expression of certain genes depends on the degree to which:

1. An individual is exposed to a particular environment
2. An individual's behavior influences the environment
3. An individual's behavior is itself subject to genetic influences.

In an extensive literature review, Kendler and Baker[48] noted that, although genes do influence the environment, for example, in the areas of life stress and parenting, the degree of influence is modest, with heritability estimates generally ranging from 15% to 35%.

Prior experience of depression

Although many factors, such as a family history of depression and a particular genotype, interact to form a depressive disorder, one risk factor for a depressive episode is a depressive episode itself. Having a prior history of depression increases the probability that another depressive disorder will develop. In fact, Lewinsohn and colleagues found that 45% of adolescents with a history of depression developed another episode of depression between the ages of 19 and 24.[49] Moreover, in a 10- to 15-year longitudinal study conducted by Weissman and colleagues, individuals who had adolescent-onset major depressive disorder (MDD) were two times more likely to develop a depressive disorder in adulthood than those with no history of depression.[18] In addition, although a history of depression increases the risk of developing another depressive disorder, those with subsyndromal symptoms of depression are also at increased risk for developing depression, even if they do not have a full-blown disorder.[49]

Depressogenic cognitive style

A number of studies have demonstrated that how a child interprets the world and the way in which he or she responds to it will affect the likelihood of developing depression.[50–52] Several cognitive explanations regarding risk of depression have been examined, such as Beck's model, which emphasizes underlying beliefs and ways of interpreting various life events (eg, depression in parents, parenting). Such perceptions of the world are often critical and extremely pessimistic, potentially leading to feelings of hopelessness and lack of self-worth, and consequently to depression. It has also been hypothesized that biases in attention or selective attention to negative events contribute to a depressogenic cognitive style, a processes that is thought to be partly heritable.[53,54]

A number of studies have bolstered such cognitive theories, demonstrating the pervasive nature of having a depressive cognitive style. Garber and Flynn,[50] for example, found that maternal depression history was positively associated with depressive cognitions in adolescent offspring, specifically hopelessness, low self-worth, and a negative attribution style. Children (aged 6–14 years) who exhibited depressogenic inferential styles were more likely to report elevated depressive symptoms after an increase in their parent's depressive symptoms than children who did not have depressogenic inferential styles.[51] Lau and colleagues found a heritability component in a depressogenic attribution style in that, although social factors clearly influence attribution style, such as feedback and modeling processes, children and adolescents may also inherit a certain attribution style from their parents.[53] Likewise, Gibb and colleagues[54] found that children of depressed parents may inherit a genetic risk factor for developing depression by way of the 5-HTTLPR alleles when paired with a negative inferential style. *Kovacs and Lopez-Duran, in Contextual Emotion Regulation Therapy: A Developmentally-Based Intervention for Pediatric Depression,* have identified positive and negative affectivity as contributing to depressogenic cognitive style.

Bereavement

As stated, a depressogenic cognitive style may predispose a child or adolescent to certain risk factors in the way they interpret various life stressors and adversities. One of the more traumatic stressors that can occur in a child's life is the loss of a parent.[55] Parentally bereaved youth have been found to have a host of functional impairments, in addition to depression, such as suicidal ideation, and post-traumatic stress disorder.[34] Studies have shown that children who had psychiatric diagnoses prior to the death of a parent are likely to fare worse than those who had no prior diagnosis.[56] Moreover, children are likely to have more psychopathology after a parent's death if the parent died traumatically, especially by suicide, or if the surviving parent has higher levels of psychopathology.[56] Cerel and colleagues[57] compared a group of bereaved children and adolescents (aged 6–17 years) to a group of depressed youth, and to a community sample of youth. They found that bereaved children were more likely to demonstrate elevated depressive symptoms than the community sample, but were not as impaired as the clinically depressed group.[57] The authors point out, however, that even though the elevated depressive symptoms in the bereaved children were somewhat modest, these children are still at risk for a number of disorders, including depression, due to a number of risk factors that may accompany a parent's death, such as parental depression and loss of income.[57]

Nonspecific Risk Factors

A comprehensive approach to the prevention of depression involves addressing both specific and nonspecific risk factors. Nonspecific risk factors are associated with increased risk for a range of disorders, including depression. Nonspecific risk factors that are documented to increase rates of youth depression include[33]:

- Poverty
- Exposure to violence
- Life stressors
- Social isolation.

In fact, reducing the burdens of poverty, exposure to violence, child maltreatment, and other forms of family instability may play an important role in the reduction of depressive disorders in youth.[33] It is important to note that some of these adverse life experiences, such as poverty, will have varying degrees of adverse effects depending on the length of exposure, as current life stressors tend to have less of an adverse impact than do lifetime stressors. In other words, living in poverty for a number of years is, on average, worse than living in poverty for 6 months.

Poverty

Exposure to poverty has been associated with many negative outcomes. Specifically, a recent study of a subsample of the US National Collaborative Perinatal Project examined the relation between lower socioeconomic status (SES) in families of young children and later rates of depression.[58] Lifetime risk for depression was related to occupational level of the parents at birth. Subjects with parents of lower SES backgrounds had significantly increased lifetime rates of depression.

In a recent longitudinal study spanning 21 years, Najman and colleagues[59] looked at the effect of exposure to poverty on long-term mental health and found that children who were exposed to family poverty were more likely to report depression and anxiety in adolescence and young adulthood. Specifically, poverty experienced when the individuals were 14 years old was the single greatest predictor of depression and anxiety in adolescence and young adulthood.[59] These findings point to the importance of examining multiple risk factors when exploring the prevention of adverse mental health outcomes, as certain age groups appear to be particularly vulnerable to a variety of risk factors.

Abuse/Violence

The link between childhood abuse, violence, and depression has long been established. A history of childhood sexual abuse has been found to be a particularly potent predictor of depression in adolescence.[60] Aslund and colleagues found that, overall, maltreatment had a strong association with adolescent depression, and on further analysis, found that maltreatment interacted with the 5-HTTLPR promoter region to predict greater risk of depression.[61] Specifically, girls, but not boys, who were homozygous for the short allele of the 5-HTTLPR promoter region were at greater risk for depression in the face of maltreatment.[61] In light of findings such as these, Harkness and colleagues postulated that abuse in childhood may sensitize individuals to the effects of adverse life events, thus accounting for the increased risk for depression in such individuals when confronted with other life stressors.[62] They use the concept of "stress sensitization" to explain their findings that adolescents with trauma history, as compared to those with no trauma history, had lower levels of threat when confronted with independent life events. Individuals with a history of abuse were more likely to develop a depressive episode in the face of a life event than were individuals without a history of abuse. The authors suggest that the maltreated individuals required lower levels of acute life events to trigger the onset of the depressive episode due to the persistent chronic stress in years prior.[62]

In a prospective longitudinal study of 676 maltreated children and 520 non-abused and non-neglected control subjects, Widom and colleagues[63] found a significant relation between child physical abuse and increased risk for lifetime MDD, and between child neglect and increased risk for current MDD. Similarly, MacMillan and colleagues found that in a community sample, women who were physically abused as children had significantly higher lifetime rates of major depression than did women with no history of abuse.[64] Gibb also looked at a community sample and found that children who experienced emotional abuse from their parents or verbal victimization from their peers underwent changes in their inferential styles and had increases in depressive symptoms.[65] The authors suggest that children who undergo emotional/verbal abuse may learn to see certain events in a negative light, and over time may generalize this pessimistic outlook to other life events, potentially contributing to an overall depressogenic cognitive style. While the exact mechanisms remain unclear, selective central nervous system (CNS) remodeling and sensitization of the hypothalamic–pituitary–adrenal (HPA) axis have been suggested. For a more detailed discussion, please see Singh and Gotlib: Developmental Risk I: Depression and the Developing Brain in this publication.

Life stressors

As is the case with low SES, children whose parents divorce are often exposed to a number of adverse life events. Children may experience increased family conflict, lack of family cohesion, and less supportive parenting.[66] In a study involving college students whose parents divorced when they were between the ages of 8 and 18, parental divorce was significantly related to current depression in the students who reported parental divorce, as opposed to students whose parents were still married.[66] Kelly, in a meta-analysis, discusses the fact that children whose parents divorce are more likely to witness a reduction in household income and resources to which they may otherwise have had access.[67] As stated earlier, low SES poses a risk for youth depression, and therefore it may be that the financial consequences of divorce contribute to this population's increased risk for depression. Moreover, Kelly found that it may not be the actual divorce that predicts child adjustment, but rather the degree of marital conflict to which the children are exposed. Consequently, children and adolescents whose parents divorce need to be monitored for a variety of adverse consequences, especially if the divorce was extremely conflictual and there was resulting household and financial instability.[67]

Social and family disruptions have also been implicated as risk factors for depression in children and adolescents. Gilman and colleagues found that frequent location changes before age 7 predicted depression onset by age 14.[68] Frequent location changes were not associated with depressive symptoms in adulthood, only in childhood; however, low SES did have a lasting impact into adulthood in this population, further demonstrating the need for poverty intervention in such vulnerable populations.[68]

Social isolation

Clearly a child or adolescent's social environment is an important factor in his or her overall well being, and like social disruption from relocations or parental divorce, social isolation or disengagement can be just as devastating. Joiner and colleagues demonstrated this in their study looking at lack of pleasurable engagement, loneliness, and the onset and recurrence of depression in adolescents.[69] They found that lack of pleasurable engagement was significantly related to the onset of depressive disorder, and hypothesized that this lack of pleasurable engagement may represent the core of loneliness for these individuals. The authors make the important point that this variable may be especially salient for youth, as they are in a developmental stage when engagement with peers in social activities is especially critical. Interestingly, lack of pleasurable social engagement was predictive of mood disorders (ie, depression), whereas it was not predictive of nonmood disorders. This distinction is important in that it demonstrates the unique vulnerabilities of those at risk for depression in childhood and adolescence.[69]

Brain imaging for social isolation–depressive link A recent study by Masten and colleagues[70] attempted to demonstrate the connection between social isolation and risk for depressive disorder using brain imaging techniques. They looked at the subgenual region of the anterior cingulate cortex (subACC), a region that has been linked to depression as well as heightened sensitivity to peer rejection in adolescence.[70] Adolescents who showed greater activity in the subACC region during social exclusion were more likely to have reported depressive symptoms a year later. The authors proposed that this heightened brain activity may act as a neural marker for depression during adolescence and may, in part, explain the sensitivity to peer rejection that is often observed in adolescence.[70]

Impoverishment as risk for depressed populations Another important aspect of social isolation or exclusion is that on a broad scale, it leaves certain populations especially vulnerable to depression.[33] For instance, many impoverished communities do not have access to the treatment and resources they may need due to factors such as racial discrimination, poverty, language barriers, and geographic isolation.[33] Although individuals who are socially isolated are at risk for developing depression, it is important to remember that entire communities are also at risk due to a compilation of adverse life events and stressors.

Adversity index

As stated, there are often certain groups of people that will be exposed to multiple risk factors due to their surrounding environment. Poverty, by itself, is a risk factor for depression but, by being exposed to poverty, an individual will likely experience additional risk factors, such as abuse and violence.[71] This is important as risk factors are additive, and it is the compilation of risk factors that confers the most risk.[30] It is the general consensus that psychopathologic risk is far greater when multiple factors are taken into consideration, as isolated risk factors tend to confer relatively low risk by themselves.[72,73] For instance, the Adverse Childhood Experiences (ACE) Study found that children who were exposed to a number of adverse experiences were more likely to have negative outcomes in adulthood than children who were exposed to fewer adversities.[74] In an earlier study, Sameroff and colleagues calculated a multiple risk score such that a family could receive a score ranging from 0 (no risk) to 8 (high risk) and were subsequently divided into a low-risk group, a moderate-risk group, and a high-risk group. Analyses showed that multiple risk was significantly associated with poorer outcomes among preschoolers, such that the more risk factors (higher risk), the worse the outcome.[73] Likewise, Espejo and colleagues found that youth who had been exposed to a number of adverse life events and who also had a history of anxiety disorder were more likely to have a severe depressive episode after a stressful event compared to youth who had experienced none or only one adverse life event.[75]

RESILIENCE AND PROTECTIVE FACTORS

Although the presence of both specific and nonspecific risk factors does indicate an increased risk for youth depression, it is important to remember that not all children and adolescents who are exposed to these risk factors develop disorder. In fact, many children who are exposed to risk factors for depression also have protective factors and exhibit resilience, which means that they have characteristics that decrease the likelihood of developing depression.[33] A classic 1988 paper by Beardslee and colleagues found that teen resilience was characterized by considerable self-understanding, a deep commitment to relationships, and the ability to think and act separately from others, specifically their parents.[76]

Since then there has been a wide expansion in the understanding of resilience and a rich array of different dimensions including self-reflection, spirituality, formation of caring relationships, and ability to understand others' worlds.[77–82] The resiliency literature has noted that there are several specific factors that universally contribute to childhood resilience.[33] These factors include[83]:

- Connection and attachment to caring adults
- Positive family systems
- Normal cognitive development (IQ)
- Adequate self-regulatory systems
- Positive outlook
- Motivation for achievement.

All of these dimensions are important to consider in a comprehensive assessment. Recently, Beardslee proposed that self-reflection and self-understanding are the felt, conscious manifestations of the larger process of self-regulation.[84]

Finally, there has been progress both in greater precision in measuring diagnoses and in some instances, in linking risk and resilience factors to underlying mechanisms. In this section, we discuss various dimensions in which progress has been made in the resilience field, such as:

- Certain gene–environment interactions
- Positive relationships
- Participation in activities
- Ability to successfully self-regulate.

Gene–Environment Interaction

Kim-Cohen and colleagues discuss an important shift in resilience research in that more research is being devoted to gene–environment interactions.[85] Certain individuals may be at risk for depression in the context of adverse life events due to various genes they have, such as the 5HT transporter polymorphism; however, this also means that certain individuals who face these same adverse life events, but who do not carry the same genes, may be resilient despite the apparent environmental risk.[85] Specifically, Cicchetti and colleagues[86] found that maltreated adolescents reported fewer internalizing symptoms if they had two of the 5HTT long allele, as opposed to two of the short allele, indicating that their genetic makeup may have promoted resilience in the face of maltreatment.

Offspring resilience to parental depression

It is now known that having a parent who is depressed is the single greatest risk factor for youth depression, and therefore in terms of prevention, it is important to elucidate what makes certain offspring resilient in the face of parental depression. In a specific study of children of depressed parents,[76] the authors studied a subset of resilient youth whose parents had experienced depression. The authors found that, within the youth, several factors contributed to resilience, including a focus on accomplishing age-appropriate developmental tasks, on relationships, and on understanding their parents' illness. Three dimensions of understanding a parents' illness were identified.

First Dimension: Youth were able to describe observable behaviors associated with the illness (withdrawn behavior or frequent crying).

Second Dimension: Although they often indicated that they wanted to cure their parents, they were aware that they could not, but that they could take certain concrete actions to help them.

Third Dimension: They took actions based on their cognitive knowledge. By observing their parents, they found that resilience was associated with a commitment to parenting and relationships, despite the depression.

In a more recent study, Brennan and colleagues found that, in a sample of offspring of depressed mothers, a number of mother–child interaction variables contributed to resilience in these youth. Specifically, they found that low levels of psychological control, high levels of maternal warmth, and low levels of maternal over involvement interacted with maternal depression to predict resiliency, meaning that the youth had no current Axis I disorders, no current symptoms or history of disorder, and had no current social functioning difficulties.[37]

Relationships

Resiliency researchers point to the early environment as especially important in creating resilience to various stressors and adversities.[80] Sensitive periods early in development, if they include responsive and supporting caregivers, can promote the development of various neural pathways in the young child that may play a role in buffering the individual from various life stressors.[87] These early supportive relationships with caregivers are especially important in environments in which a child is exposed to extreme or chronic stress, and it has been found that, not only do these supportive relationships *buffer* against negative effects of stress, but may in fact *reduce* the harmful effects.[80,88]

Relationships in later adolescence may also confer protection against depressive symptoms.[89] Desjardins and colleagues,[89] not surprisingly, found that adolescents who were relationally victimized had higher levels of depressive symptoms compared to adolescents who had not been relationally victimized. However, among those adolescents who had been relationally victimized, those with high levels of paternal emotional support reported lower levels of depressive symptoms. Interestingly, however, they also found that the victimized adolescents reported an increase in depressive symptoms when they reported high levels of maternal and peer support.[89] Helsen and colleagues also found that some form of parental support in adolescence seemed to buffer against symptoms, such that parental support was found to mediate the relation between peer support and emotional problems.[90] Specifically, adolescents who reported high levels of peer support were less likely to have emotional problems if they also reported high levels of parental support (as compared to those who reported low levels of peer support). A similar study by Young and colleagues[91] found that anticipated peer support was a protective factor for adolescents developing depressive symptoms when they also reported high levels of parental support. However, in adolescents who reported low levels of parental support, anticipated peer support did not act as a protective factor.[91] Although not empirically tested in this study, it is quite possible that current and past parental support enabled youngsters to actively engage with peers and receive support whereas in the absence of parental support, youngsters may have been preoccupied with the relationship that the parents were not open to peer support.

Activity

One area of resilience related to social relationships and support that has been found to play a role in the protection of children and adolescents from developing psychopathology is activity involvement and social interaction.[92] Babiss and colleagues examined the relationship between activity involvement and depression in adolescents.[93] They looked specifically at sports participation and found that as sports participation increased, depression and suicidal ideation decreased. Moreover, this relationship was mediated by self-esteem and social support, supporting the resiliency literature that has named these two factors as important mechanisms in which youth are protected against depression.[33] For instance, Kaufman and colleagues[94] demonstrated that maltreated adolescents were less likely to develop depression if they had a supportive relationship with an adult.

Self-Regulation

A number of studies have begun to look at how a child's ability to regulate his or her emotions and behaviors contributes to the risk for depression. In some cases, when a child is unable to self-regulate, his or her risk for depression increases whereas when a child is able to successfully regulate his or her emotions and behaviors, the child may be resilient, even in the face of other risk factors.[95–97] Silk and colleagues examined a number of possible self-regulation mechanisms by which children are protected against depression.[95] Children's emotion regulation skills, as well as other family predictors of emotion regulation (eg, maternal nurturance, parent–child relationship quality), were all found to be associated with positive adjustment in the children, despite their risk for depression via maternal depression.[95] Silk and colleagues also found that the sleep patterns of children who were at high risk for depression due to a parent having depression appear to act as a buffer against developing a depressive disorder.[95] Among the at-risk children, those who took less time falling asleep and spent more time in stage 4 sleep were less likely as young adults to be depressed. The authors propose that sleep patterns may provide resilience against depression because sleep processes are thought to play a part in self-regulation, a well-documented resilience factor.[95] For a more detailed discussion of the role of sleep, see article elsewhere in this issue.

SUMMARY

An understanding of risk and resiliency drives the development of prevention programs for youth depression, and enables researchers to make careful choices about the prevention strategies they use. A key early stage of prevention research involves understanding specific and nonspecific risk and protective factors, as prevention efforts that work benefit from a focus on decreasing risk factors and enhancing protective factors for a particular disorder. Research and clinical implications of advancements in this area are reviewed in the text that follows.

Research Implications

In the past several decades, research on the prevention of youth depression has blossomed, and as a result, much more is known about ways to maximize the efficacy of prevention efforts. That is, because more is known about risk and protective factors for depression, more is known about the variables to target, the timing of interventions, and the samples that will be most likely to benefit from depression prevention efforts. To date, researchers who have studied the effects of preventive interventions on depression in youth generally have based their prevention strategies on cognitive–behavioral or interpersonal approaches.[98] These approaches have been found to be helpful in the treatment of depression,[99] and recently have been evaluated to determine whether they may be useful in preventing youth depression.

Currently, there are a number of promising prevention strategies that are based on depression risk research. For example, Clarke and colleagues developed the Coping With Stress (CWS) course, a manual-based psychoeducational group program targeting at-risk adolescents with depressed parents.[100] A four-site effectiveness study led by Judy Garber[101] is being conducted using a variant of the CWS program developed by Clarke and colleagues.[102] The Penn Resiliency Program (PRP)[103] is perhaps the most widely evaluated depression prevention program for youth.[104] It was developed to target cognitive and behavioral risk factors for depression in school-aged children. Based on cognitive behavioral therapy, PRP is a school-based program that teaches participants the connection between life events, their beliefs about those events, and the emotional consequences of their interpretations. A number of intervention programs for children of depressed parents have incorporated the family system as an integral target of intervention. For example, Compas and colleagues assessed the efficacy of a family cognitive–behavioral preventive intervention aimed at preventing depression in the offspring of parents with a history of depression.[105] Beardslee and coworkers also have developed family-based, public health interventions for families when parents are depressed: a clinician-based program and a lecture program.[106] Both approaches emphasize a cognitive orientation, focus on building strengths and resilience in youth and their parents, and highlight the importance of treatment for parental depression. This work has been used in countrywide programs in Europe and Central America and has been adapted for use with single-parent African American families, Latino families, and for use in Head Start and Early Head Start.[107–109] Unlike other researchers examining the prevention of youth depression in teens identified based on their elevated depressive symptoms or family history of depression, Sandler and colleagues[110] focused on preventing negative outcomes in children at risk based on difficult life circumstances, including parental divorce and bereavement.

Clinical Implications

Research on risk and protective factors for youth depression should inform our clinical efforts as well. When meeting with children and families, clinicians must conduct a comprehensive assessment that views children in the multiple contexts they exist in and details past and current development difficulties, symptoms, and past and current diagnoses. In addition, a full assessment of strengths and resources in individuals and families is essential. It is in fact the presence of strengths and resources (eg, a parent's willingness to seek treatment for a child, the child's willingness to engage in treatment) that influence outcome.

It may seem obvious that the assessment of broader risk factors is important for a different reason. A child who goes to school hungry has much more difficulty learning. Some social policies have attempted to address the limited resources in both early childhood and educational programs, including a focus on providing adequate nutrition for children in need.[111] This work has met with some success but much more remains to be done. In the same way, if a child is subjected to a difficult environment (eg, a depressed, unemployed parent who is drinking), then treatment efforts must consider the effects of the adverse environments on that child's functioning. Overall, understanding the multiple dimensions of risk is central to the development of successful intervention strategies. Also, understanding the multiple dimensions affected by either depression or risks for depression heightens awareness of possible strategies for intervention by combining individual and family-based approaches or combining treatment for depression with a focus on exercise and building social relationships.

Finally, given what we know about the natural history of childhood and adolescent depression, the likelihood of recurrence, and the profound impairments that accompany youth depression, we believe in the importance of long-term follow-up, even after an episode has been resolved. Regularly scheduled follow-ups, even in the absence of illness, are now the norm for many pediatric diseases; such follow-ups allow for more rapid recognition and response. In the case of youth depression, research advances in our understanding of risk factors enable us to target treatment and prevention efforts, and to take steps to ensure the long-term success of children and families.

REFERENCES

1. Costello EJ, Pine DS, Hammen C, et al. Development and natural history of mood disorders. Biol Psychiatry 2002;52(6):529–42.
2. Kessler RC, Walters EE. Epidemiology of DSM-III-R major depression and minor depression among adolescents and young adults in the national comorbidity survey. Depression Anxiety (1091–4269) 1998;7(1):3–14.
3. Birmaher B, Ryan ND, Williamson DE, et al. Childhood and adolescent depression: a review of the past 10 years. Part I. J Am Acad Child Adolesc Psychiatry 1996;35(11): 1427–39.

4. Birmaher B, Ryan ND, Williamson DE, et al. Childhood and adolescent depression: a review of the past 10 years. Part II. J Am Acad Child Adolesc Psychiatry 1996;35(12): 1575–83.

5. Kessler RC, McGonagle KA, Zhao S, et al. Lifetime and 12-month prevalence of DSM-III-R psychiatric disorders in the United States: results from the National Comorbidity Study. Arch Gen Psychiatry 1994;51(1):8–19.

6. Treatment for Adolescents with Depression Study (TADS) Team. Fluoxetine, cognitive-behavioral therapy, and their combination for adolescents with depression. JAMA 2004;292(7):807–20.

7. Birmaher B, Brent DA, Kolko D, et al. Clinical outcome after short-term psychotherapy for adolescents with major depressive disorder. Arch Gen Psychiatry 2000;57(1): 29–36.

8. Brent DA, Kolko DJ, Birmaher B, et al. Predictors of treatment efficacy in a clinical trial of three psychosocial treatments for adolescent depression. J Am Acad Child Adolesc Psychiatry 1998;37(9):906–14.

9. Clarke G, Hops H, Lewinsohn PM, et al. Cognitive-behavioral group treatment of adolescent depression: prediction of outcome. Behav Ther 1992;23(3):341–54.

10. Emslie GJ, Rush AJ, Weinberg WA, et al. Fluoxetine in child and adolescent depression: acute and maintenance treatment. Depression Anxiety (1091–4269) 1998;7(1):32–9.

11. Kovacs M. Next steps for research on child and adolescent depression prevention. Am J Prev Med 2006;31(6 Suppl 1):S184–5.

12. Kovacs M. Depressive disorders in childhood: II. A longitudinal study of the risk for a subsequent major depression. Annu Prog Child Psychiatry Child Dev 1985:520–41.

13. Lewinsohn PM, Clarke GN, Seeley JR, et al. Major depression in community adolescents: age at onset, episode duration, and time to recurrence. J Am Acad Child Adolesc Psychiatry 1994;33(6):809–18.

14. Bardone AM, Moffitt T, Caspi A, et al. Adult mental health and social outcomes of adolescent girls with depression and conduct disorder. Dev Psychopathol 1996; 8(4):811–29.

15. Bardone AM, Moffitt TE, Caspi A, et al. Adult physical health outcomes of adolescent girls with conduct disorder, depression, and anxiety. J Am Acad Child Adolesc Psychiatry 1998;37(6):594–601.

16. Lewinsohn PM, Petit JW, Joiner TE Jr, et al. The symptomatic expression of major depressive disorder in adolescents and young adults. J Abnorm Psychol 2003; 112(2):244–52.

17. Rao U, Ryan ND, Birmaher B, et al. Unipolar depression in adolescents: clinical outcome in adulthood. J Am Acad Child Adolesc Psychiatry 1995;34(5):566–78.

18. Weissman MM, Wolk S, Goldstein RB, et al. Depressed adolescents grown up. JAMA 1999;281(18):1707–13.

19. Rubin KH, Both L, Zahn-Waxler C, et al. Dyadic play behaviors of children of well and depressed mothers. Dev Psychopathol 1991;3(3):243–51.

20. Harnish JD, Dodge KA, Valente E. Mother-child interaction quality as a partial mediator of the roles of maternal depressive symptomatology and socioeconomic status in the development of child behavior problems. Child Dev 1995;66(3):739–53.

21. Centers for Disease Control and Prevention (CDC). Web-based injury statistics query and reporting system (WISQARS). 2010. Available at: www.cdc.gov/injury/wisqars/index.html. Accessed August 23, 2010.

22. Centers for Disease Control and Prevention (CDC). Youth risk behavior surveillance—United States 2009. Surveill Summ 2010;59:1–142.

23. Bridge JA, Goldstein TR, Brent DA. Adolescent suicide and suicidal behavior. J Child Psychol Psychiatry 2006;47(3–4):372–94.

24. Brent DA, Baugher M, Bridge J, et al. Age- and sex-related risk factors for adolescent suicide. J Am Acad Child Adolesc Psychiatry 1999;38(12):1497–505.

25. Gotlib IH, Hammen CL. Handbook of depression. 2nd edition. New York: Guilford Press; 2009.

26. Brent DA, Perper JA, Moritz G, et al. Psychiatric risk factors for adolescent suicide: a case-control study. J Am Acad Child Adolesc Psychiatry 1993;32(3):521–9.

27. Shaffer D, Gould MS, Fisher P, et al. Psychiatric diagnosis in child and adolescent suicide. Arch Gen Psychiatry 1996;53(4):339–48.

28. Gould MS, Greenberg T, Velting DM, et al. Youth suicide risk and preventive interventions: a review of the past 10 years. J Am Acad Child Adolesc Psychiatry 2003;42(4):386–405.

29. McLaughlin KA, Green JG, Gruber MJ, et al. Childhood adversities and adult psychopathology in the National Comorbidity Survey Replication (NCS-R) III: associations with functional impairment related to DSM-IV disorders. Psychol Med 2010;40(5):847–59.

30. Rutter M. Psychosocial resilience and protective mechanisms. Am J Orthopsychiatry 1987;57(3):316–31.

31. Kessler RC, Davis CG, Kendler KS. Childhood adversity and adult psychiatric disorder in the US National Comorbidity Survey. Psychol Med 1997;27(5):1101–19.

32. Sadowski HS, Ugarte B, Kolvin I, et al. Early life family disadvantages and major depression in adulthood. Br J Psychiatry 1999;174:112–20.

33. England MJ, Sim LJ. Depression in parents, parenting, and children: opportunities to improve identification, treatment, and prevention. Washington, DC: National Academies Press; 2009.

34. Melhem NM, Moritz G, Walker M, et al. Phenomenology and correlates of complicated grief in children and adolescents. J Am Acad Child Adolesc Psychiatry 2007;46(4):493–9.

35. Commission on Adolescent Depression and Bipolar Disorder. Defining depression and bipolar disorder. In: Evans DL, Foa EB, Gur RE, et al, editors. Treating and preventing adolescent mental health disorders: what we know and what we don't know: a research agenda for improving the mental health of our youth. New York: Oxford University Press; 2005. p. 3–27.

36. Beardslee WR, Gladstone TRG, O'Connor EE. Transmission and prevention of mood disorders among children of affectively ill parents: a review. J Am Acad Child Adolesc Psychiatry 2011;50(11):1098–1109.

37. Brennan PA, Le Brocque R, Hammen C. Maternal depression, parent-child relationships, and resilient outcomes in adolescence. J Am Acad Child Adolesc Psychiatry 2003;42(12):1469–77.

38. Joormann J, Eugene F, Gotlib IH. Parental depression: impact on offspring and mechanisms underlying transmission of risk. In: Nolen-Hoeksema S, Hilt LM, editors. Handbook of depression in adolescents. New York: Routledge; 2009. p. 441–72.

39. Warner V, Weissman MM, Mufson L, et al. Grandparents, parents, and grandchildren at high risk for depression: a three-generation study. J Am Acad Child Adolesc Psychiatry 1999;38(3):289–96.

40. Weissman MM, Wickramaratne P, Nomura Y, et al. Families at high and low risk for depression: a 3-generation study. Arch Gen Psychiatry 2005;62(1):29–36.

41. Campbell SB, Morgan-Lopez AA, Cox MJ, et al. A latent class analysis of maternal depressive symptoms over 12 years and offspring adjustment in adolescence. J Abnorm Psychol 2009;118(3):479–93.

42. Bruder-Costello B, Warner V, Talati A, et al. Temperament among offspring at high and low risk for depression. Psychiatry Res 2007;153(2):145–51.
43. Weissman MM, Wickramaratne P, Nomura Y, et al. Offspring of depressed parents: 20 years later. Am J Psychiatry 2006;163(6):1001–8.
44. Hammen C, Brennan PA, Keenan-Miller D, et al. Chronic and acute stress, gender, and serotonin transporter gene environment interactions predicting depression symptoms in youth. J Child Psychol Psychiatry 2010;51(2):180–7.
45. Schumacher J, Jamra RA, Becker T, et al. Evidence for a relationship between genetic variants at the brain-derived neurotrophic factor (BDNF) locus and major depression. Biol Psychiatry 2005;58(4):307–14.
46. Risch N, Herrell R, Lehner T, et al. Interaction between the serotonin transporter gene (5-HTTLPR), stressful life events, and risk of depression: a meta-analysis. JAMA 2009;301(23):2462–71.
47. Munafò MR, Durrant C, Lewis G, et al. Gene × environment interactions at the serotonin transporter locus. Biol Psychiatry 2009;65(3):211–9.
48. Kendler KS, Baker JH. Genetic influences on measures of the environment: a systematic review. Psychol Med 2007;37(5):615–26.
49. Lewinsohn PM, Rohde P, Klein DN, et al. Natural course of adolescent major depressive disorder: I. Continuity into young adulthood. J Am Acad Child Adolesc Psychiatry 1999;38(1):56–63.
50. Garber J, Flynn C. Predictors of depressive cognitions in young adolescents. Cogn Ther Res 2001;25(4):353–76.
51. Abela JRZ, Skitch SA, Adams P, et al. The timing of parent and child depression: a hopelessness theory perspective. J Clin Child Adolesc Psychol 2006;35(2):253–63.
52. Jacobs RH, Reinecke MA, Gollan JK, et al. Empirical evidence of cognitive vulnerability for depression among children and adolescents: a cognitive science and developmental perspective. Clin Psychol Rev 2008;28(5):759–82.
53. Lau JYF, Rijsdijk F, Eley TC. I think, therefore I am: a twin study of attributional style in adolescents. J Child Psychol Psychiatry 2006;47(7):696–703.
54. Gibb BE, Uhrlass DJ, Grassia M, et al. Children's inferential styles, 5-HTTLPR genotype, and maternal expressed emotion-criticism: an integrated model for the intergenerational transmission of depression. J Abnorm Psychol 2009; 118(4):734–45.
55. Sandler IN, Ma Y, Tein J-Y, et al. Long-term effects of the family bereavement program on multiple indicators of grief in parentally bereaved children and adolescents. J Consult Clin Psychol 2010;78(2):131–43.
56. Dowdney L. Childhood bereavement following parental death. J Child Psychol Psychiatry 2000;41(7):819–30.
57. Cerel J, Fristad MA, Verducci J, et al. Childhood bereavement: psychopathology in the 2 years postparental death. J Am Acad Child Adolesc Psychiatry 2006;45(6): 681–90.
58. Gilman SE, Kawachi I, Fitzmaurice GM, et al. Socioeconomic status in childhood and the lifetime risk of major depression. Int J Epidemiol 2002;31(2):359–67.
59. Najman JM, Hayatbakhsh MR, Clavarino A, et al. Family poverty over the early life course and recurrent adolescent and young adult anxiety and depression: a longitudinal study. Am J Public Health 2010;100(9):1719–23.
60. Buzi RS, Weinman ML, Smith PB. The relationship between adolescent depression and a history of sexual abuse. Adolescence 2007;42(168):679–88.
61. Åslund C, Leppert J, Comasco E, et al. Impact of the interaction between the 5HTTLPR polymorphism and maltreatment on adolescent depression. A population-based study. Behav Genet 2009;39(5):524–31.

62. Harkness KL, Bruce AE, Lumley MN. The role of childhood abuse and neglect in the sensitization to stressful life events in adolescent depression. J Abnorm Psychol 2006;115(4):730–41.

63. Widom CS, DuMont K, Czaja SJ. A prospective investigation of major depressive disorder and comorbidity in abused and neglected children grown up. Arch Gen Psychiatry 2007;64(1):49–56.

64. MacMillan HL, Fleming JE, Streiner DL, et al. Childhood abuse and lifetime psychopathology in a community sample. Am J Psychiatry 2001;158(11):1878–83.

65. Gibb BE, Abela JRZ. Emotional abuse, verbal victimization, and the development of children's negative inferential styles and depressive symptoms. Cogn Ther Res 2008;32(2):161–76.

66. Short JL. The effects of parental divorce during childhood on college students. J Divorce Remarriage 2002;38(1–2):143–56.

67. Kelly JB. Children's adjustment in conflicted marriage and divorce: a decade review of research. J Am Acad Child Adolesc Psychiatry 2000;39(8):963–73.

68. Gilman SE, Kawachi I, Fitzmaurice GM, et al. Socio-economic status, family disruption and residential stability in childhood: relation to onset, recurrence and remission of major depression. Psychol Med 2003;33(8):1341–55.

69. Joiner TE Jr, Lewinsohn PM, Seeley JR. The core of loneliness: lack of pleasurable engagement—more so than painful disconnection—predicts social impairment, depression onset, recovery from depressive disorders among adolescents. J Pers Assess 2002;79(3):472–91.

70. Masten CL, Eisenberger NI, Borofsky LA, et al. Subgenual anterior cingulate responses to peer rejection: a marker of adolescents' risk for depression. Dev Psychopathol 2011;23(1):283–92.

71. Garber J. Vulnerability to depression in childhood and adolescence. In: Ingram RE, Price JM, editors. Vulnerability to psychopathology: risk across the lifespan. 2nd edition. New York: Guilford Press; 2010. p. 189–247.

72. Rutter ML. Psychosocial adversity and child psychopathology. Br J Psychiatry 1999;174:480–93.

73. Sameroff A, Seifer R, Zax M, et al. Early indicators of developmental risk: Rochester longitudinal study. Schizophrenia Bull 1987;13(3):383–94.

74. Brown DW, Anda RF, Tiemeier H, et al. Adverse childhood experiences and the risk of premature mortality. Am J Prev Med 2009;37(5):389–96.

75. Espejo EP, Hammen CL, Connolly NP, et al. Stress sensitization and adolescent depressive severity as a function of childhood adversity: a link to anxiety disorders. J Abnorm Child Psychol 2007;35(2):287–99.

76. Beardslee WR, Podorefsky D. Resilient adolescents whose parents have serious affective and other psychiatric disorders: importance of self-understanding and relationships. Am J Psychiatry 1988;145(1):63–9.

77. Roosa MW. Some thoughts about resilience versus positive development, main effects versus interactions, and the value of resilience. Child Dev 2000;71(3):567–9.

78. Luthar SS, Cicchetti D. The construct of resilience: implications for interventions and social policies. Dev Psychopathol 2000;12(4):857–85.

79. Luthar SS, Goldstein A. Children's exposure to community violence: implications for understanding risk and resilience. J Clin Child Adolesc Psychol 2004;33(3):499–505.

80. Luthar SS, Brown PJ. Maximizing resilience through diverse levels of inquiry: prevailing paradigms, possibilities, and priorities for the future. Dev Psychopathol 2007;19(3):931–55.

81. Luthar SS, Sexton CC. Maternal drug abuse versus maternal depression: vulnerability and resilience among school-age and adolescent offspring. Dev Psychopathol 2007;19(1):205–25.

82. Hauser ST, Allen JP, Golden E. Out of the woods: tales of resilient teens. Cambridge (MA): Harvard University Press; 2006.

83. Masten AS. Resilience in developing systems: progress and promise as the fourth wave rises. Dev Psychopathol 2007;19(3):921–30.

84. Beardslee WR, Ayoub C, Avery MW, et al. Family connections: an approach for strengthening early care systems in facing depression and adversity. Am J Orthopsychiatry 2010;80(4):482–95.

85. Kim-Cohen J, Gold AL. Measured gene-environment interactions and mechanisms promoting resilient development. Curr Dir Psychol Sci 2009;18(3):138–42.

86. Cicchetti D, Rogosch FA, Sturge-Apple ML. Interactions of child maltreatment and serotonin transporter and monoamine oxidase A polymorphisms: depressive symptomatology among adolescents from low socioeconomic status backgrounds. Dev Psychopathol 2007;19(4):1161–80.

87. Gunnar MR, Fisher PA. Bringing basic research on early experience and stress neurobiology to bear on preventive interventions for neglected and maltreated children. Dev Psychopathol 2006;18(3):651–77.

88. National Scientific Council on the Developing Child. Excessive stress disrupts the architecture of the developing brain: Working paper no. 3. Cambridge (MA): Center on the Developing Child, Harvard University; 2005.

89. Desjardins TL, Leadbeater BJ. Relational victimization and depressive symptoms in adolescence: moderating effects of mother, father, and peer emotional support. J Youth Adolescence 2011;40(5):531–44.

90. Helsen M, Vollebergh W, Meeus W. Social support from parents and friends and emotional problems in adolescence. J Youth Adolescence 2000;29(3):319–35.

91. Young JF, Berenson K, Cohen P, et al. The role of parent and peer support in predicting adolescent depression: a longitudinal community study. J Res Adolescence 2005;15(4):407–23.

92. Bohnert AM, Kane P, Garber J. Organized activity participation and internalizing and externalizing symptoms: reciprocal relations during adolescence. J Youth Adolescence 2008;37(2):239–50.

93. Babiss LA, Gangwisch JE. Sports participation as a protective factor against depression and suicidal ideation in adolescents as mediated by self-esteem and social support. J Dev Behav Pediatr 2009;30(5):376–84.

94. Kaufman J, Yang B-Z, Douglas-Palumberi H, et al. Brain-derived neurotrophic factor-5-HHTLPR gene interactions and environmental modifiers of depression in children. Biol Psychiatry 2006;59(8):673–80.

95. Silk JS, Vanderbilt-Adriance E, Shaw DS, et al. Resilience among children and adolescents at risk for depression: mediation and moderation across social and neurobiological context. Dev Psychopathol 2007;19(3):841–65.

96. Silk JS, Shaw DS, Forbes EE, et al. Maternal depression and child internalizing: the moderating role of child emotion regulation. J Clin Child Adolesc Psychol 2006;35(1):116–26.

97. Forbes EE, Shaw DS, Fox NA, et al. Maternal depression, child frontal asymmetry, and child affective behavior as factors in child behavior problems. J Child Psychol Psychiatry 2006;47(1):79–87.

98. Gillham JE, Shatté AJ, Freres DR. Preventing depression: a review of cognitive-behavioral and family interventions. Appl Prev Psychol 2000;9(2):63–88.

99. Kaslow NJ, Thompson MP. Applying the criteria for empirically supported treatments to studies of psychosocial interventions for child and adolescent depression. J Clin Child Psychol 1998;27(2):146–55.

100. Clarke GN, Hornbrook M, Lynch F, et al. A randomized trial of a group cognitive intervention for preventing depression in adolescent offspring of depressed parents. Arch Gen Psychiatry 2001;58(12):1127–34.

101. Garber J, Clarke GN, Weersing VR, et al. Prevention of depression in at-risk adolescents: a randomized controlled trial. JAMA 2009;301(21):2215–24.

102. Clarke GN, Hawkins W, Murphy M, et al. Targeted prevention of unipolar depressive disorder in an at-risk sample of high school adolescents: a randomized trial of group cognitive intervention. J Am Acad Child Adolesc Psychiatry 1995;34(3):312–21.

103. Gillham JE, Reivich KJ, Jaycox L, et al. The Penn Resiliency Program. Philadelphia: University of Pennsylvania; 1990.

104. Gillham JE, Brunwasser SM, Freres DR. Preventing depression in early adolescence: the Penn Resiliency Program. In: Abela JRZ, Hankin BL, editors. Handbook of depression in children and adolescents. New York: Guilford Press; 2008:309–22.

105. Compas BE, Forehand R, Keller G, et al. Randomized controlled trial of a family cognitive-behavioral preventive intervention for children of depressed parents. J Consult Clin Psychol 2009;77(6):1007–20.

106. Beardslee WR, Gladstone TRG, Wright EJ. A family-based approach to the prevention of depressive symptoms in children at risk: evidence of parental and child change. Pediatrics 2003;112:E99–111.

107. Solantaus T, Toikka S, Alasuutari M, et al. Safety, feasibility and family experiences of preventive interventions for children and families with parental depression. Int J Ment Health Promot 2009;11(4):15–24.

108. D'Angelo EJ, Llerena-Quinn R, Shapiro R, et al. Adaptation of the Preventive Intervention Program for Depression for use with predominantly low-income Latino families. Fam Process 2009;48(2):269–91.

109. Podorefsky DL, McDonald-Dowdell M, Beardslee WR. Adaptation of preventive interventions for a low-income, culturally diverse community. J Am Acad Child Adolesc Psychiatry 2001;40(8):879–86.

110. Sandler I, Wolchik S, Davis C, et al. Correlational and experimental study of resilience in children of divorce and parentally bereaved children. In: Luthar SS, editor. Resilience and vulnerability: adaptation in the context of childhood adversities. New York: Cambridge University Press; 2003. p. 213–40.

111. O'Connell ME, Boat T, Warner KE, editors. Preventing mental, emotional, and behavioral disorders among young people: progress and possibilities. Washington, DC: National Academies Press; 2009.

Developmentally Informed Evaluation of Depression: Evidence-Based Instruments

Eugene J. D'Angelo, PhD[a,b],*, Tara M. Augenstein, BA[a]

KEYWORDS

• Depression • Evidence-based assessment • Childhood
• Developmental • Diagnosis

The presence of depressive symptoms during childhood and adolescence has gained acceptance in the mental health community over the past 30 years.[1] Although professionals now agree that depression in youth occurs, several controversies remain regarding its clinical picture, how symptoms vary with age, and the best approaches toward the assessment and diagnosis of depression prior to adulthood.[2] However, points of consensus now also exist. First, the identification of depression in childhood should occur as early as possible in order to afford the opportunity for early intervention.[3] Second, given the heterogeneous presentation of depressive symptoms across different age groups, an empirically based developmental approach to diagnosis is necessary.[1]

A number of issues exist to keep in mind when approaching the diagnosis of depression in childhood:

• Nature of the diagnostic process in daily clinical practice
• Impact of depression on daily functioning
• Role of comorbidity
• Cultural variations in symptom descriptions
• Various methods and measures used to assess depression.

Each of these issues impacts the decisions made by the clinician when selecting a measure or method for use with a particular patient to enhance clinical understanding of the patient's symptoms and functioning. In addition to assessing symptoms and severity, some measures can also be used to evaluate treatment progress and to assess overall clinical outcome.

The authors have nothing to disclose.
[a] Division of Psychology, Department of Psychiatry, Children's Hospital Boston, 300 Longwood Avenue, Boston, MA 02115, USA
[b] Department of Psychiatry, Harvard Medical School, 401 Park Drive, Boston, MA 02215, USA
* Corresponding author. Division of Psychology, Department of Psychiatry, Children's Hospital Boston, 300 Longwood Avenue, Boston, MA 02115.
E-mail address: eugene.dangelo@childrens.harvard.edu

Child Adolesc Psychiatric Clin N Am 21 (2012) 279–298
doi:10.1016/j.chc.2011.12.003
1056-4993/12/$ – see front matter © 2012 Elsevier Inc. All rights reserved.

The primary aims of this article are twofold. First, a description is provided regarding how to incorporate evidence-based assessment procedures into diagnostic practice. This discussion is followed by a review of the more commonly used interview methods and clinical measures of depression among preschoolers, school-aged children, and adolescents.

THE DIAGNOSTIC PROCESS
Systematic Evaluation

The diagnostic process has long been conceptualized as an evolving component of clinical practice whose evolution is reliant on the changing standards of care in psychiatry.[4] Ideally, this diagnostic effort represents a complex decision-making process that involves the collection of an array of information about a patient from several sources and procedures, the evaluation of this data in light of its sometimes incomplete and/or contradictory nature, and the desire to reduce errors that may occur in the synthesis and interpretation of this information.[5] Similarly, the complexities of the diagnostic process and the factors that can adversely impact clinical reasoning and subsequent judgments must be considered.[6] In this process, clinical reasoning is a skill that can be enhanced through the use of systematic sources of data collection about a patient, thereby reducing some of the biases and potentially erroneous influences on clinical judgment.[7] This call for systematic evaluation converges with the increased focus on evidence-based practice in child and adolescent psychiatry.[8]

Unstructured Evaluation

Despite this focus on evidence-based practice, surveys of practicing clinicians have revealed that clinicians do not regularly follow best-practice assessment guidelines or use formal treatment outcome measures to monitor therapeutic progress.[9,10] One example of this phenomenon has been presented by Jensen-Doss,[11] who observed that the unstructured clinical interview remains the most common and often the sole method for diagnostic assessment among surveyed clinicians, despite findings that these interviews result in low clinical agreement when compared with structured diagnostic interviews. Relying on unstructured diagnostic interviews can result in a failure to fully evaluate critical aspects of symptom presentation, particularly when these symptoms are perceived to be incompatible during the initial diagnostic assessment.[12] There is likely a multiplicity of reasons behind such variation in practice, ranging from insufficient time to complete evaluations to problems with reimbursement for these practices.[5,11] However, the dilemma of reduced diagnostic accuracy due to these variations in practice remains.

Evidence-Based Assessment

Although less developed than evidence-based treatments, evidence-based assessment consists of three essential features[5]:

1. Use of research and theory to inform the target symptoms for assessment
2. Creation and selection of empirically supported methods and measures to be used during assessment
3. Continuous review of the assessment process.

An evidence-based assessment process incorporates the use of measures with strong psychometric properties in order to more systematically facilitate the decision-making efforts that are integral to meaningful diagnosis. Ideally, the use of such measures promotes incremental validity within the diagnostic process—that is, the data from these

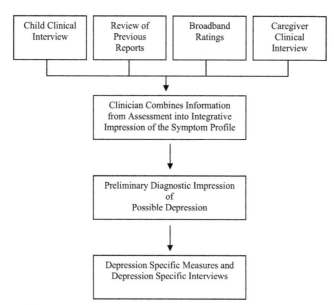

Fig. 1. Best-practice assessment.

measures serves to increase the identification of clinical problems beyond what was determined from other sources of information such as clinical interviews.[5] **Fig. 1** illustrates an example of common best-practice assessment procedures.

Previous investigations have systematically reviewed the fundamental elements of evidence-based assessment such as the use of structured interviews, family history, and relevant reports on socioemotional functioning, general behavior rating scales, and the use of depression-specific measures for appropriate age groups. Hence, these topics are not reviewed here.[1] However, two major features can impact the utility of the diagnostic process and warrant specific consideration[1]:

1. Developmental variations in symptom expression
2. Impact of comorbidities on symptom presentation.

In the construction of depression measures, the developmental process has primarily been characterized according to the age of the child, with less systematic investigation as to how depression may manifest among developmentally delayed youth. Additionally, whereas evidence suggests that the symptom picture of depressive disorders may be relatively consistent from adulthood through school-aged childhood, there is some question as to whether symptoms do vary according to a youth's cognitive level and general social development.[1] For example, there is some possibility that depressed adolescents evidence more symptoms of hopelessness, vegetative problems, and motivational difficulties than do school-aged children[2]; hence, the importance of creating measures that contain norms that can evaluate the degree of age-based symptom variations on dimensional as well as categorical bases.[13]

Comorbidities in Depression Diagnosis

Many youths also experience a combination of anxiety and mood symptoms that can impair both interpersonal relationships and functional abilities.[14] Diagnostic comorbidity between depression and other psychiatric disorders is estimated to be as high as 75% in selected clinical samples.[15] However, psychiatric comorbidity during childhood represents a complex phenomenon. For example, Garber and Weersing[16] noted that although 25% to 50% of youths in a community sample with depression also met criteria for an anxiety disorder, only 10% to 15% of those with a primary diagnosis of anxiety disorder exhibited comorbid depression.

One reason for these findings may reside in the fact that self-report measures for both anxiety and depression share a significant number of common items; however, even when these overlapping features are separated out on clinical measures, correlations between the discrete items for both symptom groups remain significant.[17] For example, the tripartite model of anxiety and depression has underscored the relative overlap of symptoms along three dimensions[18]:

1. General distress
2. Anhedonia
3. Physiological hyperarousal.

Teachman and colleagues[19] reported on the age invariance for the tripartite model among individuals 18 to 93 years old. Burke and Loeber[20] noted that symptoms of negative affect among youth diagnosed with oppositional defiant disorder were a good predictor of adult depression and hence represented homotypic continuity; that is, the affective symptoms remained similar over time.

Because of the symptom overlap and comorbidities between diagnoses, Carr[21] recommended that a stepwise approach be considered in the diagnostic assessment of depression. In this model, a "broad band" screening instrument, which measures a series of internalizing and externalizing symptoms, is used after clinical interview. If mood-related symptoms are determined to be elevated, the clinician can add more formal depression-specific measures as the next step in the process along with a more focused interview to evaluate risk and protective factors including a suicide risk assessment. As such, the clinician might use both a broad band measure and clinical interview to refine diagnostic impressions and then, depending on the results, follow up with more specific, developmentally appropriate measures of depression to further evaluate the symptoms and enhance the accuracy of the diagnosis. **Fig. 2** is a graphic summary of Carr's model.

METHODS AND MEASURES

Klein and colleagues[1] noted that the two major ways the diagnosis of depressive disorders can be enhanced is through the use of formal interviews and rating scales. These interviews can begin as unstructured and move to either semistructured or structured in nature. Rating scales can be completed by parents, youths, and/or teachers. Each approach has its merits as well as potential sources of difficulty and will be discussed here, followed by a review of some of the most common assessment measures available for the various age groups. For very detailed coverage of these issues and specific measures, see Klein and colleagues.[1]

Unstructured, Semistructured, and Structured Interviews

As previously noted, the use of unstructured interviews poses a risk for an incomplete evaluation and as a result, inaccurate diagnostic impressions and fewer diagnoses.[1,12] Semistructured and structured interviews are believed to be more comprehensive and systematic in nature. In fact, Kashner and colleagues[22] reported that diagnosis and treatment plans were changed when a semistructured interview was

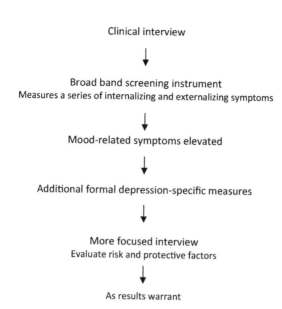

Fig. 2. Carr's model of stepwise approach. (Carr A. Depression in young people: description, assessment and evidence-based treatment. Dev Neurorehabil 2008;11:3–15.)

used by practitioners. Semistructured interviews are organized such that the clinician is required to complete the interview based on a range of clinical signs, symptoms, and functional assessments. The clinician then combines the information from the interview with any other information available and rates the findings as accurately as possible on the clinical scales provided. Ultimately the clinician rates the presence/absence of specific symptoms on operationally defined scales and is then guided by the semistructured interview process to determine the severity of the symptoms on the rating scales. The ratings in turn help facilitate diagnosis. Structured interviews are organized similarly; however, in structured interviews the clinician reads specific questions verbatim from the interview and records the responses. These recorded responses then inform any subsequent diagnoses. Although structured interviews can provide valuable clinical information during the assessment process, the time needed to complete each one is extensive; therefore, the primary use of these interviews is limited to research settings.

Rating Scales

Rating scales vary in length and format and can be clinician-administered, self-report, and/or completed by parents and teachers. This flexibility contributes to rating scales being more practical tools for assessment than the aforementioned time-intensive interviews. There are generally two types of rating scales:

1. Consistent with semistructured interviews, a number of symptoms and/or functional areas are evaluated based on the norms created for the measures.
2. Symptom-specific measures such as a depression measure seek to evaluate the respondent's answers based on its norms.

Table 1
Broad band measures by age

Measure Name	Informant (s)	Age Range (y)	Measure Design	Number of Items	Reliability
Child Behavior Checklist (CBCL)/ Youth Self-Report (YSR)/Teacher Report Form (TRF)[24,25]	Parent, Youth, Teacher	1.5–5; 6–18	Rating scale	105–120	α = .55–.90 (competence and adaptive); α = .71–.97 (empirically based); α = .67–.94 (DSM-oriented); α = .89 (preschool version)
Preschool Age Psychiatric Assessment (PAPA)[26]	Parent	2–5	Interview	Varies based on responses	κ = .72 (depression)
Behavior Assessment System for Children (BASC)[27,28]	Youth, Parent, Teacher	2.5–18	Rating scale	109–148	α = .42–.97 (across youth-, parent-, and teacher-report subscales)
Early Childhood Inventory-4 (ECI-4)[29]	Parent, Teacher	3–5	Rating scale	108 (parent) 77 (teacher)	α = .59–.68 (depressive disorders, parent); α = .42–.54 (depressive disorders, teacher)
Berkeley Puppet Interview (BPI-S)[30]	Youth	4–7	Interview	65	α = .68–.89 (clinical sample)
McArthur Health and Behavior Questionnaire (HBQ)[30]	Parent, Teacher	4–8	Rating scale	140 (parent) 115 (teacher)	α = .68–.88 (parent); α = .56–.92 (teacher)
Child Symptom Inventory-4 (CSI-4)/ Child Symptom Inventory-4 Teacher (CSI-4-T)[31]	Parent, Teacher	5–12	Rating scale	97 (parent) 77 (teacher)	α = .59 (parent); α = .75 (teacher)
Children's Interview for Psychiatric Symptoms (ChIPS)/ Parent version (P-ChIPS)[32]	Youth, Parent	6–18	Interview	Varies based on responses	κ = .452 (ChIPS and PChIPS comparison)
Diagnostic Interview for Children and Adolescents (DICA)[33]	Youth, Parent	6–12; 13–17	Interview, computerized version available	Varies based on responses	κ = .55–.90 (ages 6–12); κ = .80–.90 (ages 13–17)

Instrument	Reporter	Age	Format	Number of items	Reliability
Diagnostic Interview Schedule for Children: Youth version (DISC-Y)/Parent version (DISC-P)[34]	Youth, Parent	9–17(youth-report); 6–17 (parent)	Interview, paper-based and computerized versions available	Varies based on responses	κ = .92 (major depressive episode, youth report) κ = .66 (major depressive episode, parent report)
Dominic-R[35]	Youth	6–11	Pictorial interview, computerized version available	2 booklets	α = .83 (MDD)
Kiddie Schedule for Affective Disorders and Schizophrenia (K-SADS)[36]	Youth, Parent	6–18	Interview	Varies based on responses	α = .68–.84
Pictorial Instrument for Children and Adolescents (PICA-III-R)[37]	Youth	6–16	Pictorial interview	137	α = .84 (depression)
Child Assessment Schedule (CAS)[38]	Youth, Parent	7–16	Interview	56	α > .80 (psychiatrically ill youth) α > .77 (parents of psychiatrically ill youth)
Child and Adolescent Psychiatric Interview (CAPA)[39]	Youth, Parent	9–17	Interview	Varies based on responses	κ = .90 (major depression)
Youth's Inventory-4 (YI-4)[40]	Youth	11–18	Rating scale	128	α = .66–.87
Adolescent Symptom Inventory-4 (ASI-4)[40]	Parent, Teacher	12–18	Rating scale	120 (parent) 79 (teacher)	α = .61–.95 (parent) α = .74–.95 (teacher)
Minnesota Multiphasic Personality Inventory-Adolescent (MMPI-A)[41]	Youth	14–18	Rating scale	478	α = .35–.91 (across clinical scales)

Note: Alpha coefficients were used to describe reliability when available. When alpha coefficients were unavailable or not appropriate, kappa coefficients were used.

Abbreviations: DSM, Diagnostic and Statistical Manual of Mental Disorders; MDD, major depressive disorder.

Table 2
Affect-specific measures by age

Measure Name	Informant(s)	Age Range	Symptoms Assessed	Measure Design	Number of Items	Reliability
Preschool Feelings Checklist (PFC)	Parent	3–5.6 y	Depression-specific	Rating scale	20	$\alpha = .76$
Preschool Symptom Self-report (PRESS)[42]	Youth, Parent, Teacher	3–5 y	Depression-specific	Pictorial interview	25	$\alpha = .89$
General Behavior Inventory (GBI)/Parent version (P-GBI)[43,44]	Youth, Parent	10–17 y (youth) 5 – 17 y (parent)	Depression- and mania-specific	Rating scale	73	$\alpha = .97$ (depression)
Revised Child Anxiety and Depression Scale (RCADS)/Parent version (RCADS-P)[45]	Youth, Parent	Grades 1–12	Depression- and anxiety-specific	Rating scale	47	$\alpha_{MDD} = .80$ (youth) $\alpha_{MDD} = .84$ (parent)
Children's Depression Rating Scale–Revised (CDRS-R)[46,47]	Youth, Parent, Clinician	6–18 y	Depression-specific	Interview	17	$\alpha = .85$ (6–12 y) $\alpha = .79$–.92 (7–18 y)
Depression and Anxiety in Youth Scale (DAYS)[48]	Youth, Parent, Teacher	6–19 y	Depression- and anxiety-specific	Rating scale	20–28 per scale	$\alpha = .61$–.91
Children's Depression Inventory (CDI)/ Second Edition (CDI-2)[49,50]	Youth	7–17 y	Depression-specific	Rating scale	12–28	$\alpha = .71$–.89 (summary) $\alpha = .59$–.68 (factors) $\alpha = .76$–.92 (CDI-2)
Depression Self-Rating Scale (DSRS)[51]	Youth	7–13 y	Depression-specific	Rating scale	18	$\alpha = .90$ (psychiatrically ill sample)
Beck Depression Inventory for Youth (BDI-Y)[52]	Youth	7–14 y	Depression-specific	Rating scale	20	$\alpha = .90$–.92
Mood and Feelings Questionnaire (MFQ)/Parent version (MFQ-P)[53]	Youth, Parent	8–18 y	Depression-specific	Rating scale	32	$\alpha = .94$ (youth) $\alpha = .92$ (parent)

Measure	Reporter	Age	Type	Format	Items	Reliability
Positive and Negative Affect Schedule for Children (PANAS-C)/Parent version (PANAS-C-P)[45,54]	Youth, Parent	8–18 y	Depression- and anxiety-specific	Rating scale	27	α_{NA} = .92; α_{PA} = .89 (youth); α_{NA} = .92; α_{PA} = .92 (parent)
Reynolds Child Depression Scale (RCDS)[28]	Youth	8–13 y	Depression-specific	Rating scale	30	α = .90
Reynolds Adolescent Depression Scale, Second Edition (RADS-2)[55]	Youth	11–20 y	Depression-specific	Rating scale	30	α = .87–.96
Dysfunctional Attitudes Scale (DAS)[56]	Youth	12 + y	Feelings of self-worth	Rating scale	40	α = .93
Beck Depression Inventory (BDI)[57]	Youth	13 + y	Depression-specific	Rating scale	21	α = .76–.91 (total)

Note: Alpha coefficients were used to describe reliability when available. When alpha coefficients were unavailable or not appropriate, kappa coefficients were used.

Abbreviations: MDD, major depressive disorder; NA, negative effect; PA, positive effect.

Typically, self-rated measures are considered to have greater sensitivity than either parent or teacher rating forms, and a number of measures exist that are used to investigate specific features of depression (eg, self-esteem, depressive cognitions, suicidal ideation).[1,23] However, their specificity distinguishing between depression and anxiety remains variable in nature, with improvements noted when there is greater focus on symptoms such as anhedonia and low positive affectivity.[1]

The next section of this article identifies some of the interview schedules and rating scales that are in most common use for the identification and diagnosis of depression in childhood. The review also briefly describes each measure from a developmental framework in the context of the ages for which they are intended. For additional information on each measure, **Tables 1** and **2** list the names and associated references for each measure, the type of assessment procedure (eg, interview vs rating scale), the ages for which it is intended, the number of items contained in the measure, whether it is a broad band or symptom-specific measure, and its internal reliability. For convenience the table has been separated into broad band measures (see **Table 1**) and depression- or affect-specific measures (see **Table 2**).

BROAD BAND ASSESSMENT

In addition to the more open-ended diagnostic interviews that are characteristic of clinical practice, there are semistructured interviews that have practical utility.

The Berkeley Puppet Interview Symptomatology Scales (BPI-S)[58] use both structured and minimally structured interviewing techniques to identify the self-perceptions of children (aged 4–7 years) about their levels of distress and range of symptomatology. Initial results suggest that the BPI-S method is a reliable and valid way of obtaining children's perceptions of their competencies and emotional well-being.[59] It contains 65 items to evaluate a broad array of symptoms along nine distinct scales, namely overanxious, separation anxiety, depression (internalizing symptoms), oppositional defiant, conduct problems, overhostility, relational aggression (externalizing problems), inattention, and impulsivity. Complementing the BPI-S is the McArthur Health and Behavior Questionnaire,[60] which provides both a parent and a teacher report form.

There are additional interviews that evaluate broad band symptoms and are also specifically focused on school-aged children and/or adolescents. The Dominic-R[35] is a pictorially presented semistructured questionnaire intended for use with children aged 6 to 11 years. The Dominic-R is a unique measure, given that it appreciates the cognitive immaturity of its informants. Particularly, it takes into account that children of this age have difficulty appreciating the frequency, duration, and age-of-onset of symptoms, all of which represent information essential to *Diagnostic and Statistical Manual of Mental Disorders* (*DSM*)–based diagnostic criteria. The measure consists of pictures of a child named Dominic who is shown in a variety of individual and social situations. The pictures are accompanied by a single question about the picture that can be read to the child. The Dominic takes approximately 15 to 25 minutes to complete in either the booklet or computerized format. Computerized versions for African American, Latino, and Asian children are also available.

The Children's Interview for Psychiatric Syndromes (ChIPS)[61] is a semistructured interview used with children aged 6 to 13 years that evaluates 20 distinct Axis I disorders based on the *DSM Fourth Edition* (*DSM-IV*).[62] The potential benefits of the ChIPS include its use of shorter and less complicated sentence structure designed to enhance comprehension on the part of the child and its focus on building and maintaining rapport between the informant and clinician in order to promote more accurate responses. The Children's Interview for Psychiatric Syndromes—Parent

Version (P-ChIPS)[32] is also available and has demonstrated moderate levels of agreement with the child version and adequate psychometric properties useful in clinical settings.

The Pictorial Instrument for Children and Adolescents (PICA-III-R)[37] is a pictorial-based semistructured interview and is composed of 137 pictures organized into five different modules, each covering a range of diagnostic categories including mood disorders, anxiety disorders, psychotic disorders, disruptive behavior disorders, and substance abuse. Children and adolescents completing the interview are presented with simple pictures that depict a variety of emotions, behaviors, and thought content. After each picture the child is asked to provide a rating from a 5-point visual rating scale indicating how much the picture is similar to his or her own thoughts, feelings, and behaviors. The pictorial nature of the measure allows for a more developmentally appropriate form of assessment than the traditional question-based diagnostic interviews; however, the current version of the PICA-III-R is modeled after *DSM Third Edition, Revised (DSM-III-R)*[63] diagnostic criteria. Despite the need for the interview to be updated to match *DSM-IV* diagnostic requirements, the PICA-III-R can still be of clinical use for diagnostic purposes, especially when working with children with hearing difficulties.[37]

The Child Assessment Schedule (CAS)[38] is a semistructured interview to be completed by youths (aged 7–16 years) or their parents. The CAS is based on *DSM-III-R* diagnostic criteria and is organized around 11 different topic areas ranging from school and friends to fears, self-image, and mood. The CAS centers around three main types of information that, when combined, make it a valuable diagnostic and clinical tool. These three sections include information specific to the 11 topic areas mentioned previously, time of onset and duration for positive symptoms that are endorsed, and interviewer observations about the child for 53 target symptoms and behaviors.[38] The parent version of the CAS parallels the child version, and both have proved to have strong validity and reliability for their depression scales.

Each of these interview methods typically requires training in administration in order to establish interrater reliability. Whereas they provide excellent usage in research projects, these methods take a great deal of time for the busy clinician; however, they are particularly useful in helping to identify accurate diagnoses.

The most commonly used broad band rating scale for adolescents is the Minnesota Multiphasic Personality Inventory—Adolescent Version (MMPI-A).[41] The MMPI-A is one of the most highly developed, empirically based measures of adolescent psychopathology. It is a 478-item broad band self-report measure that yields a number of validity and basic clinical scales (including depression), along with a variety of content scales that offer important information about the adolescent's overall functioning. It is normalized for 14- to 18-year-olds and takes approximately 45 minutes to 1 hour to complete. The MMPI-A can either be hand or computer scored; however, it does require formal training in the interpretation of the arrangement of the clinical and content scales, which makes it a measure most often used in the context of a psychological testing battery.

There is also a series of related broad band rating scales that assess a range in youth functioning. The Child Symptom Inventory–4 (CSI-4)[31] is a 97-item parent and 77-item teacher report form. A preschool version, the Early Childhood Inventory—4,[29] is also available for children between ages 3 and 5 years. The upward extension to the CSI-4 is the Youth's Inventory–4 (YI-4).[40] The YI-4 is a self-report scale for adolescents (aged 11–18 years) that includes 128 items that assess symptoms across a variety of *DSM-IV* diagnoses. The respondent answers each item with one of four ratings: *never*, *sometimes*, *often*, or *very often*. Last, the Adolescent Symptom

Inventory–4 (ASI-4)[40] is a parent-report rating scale that closely mirrors the format and content found in the YI-4. The ASI-4 consists of 120 questions and demonstrates good reliability and both convergent and divergent validity.[40]

Additional broad band measures available include the Child Behavior Checklist (CBCL)[24] and the Behavior Assessment System for Children (BASC),[27] both of which offer multiple parent, child, and teacher forms across a variety of ages. Parent forms of the CBCL may be completed by parents of children aged 1.5 to 5 years or 6 to 18 years. The Youth Self-report version of the CBCL is available for use with youths aged 6 through 18 years. Last, a Teacher Report Form is also available. The BASC[27] offers similar forms for youths aged 2.5 to 18 years.

Several of the broad band structured and semistructured interviews have been used extensively in research settings to test the diagnostic utility of other clinical measures. As previously mentioned, these interview schedules are broad band diagnostic measures; however, because of the lengthy administration time needed to complete some of these interviews they are often exclusively used for research purposes. One such example can be found in the Diagnostic Interview Schedule for Children (DISC)[64]; despite its clinical utility, the DISC is considered to be most valuable for use in research as opposed to clinical settings.[1] There are also three semistructured diagnostic interviews that are commonly used to diagnose a variety of child and adolescent disorders:

1. Diagnostic Interview for Children and Adolescents (DICA)[65]
2. Child and Adolescent Psychiatric Assessment (CAPA)[39]
3. Schedule for Affective Disorders and Schizophrenia in School-Age Children (K-SADS).[66]

Both parent and youth versions of these interviews are available, although it is believed that children below the age of 8 may not be able to provide valid responses to the questions, and therefore parent report is most commonly used for children younger than 8 years old.

The DICA[65] contains separate interviews for parents, children (6–12 years), and adolescents (13–17 years). The interview evaluates lifetime symptoms, is completed in 1 to 2 hours, and yields assessments consistent with *DSM-III-R* and *DSM-IV*.[62,63]

When an interview with young children is thought to be helpful, several options exist. With respect to parent-focused structured interviews, the Preschool Age Psychiatric Assessment[26] is based on the CAPA and is used for children aged 2 to 5 years. As a broad band assessment method, it contains 25 modules to assess both preschooler symptoms and general functioning. Because it is also interviewer-based, the burden is on the interviewer to ensure that patients understand the questions being asked, provide clear examples about behaviors or feelings relevant to the symptom, and have the symptom at a prescribed severity level that is operationally defined in a glossary.

The CAPA is used with youths aged 9 to 17 years. Completed in 1 to 2 hours, it assesses symptoms over the prior 3-month period. As Klein and colleagues[1] observed, it contains an extensive glossary that defines the symptoms being assessed and also evaluates several functional domains (eg, peers, school, leisure activities, family functioning, and life events).

The K-SADS[66] is the most widely used and least structured interview for youth (aged 6–18 years). It is completed in 35 minutes to 2.5 hours. As the investigators observed, it is the least structured of these research interviews and hence requires considerable training to be used with reliability.[1]

DEPRESSION/AFFECT-SPECIFIC ASSESSMENT

As noted previously, once elevated levels of depressive symptoms are noted using broad band measures, the clinician may benefit from administering a more depression-specific measure to gain a deeper understanding of symptom presentation, duration, and severity.[1] Several interviews and rating scales focus on depression or affect-specific assessment. Similar to the broad band measures, these vary in their intended age ranges.

Preschool Assessment

The evaluation of negative affect in preschoolers is primarily undertaken using either a parental rating scale or a semistructured interview format. More specific parent report measures of depression include the Preschool Feelings Checklist (PFC),[3] a 16-item checklist designed to identify preschoolers (aged 3–5.6 years) with symptoms of depression.[3] The PFC relies on a yes/no checklist that takes only 2 to 4 minutes to complete by a parent or caregiver about the preschool child. Although the majority of items address internalizing depressive symptoms, a few items also assess disruptive behaviors known to be associated with depression.

Aside from parent-report measures, several additional assessments have been created using a more visual format to enable preschoolers the ability to more effectively act as their own informants. One example of such a measure is the Preschool Symptom Self-report (PRESS).[42] The PRESS is a 25-item pictorial self-report measure designed to assess depression in preschool children (aged 3–5 years). Each item consists of two pictures for the child to consider, one illustrating a problem behavior or emotion and one illustrating the absence of that behavior. The administrator reads an accompanying prompt for each picture, and the child is then asked to indicate "which picture is more like you?" The PRESS also includes a modified version that allows parents and teachers to respond to the same pictures about the child.

School-Age Assessment

There are a number of rating scales available in several formats to allow for completion by the clinician, parent, teacher, or child. Many of these rating scales are used for the evaluation of depressive symptoms in youths aged 6 through 17 years. As Klein and colleagues[1] observed, the most widely used clinician rating scale is the Children's Depression Rating Scale—Revised (CDRS-R),[46] a measure based on the Hamilton Rating Scale for Depression used with adults. The CDRS-R includes 17 items that review a range of functions adversely impacted by depression. It takes only 15 to 20 minutes to complete and comes in either self- or parent-report versions, with cutoff scores provided to assist in determining the severity of the depression. The CDRS-R covers a wide range of topic areas including depressed mood, self-esteem, suicidal ideation, schoolwork, capacity for fun, physical complaints, and irritability.[46]

The Children's Depression Inventory (CDI)[49] represents another of the most commonly used measures to evaluate the severity of depressive symptoms in youths. The original CDI is a 27-item self-rating scale for children aged 7 through 13 years based on the Beck Depression Inventory, which is used with adults. The CDI takes 10 to 20 minutes to complete. Once again, age-specific norms are provided to permit the determination of the severity of depressive symptoms and related functioning. Recently a revised version of the CDI was released that offers optional computerized scoring capabilities and short forms for use when assessment time is limited. The Children's Depression Inventory—Second Edition (CDI-2)[50] has between 12 and

28 items depending on the form used, and it can be used with an extended age range of 7 through 17 years. Of note, a related adolescent measure, the Beck Depression Inventory for Youth,[52] contains 20 items and is also normed for symptom severity.

The General Behavior Inventory (GBI)[43] is a 73-item self-report measure for youths (aged 10–17 years) that evaluates symptoms of depression and hypomania during the week prior to administration. A parent version of the GBI (P-GBI) also exists for the parents of youths (aged 5–17 years). The P-GBI is directly adapted from the GBI, with the questions reworded to ask the parent respondent about his or her child.[44]

The Revised Child Anxiety and Depression Scale (RCADS)[45] is a 47-item self-report measure for youths (grades 1–12) with subscales spanning several diagnostic categories including separation anxiety disorder, social phobia, generalized anxiety disorder, panic disorder, obsessive–compulsive disorder, and major depressive disorder. A parent version (RCADS-P) is also available and consists of 47 items covering the same diagnostic subscales as the RCADS.[45]

The Depression and Anxiety in Youth Scale (DAYS)[48] is a *DSM-III*–based measure that consists of three rating scales used to identify symptoms of depression and anxiety in youths (aged 6–19 years). Each of the three scales is completed by the youth, parent, or teacher and contains 20 to 28 items. The three scales may be completed together or individually, and administration time for the DAYS is approximately 30 minutes.

The Positive and Negative Affect Schedule for Children (PANAS-C)[45] is a 27-item self-report scale of positive and negative affect for youths (aged 8–18 years). The respondent is given a list of adjectives describing several mood states and is then asked to rate how much that mood corresponds to how they have felt for the past few weeks. The results are divided into two subscales: positive and negative effect. The PANAS-C has demonstrated good validity and internal consistency. A parent version of the PANAS-C (PANAS-C-P) is also available and mirrors the PANAS-C closely from the parent's perspective.[45]

The Reynolds Child Depression Scale[28] is a 30-item measure for use with children 8 to 12 years of age. It takes roughly 10 minutes to complete and evaluates depressive symptoms consistent with the *DSM-IIIR*.[63] An adolescent version of the measure, the Reynolds Adolescent Depression Scale,[67] is also available for use with 13- to 18-year-olds.

The Mood and Feelings Questionnaire[53] is a 32-item questionnaire that assesses depression during the 2 weeks prior to assessment in 13- to 18-year-olds. A child version is also available for use with children as young as 8 years old. It reportedly has good convergent validity with other diagnostic measures including the CDI, DISC, and K-SADS.[1]

The Depression Self-rating Scale (DSRS)[51] is a self-report measure of depression designed for children (aged 7–13 years) that consists of 18 statements about mood and motivation. Each respondent is asked to rate how much each statement matches to his or her mood in the past few weeks. The respondents rate each item with *most of the time*, *sometimes*, or *never*. The DSRS offers short administration time as well as simple wording for each prompt, making it appropriate for use with young children, and the DSRS has demonstrated good internal consistency and validity.[51]

Fristad and colleagues[68] have been clear that measures such as the CDI and similar rating scales listed previously should not be used independently of a clinical or semistructured interview to formally diagnose depression. As such, these measures are used to systematically enhance the understanding of the severity of depressive symptoms and the impact that depressive disorder may have on related areas of functioning.

Adolescent Assessment

Several depression-specific interviews and rating scales appropriate for use with adolescents have been mentioned in previous sections; however the Dysfunctional Attitudes Scale (DAS)[56] also provides an additional option for assessment. It is a self-report measure used with 12- to 17-year-olds who have a diagnosis of depression to evaluate their self-worth. The measure contains 7 subscales based on personal values. The subscales are each based on a separate value system: perfectionism, approval, love, entitlement, achievement, omnipotence, and autonomy. The DAS does not necessarily provide symptom information regarding diagnosis; however, it reflects the impact of depression on overall self-worth.

DEPRESSION AND DEVELOPMENTAL DISORDERS

It is estimated that approximately 40% of individuals diagnosed with mental retardation also exhibit a significant mental health problem.[69] Until the emergence of the literature on dual diagnosis, developmental disorders were often considered incompatible with psychiatric disorders. As such, diagnostic overshadowing often occurred with the risk of underidentifying the presence of a mental health problem among developmentally delayed individuals.[69]

As Dykens[70] observed, the norms for many of the more traditional broad band measures used with children do not necessarily apply to youth experiencing developmental delays. Among the measures created for use with these youths, the majority of assessment instruments are caregiver report measures. Several of these broad band measures are discussed as follows.

The Aberrant Behavior Checklist[71] contains 58 items, each scored on a 4-point scale by the caregiver. The items factor into five subscales:

1. Irritability, agitation, crying
2. Lethargy, social withdrawal
3. Stereotypic behavior
4. Hyperactivity, noncompliance
5. Inappropriate speech.

The Behavior Problems Inventory[72] is a 49-item informant-based behavior rating scale that contains three subscales:

1. Self-injurious behavior
2. Stereotyped behavior
3. Aggressive/destructive behavior.

The Developmental Behavior Checklist (DBC)[73] is a 96-item measure completed by caregivers and provides five subscales:

1. Disruptive and antisocial behaviors
2. Self-absorbed
3. Communication disturbance
4. Anxiety
5. Social relating disturbance.

In addition, the DBC provides a total behavior problem score. Although these measures have been normed for use with developmentally delayed youth, the symptom pictures that emerge are not necessarily consistent with those traditionally found in psychiatric diagnoses; hence, the importance of caution when using these measures. Consequently there is a need to create more specific assessment measures for use with these youths in order for a more accurate diagnostic impression to be established.

One measure that seems to be specific to depression among the developmentally delayed population is the Marston 30 Symptoms Checklist[74]; however, it has primarily been used with an older (20 to 55 years) intellectually disabled population to identify depression equivalents. It has not generally been used with youth.

There seems to be an increased emphasis on evaluation of comorbid psychiatric disorders among children with an autistic spectrum disorder.[75] The Autism Comorbidity Interview—Present and Lifetime Version (ACI-PL)[76] is an adaptation of the structured K-SADS that includes some additional screening questions and coding options for behaviors that are associated with psychiatric disorders in autistic spectrum disorders. As such, although there is recognition of the more prominent characteristics of depressive disorders, the ACI-PL also codes symptoms such as increased agitation, self-injury, and temper outbursts. It is a broad band measure that covers a range of commonly described youth symptoms of psychiatric disorder. In the initial study, 25% of the autistic children were diagnosed with major depressive disorder and 14% were just subthreshold for the diagnosis using *DSM-IV* criteria based on the ACI-PL.[75] The Autism Spectrum Disorders—Comorbid for Children[76] measure is a 49-item rating scale completed by caregivers.

SUMMARY

As noted, there are a variety of measures and interview methods available to the practicing psychiatrist and other mental health professionals to evaluate depression in children and adolescents. However, as described, there are still barriers to the use of more standardized methods for systematically gathering clinical information to facilitate diagnosis.[77] Clinicians do not regularly make use of evidence-based assessment methods to facilitate diagnosis.[5] There are likely several reasons for this occurrence[77]:

1. Increasing attention is focused on evidence-based treatment in daily practice; however, limited focus exists on use of evidence-based assessment
2. Practical issues come to bear on a busy clinical practice—although the administration, scoring, and review of standardized measures and completion of semistructured interviews may result in improved diagnostic accuracy, they take time
3. As Klein and colleagues[1] noted, the true incremental validity of standardized assessment measures as they complement the unstructured diagnostic interview has yet to be defined.

It is presumed that such data provide additive and clinically useful information, particularly in the monitoring of treatment progress and clinical outcome. However, the use of developmentally informed assessments of depression provides unquestionable benefit to the overall diagnostic decision-making and treatment planning process. It remains the hope that developmental sensitivity, usefulness, practicality, and the defined benefit to the clinical process from using evidence-based assessments will remain the focus of future diagnostic measures and methods. To that end, clinicians would undertake evaluation of depression using a deliberative model in which clinical interviews with the child and family members, record review, and use of initial broad band assessment measures would result in a preliminary diagnostic impression. Subsequently, more refined diagnostic interviewing and depression-specific measures would be used that seek to improve the clinical impression and, ideally, point the treatment in a more accurate and effective direction.

REFERENCES

1. Klein DN, Dougherty LR, Olino TM. Toward guidelines for evidence-based assessment of depression in children and adolescents. J Clin Child Adolesc Psychol 2005;34:412–32.
2. Weiss B, Garber J. Developmental differences in the phenomenology of depression. Dev Psychopathol 2003;15:403–30.
3. Luby JL, Heffelfinger A, Koenig-McNaught AL, et al. The Preschool Feelings Checklist: a brief and sensitive screening measure for depression in young children. J Am Acad Child Adolesc Psychiatry 2004;43:708–17.
4. Strahl MO, Lewis ND. Differential diagnosis in clinical psychiatry: the lectures of Paul H. Hoch, M.D. New York: Science House; 1972.
5. Hunsley J, Mash EJ. Evidence-based assessment. Ann Rev Clin Psychol 2007;3:29–51.
6. Gambrill E. Critical thinking in clinical practice: improving the accuracy of judgments and decisions about clients. San Francisco: Jossey-Bass; 1990.
7. Garb HN. Studying the clinician: judgment research and psychological assessment. Washington, DC: American Psychological Association; 1998.
8. Hamilton J. The answerable question and a hierarchy of evidence. J Am Acad Child Adolesc Psychiatry 2005;44:596–600.
9. Basco MR, Bostic JQ, Davies D, et al. Methods to improve diagnostic accuracy in a community mental health setting. Am J Psychiatry 2000;157:1599–605.
10. Hatfield DR, Ogles BM. Why some clinicians use outcome measures and others do not. Admin Pol Mental Health 2007;34:283–91.
11. Jensen-Doss A. Practice involves more than treatment: how can evidence-based assessment catch up to evidence-based treatment? Clin Psychol 2011;18:173–7.
12. Angold A, Fisher PW. Interviewer-based interviews. In: Shaffer D, Lucas CP, Richters JE, editors. Diagnostic assessment in child and adolescent psychopathology. New York: Guilford; 1999. p. 34–64.
13. Widiger TA, Clark LA. Toward *DSM-V* and the classification of psychopathology. Psych Bull 2000;126:946–63.
14. Costello EJ, Mustillo S, Erkanli A, et al. Prevalence and development of psychiatric disorders in childhood and adolescence. Arch Gen Psychiatry 2003;60:837–44.
15. Sorensen MJ, Nissen JB, Mors O, et al. Age and gender differences in depressive symptomatology and comorbidity: an incident sample of psychiatrically admitted children. J Affect Disord 2005;84:85–91.
16. Garber J, Weersing VR. Comorbidity of anxiety and depression in youth: implications for treatment and prevention. Clin Psychol 2010;17:293–306.
17. Stark KD, Laurent J. Joint factor analysis of the Children's Depression Inventory and the Revised Children's Manifest Anxiety Scale. J Clin Child Psychol 2001;30:552–67.
18. Clark LA, Watson D. Tripartite model of anxiety and depression: evidence and taxonomic implications. J Abnorm Psychol 1991;100:316–36.
19. Teachman BA, Siedlecki KL, Magee JC. Aging and symptoms of anxiety and depression: structural invariance of the tripartite model. Psychol Aging 2007;22:160–70.
20. Burke J, Loeber R. Oppositional defiant disorder and the explanation of comorbidity between behavioral disorders and depression. Clin Psychol 2010;17:319–26.
21. Carr A. Depression in young people: description, assessment and evidence-based treatment. Dev Neurorehabil 2008;11:3–15.
22. Kashner TM, Rush AJ, Suris A, et al. Impact of structured clinical interviews on physicians; practices in community mental health settings. Psychiatr Serv 2003;54:712–8.

23. Winters NC, Myers K, Proud L. Ten-year review of rating scales: III. Scales assessing suicidality, cognitive style, and self-esteem. J Am Acad Child Adolesc Psychiatry 2002;41:1150–81.

24. Achenbach T, Rescorla L. Manual for the ASEBA preschool forms and profiles. Burlington (VT): University of Vermont, Research Center for Children, Youth, and Families; 2000.

25. Achenbach TM, Rescorla LA. Manual for the ASEBA school-age forms and profile. Burlington (VT): University of Vermont, Research Center for Children, Youth, & Families; 2001.

26. Egger HL, Erkanli A, Keeler G, et al. Test-retest reliability of the Preschool Age Psychiatric Assessment (PAPA). J Am Acad Child Adolesc Psychiatry 2006;45: 538–49.

27. Reynolds CR, Kamphaus RW. Behavioral assessment system for children manual. Circle Pines (MN): American Guidance Service; 1992.

28. Reynolds CR, Kamphaus RW. Behavioral assessment system for children manual. Circle Pines (MN): American Guidance Service; 1998.

29. Sprafkin J, Volpe RJ, Gadow KD, et al. A DSM-IV–referenced screening instrument for preschool children: The Early Childhood Inventory-4. J Am Acad Child Adolesc Psychiatry 2002;41:604–12.

30. Ablow JC, Measelle JR, Kraemer HC, et al. The MacArthur Three-City Outcome Study: evaluating multi-informant measures of young children's symptomatology. J Am Acad Child Adolesc Psychiatry 1999;38:1580–90.

31. Gadow KD, Sprafkin J. Child Symptom Inventory-4: Screening and norms manual. Stony Brook (NY): Checkmate Plus; 2002.

32. Fristad MA, Teare M, Weller EB, et al. Study III: development and concurrent validity of the Children's Interview for Psychiatric Syndromes–Parent Version (P-ChIPS). J Child Adolesc Psychopharmacol 1998;8:221–6.

33. Reich W. Diagnostic interview for children and adolescents (DICA). J Am Acad Child Adolesc Psychiatry 2000;39:59–66.

34. Fisher PW, Lucas C, Shaffer D, et al. Diagnostic Interview Schedule for Children, Version IV (DISC IV): test-retest reliability in a clinical sample. Presented at the 44th Annual Meeting of the American Academy of Child and Adolescent Psychiatry. Toronto, October 14–19, 1997.

35. Valla JP, Bergeron L, Smolla N. The Dominic-R: A pictorial interview for 6- to 11-year-old children. J Am Acad Child Adolesc Psychiatry 2000;39:85–93.

36. Orvaschel H, Puig-Antich J, Chambers W, et al. Retrospective assessment of prepubertal major depression with the Kiddie-SADS-E. J Am Acad Child Psychiatry 1982; 21:392–7.

37. Ernst M, Cookus BA, Moravec BC. Pictorial Instrument for Children and Adolescents (PICA-III-R). J Am Acad Child Adolesc Psychiatry 2000;39:94–9.

38. Hodges K, Saunders WB, Kashani J, et al. Internal consistency of DSM-III diagnoses using the symptom scales of the Child Assessment Schedule. J Am Acad Child Adolesc Psychiatry 1990;29:635–41.

39. Angold A, Costello EJ. A test-retest reliability study of child-reported psychiatric symptoms and diagnoses using the Child and Adolescent Psychiatric Assessment (CAPA-C). Psychol Med 1995;25:755–62.

40. Gadow KD, Sprafkin J, Carlson GA, et al. A DSM-IV-referenced, adolescent self-report rating scale. J Am Acad Child Adolesc Psychiatry 2002;41:671–9.

41. Butcher JN, Williams CL, Graham JR, et al. Manual for administration, scoring, and interpretation of the Minnesota Multiphasic Personality Inventory-Adolescent. Minneapolis (MN): University of Minnesota Press; 1992.

42. Martini DR, Strayhorn JM, Puig-Antich J. A symptom self-report measure for pre-school children. J Am Acad Child Adolesc Psychiatry 1990;29:594–600.

43. Danielson CK, Youngstrom EA, Findling RL, et al. Discriminative validity of the General Behavior Inventory using youth report. J Abnorm Child Psychol 2003;31:29–39.

44. Youngstrom EA, Findling RL, Danielson CK, et al. Discriminative validity of parent report of hypomanic and depressive symptoms on the General Behavior Inventory. Psychol Assess 2001;13:267–76.

45. Ebesutani C, Okamura K, Higa-McMillan C, et al. A psychometric analysis of the Positive and Negative Affect Schedule for Children–Parent Version in a school sample. Psychol Assess 2011;23:406–16.

46. Poznanski E, Mokros H. Children's Depression Rating Scale–Revised (CDRS-R). Los Angeles (CA): WPS; 1996.

47. Mayes TL, Bernstein IH, Haley CL, et al. Psychometric properties of the Children's Depression Rating Scale- Revised in adolescents. J Child Adolesc Psychopharmacol 2010;20:513–6.

48. Newcomer PL, Barenbaum EM, Bryant BR. Depression and Anxiety in Youth Scale. Austin (TX): PRO-ED; 1994.

49. Kovacs M. The Children's Depression Inventory (CDI). Psychopharmacol Bull 1985; 21:995–8.

50. Kovacs M, Multi-Health Systems Staff. CDI-2: Children's Depression Inventory 2nd edition technical manual. Toronto (ON): Multi-Health Systems Inc; 2011.

51. Ivarsson T, Lidberg A, Gillberg C. The Birleson Depression Self-rating Scale (DSRS). Clinical evaluation in an adolescent inpatient population. J Affect Disord 1994;32: 115–25.

52. Beck JS, Beck AT, Jolly JB. Beck Youth Inventories. San Antonio (TX): Psychological Corporation; 2001.

53. Wood A, Kroll L, Moore A, et al. Properties of the Mood and Feelings Questionnaire in adolescent psychiatric outpatients: a research note. J Child Psychol Psychiatry 1995;36:327–34.

54. Laurent J, Cantanzaro S, Rudolph K, et al. A measure of positive and negative affect for children: scale development and preliminary validation. Psychol Asses 1999;11: 326–38.

55. Reynolds WM. Reynolds adolescent depression scale: professional manual. 2nd edition. Lutz (FL): Psychological Assessment Resources; 2002.

56. Rogers SG, Hoyle RH, Curry JF, et al. The Dysfunctional Attitudes Scale: Psychometric properties in depressed adolescents. J Clin Child Adolesc Psychol 2009;38: 781–9.

57. Beck A, Ward CH, Mendelson M, et al. An inventory for measuring depression. Arch Gen Psychiatry 1961;4:53–63.

58. Ablow JC, Measelle JR. Berkeley Puppet Interview: administration and scoring system manuals. Berkeley (CA): University of California; 1993.

59. Measelle JR, Ablow JC, Cowan PA, et al. Assessing young children's views of their academic, social, and emotional lives: an evaluation of the self-perception scales of the Berkeley Puppet Interview. Child Dev 1998;69:1556–76.

60. Essex MJ, Boyce WT, Goldstein LH, et al. The confluence of mental, physical, social, and academic difficulties in middle childhood. II: Developing the MacArthur Health and Behavior Questionnaire. J Am Acad Child Adolesc Psychiatry 2002;41:588–603.

61. Teare M, Fristad MA, Weller EB, et al. Study I: development and criterion validity of the Children's Interview for Psychiatric Syndromes (ChIPS). J Child Adolesc Psychopharmacol 1998;8:205–11.

62. American Psychiatric Association. Diagnostic and statistical manual of mental disorders. 4th edition. Washington, DC: American Psychiatric Association; 2000.

63. American Psychiatric Association. Diagnostic and statistical manual of mental disorders. 3rd edition, revised. Washington, DC: American Psychiatric Association; 1987.

64. Shaffer D, Fisher P, Lucas CP, et al. NIMH Diagnostic Interview Schedule for Children version IV (NIMH DISC-IV): description, differences from previous versions, and reliability of some common diagnoses. J Am Acad Child Adolesc 2000;39:28–38.

65. Herjanic B, Reich W. Development of a structured psychiatric interview for children: agreement between child and parent on individual symptoms. J Abnorm Child Psychol 1982;10:307–24.

66. Puig-Antich J, Chambers W. The Schedule for Affective Disorders and Schizophrenia for School-age Children (Kiddie-SADS). New York: New York State Psychiatric Institute; 1978.

67. Reynolds WM. Reynolds Adolescent Depression Scale: Professional manual. Odessa (FL): Psychological Assessment Resources; 1987.

68. Fristad MA, Emery BL, Beck SJ. Use and abuse of the Children's Depression Inventory. J Consult Clin Psychol 1997;65:699–702.

69. Hodapp RM, Dykens EM. Measuring behavior in genetic disorders of mental retardation. Ment Retard Dev Disabil Res Rev 2005;11:340–6.

70. Dykens EM. Psychopathology in children with intellectual disability. J Child Psychol Psychiatry 2000;41:407–14.

71. Aman MG, Singh NN, Stewart AW, et al. The Aberrant Behavior Checklist: a behavior rating scale for the assessment of treatment effects. Am J Mental Defic 1985;89:485–91.

72. Rojahn J, Matson JL, Lott D, et al. The Behavior Problems Inventory: an instrument for the assessment of self-injury, stereotyped behavior, and aggression/destruction in individuals with developmental disabilities. J Autism Dev Disord 2001;31:577–88.

73. Clarke AR, Tone BJ, Einfeld SL, et al. Assessment of change with the developmental behavour checklist. J Intellect Disabil Res 2003;47:210–2.

74. Tsiouris JA. Diagnosis of depression in people with severe/profound intellectual disability. J Intellect Disabil Res 2001;45:115–20.

75. Leyfer OT, Folstein SE, Bacalman S, et al. Comorbid psychiatric disorders in children with autism: interview development and rates of disorders. J Autism Dev Disord 2006;36:849–61.

76. Matson JL, LoVullo SV, Rivet TT, et al. Validity of the Autism Spectrum Disorder–Comorbid for Children (ASD-CC). Res Autism Spectr Disord 2009;3:345–57.

77. Jensen-Doss A, Hawley KM. Understanding barriers to evidence-based assessment: clinician attitudes toward standardized assessment tools. J Clin Child Adolesc Psychol 2010;39:885–96.

Child and Adolescent Depression Intervention Overview: What Works, for Whom and How Well?

Fadi T. Maalouf, MD[a,b,]*, David A. Brent, MD[c]

KEYWORDS

- Depression • Children • Adolescents • Psychotherapy
- Selective serotonin reuptake inhibitors

The choice of child and adolescent depression treatment is governed by developmental factors such as age and cognitive development (see discussions elsewhere in this issue on developmental epidemiology by Goldman S, and depression and the developing brain by Weir, Zakama, and Rao). In addition, family psychiatric history, family and social environment, family and patient treatment preference and expectation, and ethnic and cultural issues need to be taken into consideration (see discussion elsewhere in this issue on role of experience and life events in developmental risk by Breardslee). In this article, the authors review the evidence supporting the use of cognitive behavior therapy (CBT), interpersonal psychotherapy (IPT), and antidepressants. The authors discuss the role of these different agents in the acute, maintenance, and continuation treatment phases, as well as the predictors and moderators of treatment response.

The main goal of the acute treatment phase is to achieve response, which is defined as an at least 50% reduction in depressive symptoms, or more ideally symptomatic remission, which in turn is defined as a period of at least 2 weeks and up to 2 months with no or minimal depressive symptoms. The goal of continuation treatment is to consolidate response and prevent relapse, which is defined as an episode of depression during the period of remission. Recovery should be the

Dr Maalouf is on the speaker bureau of Eli Lilly. Dr Brent receives research support from the National Institute of Mental Health, receives royalties from Guilford Press, and is UpToDate Psychiatry Editor.

[a] Department of Psychiatry, American University of Beirut Medical Center, Beirut, Lebanon
[b] University of Pittsburgh School of Medicine, Pittsburgh, PA USA
[c] Western Psychiatric Institute and Clinic, Department of Psychiatry, University of Pittsburgh School of Medicine, 3811 O'Hara Street, Pittsburgh, PA 15213 USA
* Corresponding author. AUBMC/Psychiatry, 3 Dag Hammarskjold Plaza, 8th floor, New York, NY 10017–2303.
Email address: fm38@aub.edu.lb

Child Adolesc Psychiatric Clin N Am 21 (2012) 299–312
doi:10.1016/j.chc.2012.01.001
1056-4993/12/$ – see front matter © 2012 Elsevier Inc. All rights reserved.

childpsych.theclinics.com

ultimate treatment goal and it is defined as absence of symptoms of depression for at least 2 months. Treatment during the maintenance phase is required to avoid any recurrence of a new depressive episode during the period of recovery.

Discussion in this article will primarily cover the treatment of major depressive disorder (MDD), because there are no controlled trials for the treatment of other depressive disorders (ie, dysthymic disorder or depressive disorder not otherwise specified). However, in clinical practice, treatment recommendations for MDD are successfully used in the management of dysthymic disorder and depressive disorder not otherwise specified.[1]

Acute treatments of MDD that have shown superiority over placebo or "nondirective usual care" as monotherapies include selective serotonin reuptake inhibitors (SSRIs), CBT, and IPT. Combination treatment of medication and CBT has also demonstrated superiority over monotherapies as evidenced by some but not all clinical trials. The roles of augmentation with a second medication and other novel approaches are potentially helpful in achieving early response in certain individuals and targeting resistant symptoms in others. It is important to note, however, that evidence for the efficacy of SSRIs, CBT, and IPT is based on data available from clinical trials that included children between the ages of 6 and 17, but these trials have limited data on the preadolescent age group. For this reason the authors discuss the specificities of the treatment of preadolescent depression under a separate heading.

MONOTHERAPIES
Psychotherapies

Although CBT and IPT are the only two types of therapies that have evidence for efficacy as supported by randomized controlled trials (RCTs), other types of psychotherapies are also used clinically for the treatment of depression in youth. Supportive psychotherapy may be a reasonable first step in patients who present with mild depression, mild psychosocial impairment, and absence of suicidality and psychosis. Here, the clinician may begin treatment with education, support, and case management regarding family and school stressors.[1] However, when patients do not respond to supportive management, are more severely depressed, or have suicidal ideation/behavior, a trial of a specific evidence-based psychotherapy and/or medication is warranted. Psychodynamic psychotherapy is widely used in clinical practice despite the lack of RCT evidence for efficacy. Although family therapy, when available, is widely used because the improvement in family environment is a logical treatment target in youth with depression, there has been only one RCT that studied family therapy and found that CBT was superior to family therapy in short treatment of adolescent depression. (Please see discussion by Tompson elsewhere in this issue for more details and ongoing studies).[2]

CBT

There is strong evidence to support the efficacy of CBT as monotherapy in depression in youth as shown in clinical trials of acute treatments.[2–5] Its effects in depression are significant, but modest (effect size, Cohen's d = 0.35).[6,7] CBT focuses on identifying cognitive distortions that may lead to depressed mood and also utilizes problem-solving, behavior activation, and emotion regulation skills to help manage and combat depression. Although CBT performed better than supportive, family, and relaxation therapies in acute trials, importantly, the other treatments seem to catch up during longer term follow-ups.[3,4]

In the Treatment of Adolescent Depression Study (TADS), a National Institute of Mental Health–funded multicenter study that randomized 439 depressed adolescents to CBT alone, fluoxetine alone, CBT with fluoxetine, and pill-placebo, CBT did not perform better in acute treatment than placebo and less well than medication only. At 12 weeks the corresponding rates of response were 61% for fluoxetine, 43% for CBT, and 35% for placebo.[8] Over time, however, in open follow-up, all the different treatment options converged (at week 36, the estimated remission rates were 55% for fluoxetine and 64% for CBT).[9]

In a recent study that randomized depressed youths with MDD and other depressive disorders (dysthymia and minor depression) to manualized CBT versus usual care by community therapists, CBT showed advantages over usual care in engaging parents, shortening time to remission, and requiring less additional medications. In this study, CBT and usual care had similar remission rates of 75% at the end of treatment.[5]

Across studies, CBT is more effective than comparator treatments in patients with comorbidity (especially anxiety and attention-deficit/hyperactivity disorder) or suicidal ideation, and either no better or worse than comparators in the presence of parent-child discord, parental depression, and history of abuse.[3,10–15] Whereas the TADS study suggested that CBT, either alone or in combination with medication, was more effective than medication alone in reducing suicidal ideation and preventing suicidal events, other clinical trials of adolescent depression did not find that CBT was more advantageous than medication or other psychotherapy monotherapies in reducing suicidal events.[2,16–18]

Last, CBT has also been shown to be effective in preventing the onset of depression in offspring of parents with history of depression and in adolescents at high risk because of subthreshold depressive symptoms.[19,20] In the latter study, the risk reduction as translated into a number needed to prevent was nine; that is, for every nine adolescents who received the intervention, one was prevented from developing a depressive episode. It is important to note that the intervention was not effective if the caretaking parent was depressed at the time of the intervention.[19] Continuation treatment with CBT seems to be successful in preventing the recurrence of depression,[21] and the addition of 12 weekly sessions of CBT focused on preventing relapse to continuation treatment with fluoxetine (in fluoxetine responders) was superior to fluoxetine alone in preventing depressive relapse and recurrence.[22] Here, adolescents who did not receive continuation phase CBT had an eightfold greater risk for relapse than those who received it.

IPT

IPT is another form of psychotherapy that has proved to be an effective monotherapy in the treatment of pediatric depression. The focus of IPT is to help individuals decrease interpersonal conflicts by teaching them interpersonal problem-solving skills and helping them modify communication patterns. This is a particularly valuable approach because conflictual relationships with family members and peers are often significant stressors contributing to the level of symptomatology in depressed adolescents. IPT performs better than treatment as usual in mental health settings but has not been tested against pill-placebo or medication only.[23] Although one clinical trial showed that IPT performed better than CBT in a sample of depressed adolescents, a later study by the same group found that CBT showed some advantage over IPT in a similar sample.[24,25] IPT is especially effective for depressed adolescents who have high levels of interpersonal conflict with parents, higher depressive severity, and comorbid anxiety.[26]

In prevention studies, CBT and IPT perform similarly with effect sizes of Cohen's d = 0.37 and 0.26, for CBT and IPT, respectively. Effect sizes increase to 0.89 and

0.84 for IPT and CBT, respectively, in high-risk groups. In addition, adolescents who placed high value on interpersonal relationships seem to benefit more from IPT as compared with CBT.[27]

MEDICATION MONOTHERAPY
SSRIs

Fluoxetine and escitalopram are the only antidepressants approved by the US Food and Drug Administration (FDA) for the treatment of adolescent depression. Fluoxetine is the only antidepressant that is FDA-approved for depressed preadolescents. Other SSRIs such as sertraline or fluvoxamine are often prescribed based on factors such as comorbidity, side effect profiles, or personal or family history of response to a specific medication. For example, both of these agents have been established as efficacious treatments for pediatric anxiety disorder, which often is comorbid with depression, and sertraline has also been established as an efficacious treatment for obsessive-compulsive disorder.[8,28] Paroxetine is rarely used in the pediatric age group because combined analyses of the extant clinic trials in adolescent depression do not show superiority of drug over placebo.[29,30]

The number of children and adolescents with MDD who participated in antidepressant RCTs has exceeded 3000,[29,31] and overall, the rate of response is 61% for antidepressant versus 50% for placebo yielding a number needed to treat (NNT) of 10,[29] although fluoxetine showed greater efficacy, with an NNT of 5. Hypothesized reasons for this result include that the studies that used fluoxetine were better designed and used mainly sites at academic medical centers or because fluoxetine has a longer half-life, and therefore effects are less vulnerable to occasional nonadherence.[32] In addition, all RCTs of antidepressants in pediatric depression are hampered by very high placebo response rates, which overall were 49%.[33] Study characteristics that are associated with a higher placebo response rate include higher number of study sites, lower baseline illness severity, and younger age of participants.[33]

To date, there have been no planned head-to-head comparisons of different SSRIs for the acute treatment of depression. In The Treatment of Resistant Depression in Adolescents (TORDIA) trial, however, adolescents who had not shown a response to an adequate trial with one SSRI were randomly assigned to either a switch to another SSRI or a switch to venlafaxine. For those within the SSRI switch group, participants were changed to the complementary antidepressant or, if they had previously been treated with an antidepressant other than one of the treatment options, then they were randomly assigned to either fluoxetine or paroxetine (for the first 181 participants) or fluoxetine or citalopram (for the last 153 participants who were recruited after concerns about the efficacy and safety of paroxetine arose midway through the study). In this study of resistant depression, fluoxetine and citalopram performed similarly (response rate around 55%) and better than paroxetine (response rate 38%), although the difference was not statistically significant.[34]

Other Antidepressants

The data on other antidepressants are mixed and rather limited. The only two non-SSRI antidepressants found to be more efficacious than placebo for pediatric depression have been nefazodone and venlafaxine. Neither agent is FDA-approved for pediatric depression. Nefazodone was only examined in one study, and although the generic compound is still available, the drug is no longer marketed because of an increased risk of hepatoxicity.[29] Post hoc analyses of two clinical trials found that venlafaxine was more efficacious than placebo for adolescent, but not preadolescent, depression.[35] Also, the TORDIA study found that, in depressed adolescents who had not responded to an initial treatment with an SSRI, venlafaxine was as efficacious as SSRIs in achieving response at 12 weeks and remission at 24 weeks,[34,36] albeit with more side effects. In addition, venlafaxine was associated with a higher rate of suicidal events in those who entered the study with high suicidal ideation .[17] Mirtazapine has not demonstrated efficacy in clinical trials[29,31] but is used clinically in low doses as a sleep aid. Tricyclic antidepressants have also been shown to be no more efficacious than placebo in depressed children and adolescents through metaanalyses and head-to-head clinical trials.[37] The one exception to this result is clomipramine, which has been shown to be efficacious in the treatment of pediatric obsessive-compulsive disorder,[38] and in one small trial, intravenous infusion was demonstrated to be superior to saline infusion in treating resistant depression in adolescents.[39] Open-label studies have suggested that bupropion and duloxetine are efficacious in treating adolescents with MDD.[40-42] A dose-response relationship has been demonstrated between response and both bupropion and active metabolites.[43]

Predictors of Response

Clinical severity, comorbidity, and family conflict have all been reported to be related to resistance to treatment with SSRIs.[10,11,44] In addition, there may be a relationship between drug concentration and response in patients treated with fluoxetine or citalopram but not those treated with paroxetine or venlafaxine.[45] Furthermore, in patients who do not respond to a lower dose of an SSRI, a higher dose is associated with an increased rate of response compared with continuing to treat at the same dosage, especially if there is an increase in drug concentration.[45,46] Nonadherence, as determined by clinician pill count remainder of greater than 30%, has also been associated with a lower response rate.[47,48] Certain symptoms clusters such as anhedonia or poor sleep may also make response to treatment (either medication monotherapy or combined treatment) less likely. (McMakin D, Olino T, Porta G, et al. Anhedonia predicts poorer recovery among youth with SSRI-treatment resistant depression. Under review.) Further studies are needed in all these areas.

Suicidal Adverse Events

In metaanalyses of all available RCTs, antidepressants increase the risk of spontaneously reported suicidal adverse events by about twofold. The pooled absolute rates of suicidal ideation/suicide attempt were 3% (95% confidence interval (CI), 2%–4%) in antidepressant-treated depressed participants and 2% (95% CI, 1%–2%) in those receiving placebo with estimates of the risk difference ranging between 0.9% and 2% yielding a number needed to harm of 112.[29] A suicidal event was defined as new-onset or increased suicidal ideation or suicidal behavior; the majority of suicidal events reported in these studies were increases in ideation rather than actual behavior, with no suicide completions in any pediatric trials.[49] Predictors of suicidal adverse events include higher suicidal ideation at baseline, greater severity of depression, family conflict, and drug and alcohol use.[16,17,50] These events tend to occur early (3–5 weeks) in treatment and are most common in those who do not respond to treatment.[17,50] Hence, the achievement of early response and targeting risk factors such as family conflict and drug and alcohol use may help mitigate the risk of suicidal adverse events when treating adolescents with MDD. In addition, as discussed above, in the treatment of resistant depression, the use of venlafaxine as compared with SSRIs was associated with more suicidal adverse events in individuals with higher suicidal ideation at baseline and higher suicidal ideation over the course of treatment.[17,51] The TADS study found some evidence that combination treatment of CBT and fluoxetine reduced the rate of suicidal events compared with fluoxetine monotherapy,[50,52] but it was no more efficacious than medication alone in reducing the rate of suicidal events or suicide attempts in TORDIA.[17] One surprising finding from longitudinal studies is that nonsuicidal self-injury is a stronger predictor of a future suicide attempt compared with a history of a suicide attempt.[11,53]

COMBINATION TREATMENT
Medications with Psychotherapy

The combination of medications and CBT has been shown to be more efficacious in acute treatment of adolescent MDD than either monotherapy in two large US trials. The TADS study found that the combination of CBT and fluoxetine was associated with the most rapid and complete response compared with other interventions.[8,9] Specifically, at 12 weeks, the combination of CBT and fluoxetine led to the highest response rate (71%) as compared with CBT monotherapy (43%), fluoxetine monotherapy (61%), and placebo (35%). Whereas the difference in response between fluoxetine monotherapy and combination treatment was not statistically significant, combination treatment *was* superior to the other interventions with respect to the pace of decline in suicidal ideation, improvement in functional impairment, and achievement of remission by 12 weeks.[8,9,54] Consistent with TADS, the TORDIA study found that in treatment-resistant depressed adolescents, switching antidepressants and adding CBT was superior to a medication switch alone (55% for the combination of medication switch and addition of CBT and 41% for medication switch alone) with respect to clinical response, although not pace of response or attainment of remission.[34,36] In TADS, combination treatment did not outperform medication alone though in the subgroup with severe depression. This result is consistent with the British Antidepressant and Psychotherapy Treatment (ADAPT) study, which recruited participants who were severely depressed and who did not respond to a brief psychosocial intervention. In ADAPT, there was a 61% response rate by week 28 for SSRI alone and 53% for the combination of SSRI and CBT.[18,55] A recent metaanalysis of all available studies of combination treatment for adolescent depression concluded that combination treatment offered no superiority over antidepressants alone for depressive symptom improvement (pooled odds ratio of improvement on the Clinical Global Improvement scale for combination vs SSRI alone was 1.35 but was not statistically significant) and suicidality (standardized mean difference = 0.05). Combination therapy showed superiority, however, over medication monotherapy on improvement in functional status (weighted mean difference = -2.32 on impairment scale).[55] Some reported moderators that predicted superiority of combination treatment over medication monotherapy included high level of cognitive distortion in TADS[10] and number of comorbid diagnoses in the TORDIA study.[11] Abuse was associated with a less vigorous response to CBT with or without medication in both studies.[15,56]

The superiority of combination treatment over monotherapy in both TADS and TORDIA seems to disappear over time. This result may be due to spontaneous remission, because all treatment options ultimately catch up with each other, or because of additional open treatments received after the end of the formal portion of the trial. Remission rates were 60% for combination treatment, 55% for fluoxetine, and 64% for CBT by week 36 in TADS,[9] and total remission rate was 60% by week 72 independent of initial treatment in TORDIA.[51] Because treatment was not controlled after the acute phase in both TADS and TORDIA, it would be difficult to differentiate between the course of the depressive illness, long-term efficacy of the interventions, and the impact of additional treatments available to participants in the follow-up phases of these studies. Both of these follow-up studies had significant attrition, with differential attrition by those who did not show early symptomatic improvement; hence, the estimates of the rates of remission may be overly optimistic.

Augmentation with a Second Medication

One may augment a current antidepressant regimen with an additional antidepressant in those who have improved and have residual symptoms in order to accelerate initial treatment response, or in nonresponders. Although polypharmacy is common in clinical practice among clinically referred youth, combination treatments have not been systematically studied in depressed youth. For patients with residual fatigue, the authors recommend consideration of augmentation with bupropion, an activating antidepressant; for those with sleep difficulties, mirtazapine or melatonin; and for patients with subsyndromal manic symptoms, which have been associated with treatment resistance, one can consider augmentation with a mood stabilizer.[57] However, none of these strategies have been critically evaluated.

Because early response patterns are strongly predictive of eventual outcome, recent research in adults has focused on interventions that accelerate initial response.[58] Combinations of venlafaxine and mirtazapine, sertraline and T3, and open trials with the addition of ketamine have been reported to accelerate treatment response.[59–61] However, a recent report of the Combining Medications to Enhance Depression Outcomes (CO-MED) study did not find that medication combination outperformed medication monotherapy in acute and long-term treatment of adult MDD.[62] Augmentation of antidepressant with antipsychotics in adult nonresponders has been reported to be successful compared with antidepressant plus placebo in clinical trials.[63,64] The STAR*D (Sequenced Treatment Alternatives to Relieve Depression) study found that augmentation of an antidepressant with lithium, T3, or bupropion was equivalent, although those augmented with T3 had the lowest rate of side effects.[64] However, these combinations have not been studied for resistant depression in adolescents. In adolescents, in open treatment, augmentation with antipsychotics was supported by post hoc analyses of the TORDIA study[36] and some case studies.[65] Disadvantages of the use of atypical antipsychotics in this population include risk of weight gain, obesity, and metabolic syndrome.[66]

Low Remission Rates, High Relapse Rates

Whereas response occurs in more than half of depressed adolescents after acute treatment, complete symptomatic remission remains low: 37% of those who received combination treatment achieved remission by 12 weeks in TADS, as compared with 23% of those who received fluoxetine, 16% of those treated with CBT, and 17% of those treated with placebo, and patients who improve continue to have significant residual symptoms.[9] The results of longer term treatment are more promising; for instance, in TADS, follow-up at week 36 showed remission rates as high as 60% in all treatment groups, and in TORDIA, nearly 40% achieved remission at week 24, with 60% attaining remission by weeks 48 or 72.[51]

Early trajectory of treatment response predicts longer term remission. Indeed, in TADS, residual symptoms at the end of acute treatment predicted failure to achieve remission at weeks 18 and 36,[67] and in TORDIA, initial response at 12 weeks predicted a greater than threefold increased likelihood of remission by 6 months of treatment.[36] These findings suggest that obtaining a rapid and robust response early in treatment is key to achieving remission later.

Longer term naturalistic follow-up showed that close to 40% of participants did not achieve remission by week 72 in TORDIA and TADS, with the most common residual symptoms of depression being irritability, fatigue, anhedonia, and sleep difficulties.[51,68] As stated earlier, because the naturalistic follow-up of both TORDIA and TADS was not controlled, it is difficult to distinguish the effects of initial treatment from natural recovery and subsequent open treatment. In addition, relapse rates remain substantial even with continuation of treatment. In TORDIA, 25% of participants who remitted by week 24 relapsed in the subsequent year. In addition, 1-year follow-up after treatment discontinuation in TADS revealed that 30% of those who had remitted during the first 9 months of treatment lost their remission status.[68] These results indicate a need for further improvements in long-term treatment of major depressive disorder in youth. Even more discouraging, on a longer term follow-up of the TADS sample, the recurrence rate was close to 50% in youths who had recovered from their index depressive episode, and recurrence was not predicted by previous remission or residual symptoms.[69]

NOVEL INTERVENTIONS
Improving Sleep

Disrupted sleep predicts onset and recurrence of depression and a poorer response to treatment.[70,71] Disturbed sleep is also one of the most common residual symptoms of depression in adolescents[72] and has been shown to be an independent predictor of risk for suicide in adolescents.[73] In TORDIA, participants who were cotreated with diphenhydramine or zolpidem for sleep, based on clinician's discretion, responded as well as those without sleep medications, and much better than those treated with trazodone.[74] None of the participants (0 of 13) who were cotreated with trazodone and either fluoxetine or paroxetine responded, perhaps because these two agents are potent inhibitors of CYP 2D6. This cytochrome enzyme is responsible for breaking down methyl-chloro-piperazine (mCPP), which is a metabolite of trazodone; mCPP can induce dysphoria and anxiety, and it is possible that the poor response found in TORDIA in those cotreated with trazodone is due to the previously posited drug-drug interaction.[74] Taken together, these findings highlight the need to assess and manage sleep difficulties in adolescents with depression and support further empirical work in this area. Indeed, interventions that improve sleep have been shown to improve response to antidepressants in adults,[75] but no such interventions have been carefully investigated in children and adolescents. (See discussion by Harvey and Clarke elsewhere in this issue.).

Improving Environmental/Contextual Factors

Past history of abuse, current family conflict, and parental depression can all contribute to a less than optimal response to evidence-based treatments in depressed adolescents.[12,15,76] In TORDIA, youth with a history of abuse showed a markedly better response to medication alone than to the combination of CBT with medication, which is exactly the opposite of what was found for the remainder of the sample. Post hoc analyses did not explain why abuse is related to such a poor response to combination treatment. Some adaptations of CBT that specifically target depressive cognitions and schema associated with a history of maltreatment have looked promising.[77] In the case of parental depression, there is some evidence that concurrent treatment of the depressed parent and child with mental health problems will result in a better outcome than if the child is treated alone.[76,78] Improvement in child's mental health through treatment of the mother was mediated in part by improvements in the quality of the parent-child interaction. Other less well-studied environmental factors may affect youths' response to treatment and need to be clinically addressed. The authors' clinical experience has informed them that youth who are being bullied at school are less likely to respond to evidence-based treatments unless this issue is addressed. In addition, youth who experience same-sex attraction, particularly if there is accompanying peer victimization or parental rejection, are also at risk for persistence of depressive symptoms. Specific research needs to be conducted in the future on the role of amelioration of many of the previously described factors in improving depressive illness outcome.

Addressing Subsyndromal Manic Symptoms

Although the effect of subsyndromal bipolar symptoms on outcome of depression treatment has not been systematically investigated in children and adolescents, there is growing evidence that treatment-resistant depression in adult populations is associated with high rates of bipolar symptoms.[79] Recent evidence from the TORDIA study suggests that subsyndromal manic symptoms both at baseline and over time emerge as predictors of poor outcome in adolescent resistant-depression.[57] These symptoms were not considered clinically significant and were far below the cut point on the Mania Rating Scale for probable hypomania. Future studies should look at investigating the clinical importance of subsyndromal manic symptoms systematically in pediatric depression and the potential role of mood stabilizing agents in this clinical subpopulation as augmenting agents.

PREPUBERTAL DEPRESSION

Antidepressants, with the exception of fluoxetine, are less efficacious in children than in adolescents (NNT of 7 vs 15 for prepubertal children and adolescents, respectively, according to a recent metaanalysis).[29] The pharmacokinetic properties of paroxetine, sertraline, citalopram, and venlafaxine may explain their lower performance as compared with fluoxetine in the treatment of prepubertal depression.[32] Indeed, the half-lives of most antidepressants are much lower in children than in adolescents,[32,80] and because there is some evidence that inadequate exposure to antidepressants is associated with lower response rate, prepubertal children may require higher doses to achieve adequate blood concentration and optimal response.[45] However, sertraline and venlafaxine have been shown to be efficacious in pediatric anxiety and obsessive-compulsive disorder despite their pharmacokinetic profiles.[29]

Use of antidepressants in young populations may be associated with an increased risk of mania, suggesting that there may be differing vulnerability of the developing brain to the adverse effects of antidepressants according to the developmental stage during which exposure occurs.[81]

In addition, although there has been no head-to-head comparison or large scale trials of CBT and IPT in the treatment of prepubertal depression, versions of CBT have been adapted to high-risk prepubertal children and shown efficacy.[82,83] Larger studies that include different versions of CBT and modification of its different components (engaging in enjoyable activities tailored to school-aged children) are therefore needed. One open study of family-based IPT for preadolescent youth with depression and their families suggests that this is also a promising approach.[84]

The scarcity of intervention data in this group suggests that there is a need for age-specific intervention research in youth with MDD (see discussions by Nestor-Lopez/Kovacs and Tompson elsewhere in this issue).

SUMMARY

In this review, the authors provide a summary of the currently available research evidence on interventions in pediatric depression. The use of SSRIs as an effective intervention in the treatment of depression in childhood and adolescence is supported by numerous large clinical trials including TADS and TORDIA. There is also evidence that the combination of medication and CBT is superior to medication alone for accelerating the pace of treatment response and remission, despite some negative studies. For mild to moderate depression, CBT and IPT are reasonable options, although the rate of improvement is much slower with psychotherapy (CBT) alone. Response rates after acute treatment remain modest at best, with significant residual symptoms, and remission rates over long-term follow-ups are not more promising. In order to improve the risk-to-benefit ratio for patients treated for pediatric depression, future studies should examine how to accelerate initial treatment response; target residual symptoms, especially sleep and anhedonia; improve adherence; and target contextual environmental risk factors that may lead to an unfavorable response to treatment.

REFERENCES

1. Birmaher B, Brent D, Bernet W, et al. Practice parameter for the assessment and treatment of children and adolescents with depressive disorders. J Am Acad Child Adolesc Psychiatry 2007;46(11):1503–26.
2. Brent DA, Holder D, Kolko D, et al. A clinical psychotherapy trial for adolescent depression comparing cognitive, family, and supportive therapy. Arch Gen Psychiatry 1997;54(9):877–85.
3. Birmaher B, Brent DA, Kolko D, et al. Clinical outcome after short-term psychotherapy for adolescents with major depressive disorder. Arch Gen Psychiatry 2000;57(1):29–36.
4. Wood A, Harrington R, Moore A. Controlled trial of a brief cognitive-behavioural intervention in adolescent patients with depressive disorders. J Child Psychol Psychiatry 1996;37(6):737–46.
5. Weisz JR, Southam-Gerow MA, Gordis EB, et al. Cognitive-behavioral therapy versus usual clinical care for youth depression: an initial test of transportability to community clinics and clinicians. J Consult Clin Psychol 2009;77(3):383–96.
6. Harrington R, Campbell F, Shoebridge P, et al. Meta-analysis of CBT for depression in adolescents. J Am Acad Child Adolesc Psychiatry 1998;37(10):1005–7.
7. Weisz JR, McCarty CA, Valeri SM. Effects of psychotherapy for depression in children and adolescents: a meta-analysis. Psychol Bull 2006;132(1):132–49.
8. March J, Silva S, Petrycki S, et al. Fluoxetine, cognitive-behavioral therapy, and their combination for adolescents with depression: Treatment for Adolescents With Depression Study (TADS) randomized controlled trial. JAMA 2004;292(7):807–20.
9. Kennard B, Silva S, Vitiello B, et al. Remission and residual symptoms after short-term treatment in the Treatment of Adolescents with Depression Study (TADS). J Am Acad Child Adolesc Psychiatry 2006;45(12):1404–11.
10. Curry J, Rohde P, Simons A, et al. Predictors and moderators of acute outcome in the Treatment for Adolescents with Depression Study (TADS). J Am Acad Child Adolesc Psychiatry 2006;45(12):1427–39.
11. Asarnow JR, Emslie G, Clarke G, et al. Treatment of selective serotonin reuptake inhibitor-resistant depression in adolescents: predictors and moderators of treatment response. J Am Acad Child Adolesc Psychiatry 2009;48(3):330–9.

12. Feeny NC, Silva SG, Reinecke MA, et al. An exploratory analysis of the impact of family functioning on treatment for depression in adolescents. J Clin Child Adolesc Psychol 2009;38(6):814–25.

13. Brent DA, Kolko DJ, Birmaher B, et al. Predictors of treatment efficacy in a clinical trial of three psychosocial treatments for adolescent depression. J Am Acad Child Adolesc Psychiatry 1998;37(9):906–14.

14. Barbe RP, Bridge JA, Birmaher B, et al. Lifetime history of sexual abuse, clinical presentation, and outcome in a clinical trial for adolescent depression. J Clin Psychiatry 2004;65(1):77–83.

15. Shamseddeen W, Asarnow JR, Clarke G, et al. Impact of Physical and Sexual Abuse on Treatment Response in the Treatment of Resistant Depression in Adolescent Study (TORDIA). J Am Acad Child Adolesc Psychiatry 2011;50(3):293–301.

16. Emslie G, Kratochvil C, Vitiello B, et al. Treatment for Adolescents with Depression Study (TADS): safety results. J Am Acad Child Adolesc Psychiatry 2006;45(12):1440–55.

17. Brent DA, Emslie GJ, Clarke GN, et al. Predictors of spontaneous and systematically assessed suicidal adverse events in the treatment of SSRI-resistant depression in adolescents (TORDIA) study. Am J Psychiatry 2009;166(4):418–26.

18. Goodyer I, Dubicka B, Wilkinson P, et al. Selective serotonin reuptake inhibitors (SSRIs) and routine specialist care with and without cognitive behaviour therapy in adolescents with major depression: randomised controlled trial. BMJ 2007;335(7611):142.

19. Garber J, Clarke GN, Weersing VR, et al. Prevention of depression in at-risk adolescents: a randomized controlled trial. JAMA 2009;301(21):2215–24.

20. Clarke GN, Hornbrook M, Lynch F, et al. A randomized trial of a group cognitive intervention for preventing depression in adolescent offspring of depressed parents. Arch Gen Psychiatry 2001;58(12):1127–34.

21. Kroll L, Harrington R, Jayson D, et al. Pilot study of continuation cognitive-behavioral therapy for major depression in adolescent psychiatric patients. J Am Acad Child Adolesc Psychiatry 1996;35(9):1156–61.

22. Kennard BD, Emslie GJ, Mayes TL, et al. Cognitive-behavioral therapy to prevent relapse in pediatric responders to pharmacotherapy for major depressive disorder. J Am Acad Child Adolesc Psychiatry 2008;47(12):1395–404.

23. Klomek AB, Mufson L. Interpersonal psychotherapy for depressed adolescents. Child Adolesc Psychiatr Clin N Am 2006;15(4):959–75, ix.

24. Rossello J, Bernal G. The efficacy of cognitive-behavioral and interpersonal treatments for depression in Puerto Rican adolescents. J Consult Clin Psychol 1999;67(5):734–45.

25. Rossello J, Bernal G, Rivera-Medina C. Individual and group CBT and IPT for Puerto Rican adolescents with depressive symptoms. Cultur Divers Ethnic Minor Psychol 2008;14(3):234–45.

26. Mufson L, Dorta KP, Wickramaratne P, et al. A randomized effectiveness trial of interpersonal psychotherapy for depressed adolescents. Arch Gen Psychiatry 2004;61(6):577–84.

27. Horowitz JL, Garber J, Ciesla JA, et al. Prevention of depressive symptoms in adolescents: a randomized trial of cognitive-behavioral and interpersonal prevention programs. J Consult Clin Psychol 2007;75(5):693–706.

28. Walkup JT, Albano AM, Piacentini J, et al. Cognitive behavioral therapy, sertraline, or a combination in childhood anxiety. N Engl J Med 2008;359(26):2753–66.

29. Bridge JA, Iyengar S, Salary CB, et al. Clinical response and risk for reported suicidal ideation and suicide attempts in pediatric antidepressant treatment: a meta-analysis of randomized controlled trials. JAMA 2007;297(15):1683–96.

30. Apter A, Lipschitz A, Fong R, et al. Evaluation of suicidal thoughts and behaviors in children and adolescents taking paroxetine. J Child Adolesc Psychopharmacol 2006; 16(1/2):77–90.

31. Cheung AH, Emslie GJ, Mayes TL. Review of the efficacy and safety of antidepressants in youth depression. J Child Psychol Psychiatry 2005;46(7):735–54.

32. Findling RL, McNamara NK, Stansbrey RJ, et al. The relevance of pharmacokinetic studies in designing efficacy trials in juvenile major depression. J Child Adolesc Psychopharmacol 2006;16(1/2):131–45.

33. Bridge JA, Birmaher B, Iyengar S, et al. Placebo response in randomized controlled trials of antidepressants for pediatric major depressive disorder. Am J Psychiatry 2009;166(1):42–9.

34. Brent D, Emslie G, Clarke G, et al. Switching to another SSRI or to venlafaxine with or without cognitive behavioral therapy for adolescents with SSRI-resistant depression: the TORDIA randomized controlled trial. JAMA 2008;299(8):901–13.

35. Emslie GJ, Findling RL, Yeung PP, et al. Venlafaxine ER for the treatment of pediatric subjects with depression: results of two placebo-controlled trials. J Am Acad Child Adolesc Psychiatry 2007;46(4):479–88.

36. Emslie GJ, Mayes T, Porta G, et al. Treatment of Resistant Depression in Adolescents (TORDIA): week 24 outcomes. Am J Psychiatry 2010;167(7):782–91.

37. Hazell P, O'Connell D, Heathcote D, et al. Tricyclic drugs for depression in children and adolescents. Cochrane Database Syst Rev 2002;2:CD002317.

38. DeVeaugh-Geiss J, Moroz G, Biederman J, et al. Clomipramine hydrochloride in childhood and adolescent obsessive-compulsive disorder–a multicenter trial. J Am Acad Child Adolesc Psychiatry 1992;31(1):45–9.

39. Sallee FR, Vrindavanam NS, Deas-Nesmith D, et al. Pulse intravenous clomipramine for depressed adolescents: double-blind, controlled trial. Am J Psychiatry 1997; 154(5):668–73.

40. Glod CA, Lynch A, Flynn E, et al. Open trial of bupropion SR in adolescent major depression. J Child Adolesc Psychiatr Nurs 2003;16(3):123–30.

41. Daviss WB, Bentivoglio P, Racusin R, et al. Bupropion sustained release in adolescents with comorbid attention-deficit/hyperactivity disorder and depression. J Am Acad Child Adolesc Psychiatry 2001;40(3):307–14.

42. March J, Graham E, Kratochvil C, et al. An open-label study of tolerability, safety, and pharmacokinetics of duloxetine in children (7–11 years) and adolescents (12–17 years) with MDD. Presented at the 49th annual New Clinical Drug Evaluation Unit (NCDEU) Meeting. Hollywood, Florida, June 29 to July 2, 2009.

43. Daviss WB, Perel JM, Brent DA, et al. Acute antidepressant response and plasma levels of bupropion and metabolites in a pediatric-aged sample: an exploratory study. Ther Drug Monit 2006;28(2):190–8.

44. Emslie GJ, Rush AJ, Weinberg WA, et al. Fluoxetine in child and adolescent depression: acute and maintenance treatment. Depress Anxiety 1998;7(1):32–9.

45. Sakolsky DJ, Perel JM, Emslie GJ, et al. Antidepressant exposure as a predictor of clinical outcomes in the Treatment of Resistant Depression in Adolescents (TORDIA) study. J Clin Psychopharmacol 2011;31(1):92–7.

46. Heiligenstein JH, Hoog SL, Wagner KD, et al. Fluoxetine 40–60 mg versus fluoxetine 20 mg in the treatment of children and adolescents with a less-than-complete response to nine-week treatment with fluoxetine 10–20 mg: a pilot study. J Child Adolesc Psychopharmacol 2006;16(1/2):207–17.

47. Woldu H, Porta G, Goldstein T, et al. Pharmacokinetically and clinician-determined adherence to an antidepressant regimen and clinical outcome in the TORDIA trial. J Am Acad Child Adolesc Psychiatry 2011;50(5):490–8.

48. Nakonezny PA, Hughes CW, Mayes TL, et al. A comparison of various methods of measuring antidepressant medication adherence among children and adolescents with major depressive disorder in a 12-week open trial of fluoxetine. J Child Adolesc Psychopharmacol 2010;20(5):431–9.

49. Brent D, Melhem N, Turecki G. Pharmacogenomics of suicidal events. Pharmacogenomics 2010;11(6):793–807.

50. Vitiello B, Silva SG, Rohde P, et al. Suicidal events in the Treatment for Adolescents With Depression Study (TADS). J Clin Psychiatry 2009;70(5):741–7.

51. Vitiello B, Emslie G, Clarke G, et al. Long-term outcome of adolescent depression initially resistant to selective serotonin reuptake inhibitor treatment: a follow-up study of the TORDIA sample. J Clin Psychiatry 2010;72(3):388–96.

52. March JS, Silva S, Petrycki S, et al. The Treatment for Adolescents With Depression Study (TADS): long-term effectiveness and safety outcomes. Arch Gen Psychiatry 2007;64(10):1132–43.

53. Wilkinson P, Kelvin R, Roberts C, et al. Clinical and psychosocial predictors of suicide attempts and nonsuicidal self-injury in the Adolescent Depression Antidepressants and Psychotherapy Trial (ADAPT). Am J Psychiatry 2011;168(5):495–501.

54. Vitiello B, Rohde P, Silva S, et al. Functioning and quality of life in the Treatment for Adolescents with Depression Study (TADS). J Am Acad Child Adolesc Psychiatry 2006;45(12):1419–26.

55. Dubicka B, Elvins R, Roberts C, et al. Combined treatment with cognitive-behavioural therapy in adolescent depression: meta-analysis. Br J Psychiatry 2010;197:433–40.

56. Lewis CC, Simons AD, Nguyen LJ, et al. Impact of childhood trauma on treatment outcome in the Treatment for Adolescents with Depression Study (TADS). J Am Acad Child Adolesc Psychiatry 2010;49(2):132–40.

57. Maalouf FT, Porta G, Vitiello B, et al. Do sub-syndromal manic symptoms influence outcome in treatment resistant depression in adolescents? A latent class analysis from the TORDIA study J Affect Disord 2012 Jan 26 [epub ahead of print].

58. Tao R, Emslie G, Mayes T, et al. Early prediction of acute antidepressant treatment response and remission in pediatric major depressive disorder. J Am Acad Child Adolesc Psychiatry 2009;48(1):71–8.

59. Blier P, Ward HE, Tremblay P, et al. Combination of antidepressant medications from treatment initiation for major depressive disorder: a double-blind randomized study. Am J Psychiatry 2010;167(3):281–8.

60. Cooper-Kazaz R, Apter JT, Cohen R, et al. Combined treatment with sertraline and liothyronine in major depression: a randomized, double-blind, placebo-controlled trial. Arch Gen Psychiatry 2007;64(6):679–88.

61. Diazgranados N, Ibrahim L, Brutsche NE, et al. A randomized add-on trial of an N-methyl-D-aspartate antagonist in treatment-resistant bipolar depression. Arch Gen Psychiatry 2010;67(8):793–802.

62. Rush AJ, Trivedi MH, Stewart JW, et al. Combining medications to enhance depression outcomes (CO-MED): acute and long-term outcomes of a single-blind randomized study. Am J Psychiatry 2011;168(7):689–701.

63. Nelson JC, Papakostas GI. Atypical antipsychotic augmentation in major depressive disorder: a meta-analysis of placebo-controlled randomized trials. Am J Psychiatry 2009;166(9):980–91.

64. Rush AJ, Warden D, Wisniewski SR, et al. STAR*D: revising conventional wisdom. CNS Drugs 2009;23(8):627–47.

65. Pathak S, Johns ES, Kowatch RA. Adjunctive quetiapine for treatment-resistant adolescent major depressive disorder: a case series. J Child Adolesc Psychopharmacol 2005;15(4):696–702.

66. Correll CU, Manu P, Olshanskiy V, et al. Cardiometabolic risk of second-generation antipsychotic medications during first-time use in children and adolescents. JAMA 2009;302(16):1765–73.

67. Kennard BD, Silva SG, Tonev S, et al. Remission and recovery in the Treatment for Adolescents with Depression Study (TADS): acute and long-term outcomes. J Am Acad Child Adolesc Psychiatry 2009;48(2):186–95.

68. March J, Silva S, Curry J, et al. The Treatment for Adolescents With Depression Study (TADS): outcomes over 1 year of naturalistic follow-up. Am J Psychiatry 2009;166(10):1141–9.

69. Curry J, Silva S, Rohde P, et al. Recovery and recurrence following treatment for adolescent major depression. Arch Gen Psychiatry 2011;68(3):263–9.

70. Thase ME, Fasiczka AL, Berman SR, et al. Electroencephalographic sleep profiles before and after cognitive behavior therapy of depression. Arch Gen Psychiatry 1998;55(2):138–44.

71. Roane BM, Taylor DJ. Adolescent insomnia as a risk factor for early adult depression and substance abuse. Sleep 2008;31(10):1351–6.

72. Tao R, Emslie GJ, Mayes TL, et al. Symptom improvement and residual symptoms during acute antidepressant treatment in pediatric major depressive disorder. J Child Adolesc Psychopharmacol 2010;20(5):423–30.

73. Goldstein TR, Bridge JA, Brent DA. Sleep disturbance preceding completed suicide in adolescents. J Consult Clin Psychol 2008;76(1):84–91.

74. Shamseddeen W, Clarke G, DeBar L, et al. Insomnia medications and outcomes in the Treatment of SSRI-Resistant Depression in Adolescents (TORDIA) study. J Child Adolesc Psychopharmacol 2012. [Epub ahead of print]

75. Manber R, Edinger JD, Gress JL, et al. Cognitive behavioral therapy for insomnia enhances depression outcome in patients with comorbid major depressive disorder and insomnia. Sleep 2008;31(4):489–95.

76. Weissman MM, Pilowsky DJ, Wickramaratne PJ, et al. Remissions in maternal depression and child psychopathology: a STAR*D-child report. JAMA 2006;295(12):1389–98.

77. Eltz MJ, Shirk SR, Sarlin N. Alliance formation and treatment outcome among maltreated adolescents. Child Abuse Negl 1995;19(4):419–31.

78. Swartz HA, Frank E, Zuckoff A, et al. Brief interpersonal psychotherapy for depressed mothers whose children are receiving psychiatric treatment. Am J Psychiatry 2008;165(9):1155–62.

79. Correa R, Akiskal H, Gilmer W, et al. Is unrecognized bipolar disorder a frequent contributor to apparent treatment resistant depression? J Affect Disord 2010;127(1–3):10–8.

80. Axelson DA, Perel JM, Birmaher B, et al. Sertraline pharmacokinetics and dynamics in adolescents. J Am Acad Child Adolesc Psychiatry 2002;41(9):1037–44.

81. Martin A, Young C, Leckman JF, et al. Age effects on antidepressant-induced manic conversion. Arch Pediatr Adolesc Med 2004;158(8):773–80.

82. De Cuyper S, Timbremont B, Braet C, et al. Treating depressive symptoms in schoolchildren: a pilot study. Eur Child Adolesc Psychiatry 2004;13(2):105–14.

83. Weisz JR, Thurber CA, Sweeney L, et al. Brief treatment of mild-to-moderate child depression using primary and secondary control enhancement training. J Consult Clin Psychol 1997;65(4):703–7.

84. Dietz LJ, Mufson L, Irvine H, et al. Family-based interpersonal psychotherapy for depressed preadolescents: an open-treatment trial. Early intervention in psychiatry 2008;2(3):154–61.

Developmentally Informed Pharmacotherapy for Child and Adolescent Depressive Disorders

Dara Sakolsky, MD, PhD*, Boris Birmaher, MD

KEYWORDS

- Major depressive disorder • Adolescents • Children
- Selective serotonin reuptake inhibitors • Venlafaxine

Approximately 20% of youth will experience at least one episode of depression by age 18.[1] If left untreated, major depressive disorder (MDD) can affect the youth's development of social, emotional, and cognitive skills.[2–4] Children and adolescents with depression are also at high risk for early pregnancy, legal problems, substance abuse, or suicide. Evidence-based treatments have emerged in both psychotherapy and pharmacotherapy for the treatment of adolescent depression. However, the literature on effective treatments for depression in children between the ages of 6 and 11 is limited.

INTERVENTION OPTIONS FOR MAJOR DEPRESSION IN YOUTH

Many treatments (supportive therapy, cognitive–behavioral therapy [CBT], interpersonal therapy, contextual emotional regulation therapy, and pharmacotherapy) can be helpful for youth with major depression.[5] This article discusses the role of evidence-based pharmacotherapy in the treatment for child and adolescent depression.

The choice of treatment intervention should be influenced by developmental stage, severity of depression, duration of illness, prior treatment response, availability of interventions, comorbid disorders, familial and environmental dynamics, as well as family preference. Please see "Intervention Overview" (Maalouf and Brent) in this

Disclosures: Dr Sakolsky has received funding and support from the National Institute of Mental Health and NARSAD, the World's leading Charity Dedicated to Mental Health Research. Dr Brimaher has received research support from the National Institute of Mental Health, and served as a consultant for Scherring Plough. He has participated in forums sponsored by Dey Pharma, L.P. and Forest Laboratories, Inc. He has received royalties for publications from Random House, Inc and Lippnicott Williams and Wilkins.
Western Psychiatric Institute and Clinic, University of Pittsburgh Medical Center, 100 North Bellefield Avenue, Pittsburgh, PA 15213, USA
* Corresponding author.
E-mail address: sakolskydj@upmc.edu

issue of *Child and Adolescent Psychiatric Clinics of North America* for a complete discussion of the current range of treatment options for MDD in youth. For children and adolescents with mild or brief depression, slight impairment, and the absence of suicidal ideation or psychosis, pharmacotherapy is usually not needed. In these cases, intervention often starts with education and supportive therapy to target family or school stressors. If improvement in depressive symptoms is not achieved after 2 to 4 weeks, a more specific type of psychotherapy (eg, CBT, interpersonal psychotherapy, contextual emotional regulation therapy) should be utilized.[5] For children and adolescents with moderate, chronic, or significant impairment, the combination of psychotherapy and pharmacotherapy is often needed.[5] Nevertheless, CBT, interpersonal therapy, or contextual emotional regulation therapy alone may be helpful. Some depressive symptoms (eg, agitation, low motivation, or psychosis) can limit participation in psychotherapy; thus beginning treatment with only an antidepressant may be desirable in some cases. For children and adolescents with severe depression, depression with psychosis, or treatment-resistant depression, pharmacotherapy is usually needed.[5] In these cases, treatment often comprises both medication and psychotherapy. Youth with depression and psychosis may need treatment with an antipsychotic medication alone or in combination with an antidepressant.[5]

ACUTE EFFICACY OF SELECTIVE SEROTONIN REUPTAKE INHIBITORS FOR MDD

Treatment outcomes in depressive disorders have been described using specific terminology. Response is often defined at a significant reduction in depressive symptoms for at least 2 weeks while remission is defined as a period of at least 2 weeks and less than 2 months with no or few depressive symptoms. One measure of treatment effectiveness is the number needed to treat (NNT) or the number of patients who must receive treatment to get one response that is attributable to active treatment. A meta-analysis of published and unpublished randomized controlled trials (RCTs) of antidepressants (selective serotonin reuptake inhibitors [SSRIs] and serotonin norepinephrine reuptake inhibitors [SNRIs])[6] reported the NNT to benefit from an antidepressant was 10 (95% confidence interval [CI], 7–15) for depression in youth. These data suggest that SSRIs and SNRIs should be considered among the treatment options for childhood and adolescent depression.

Fluoxetine

At present, both fluoxetine and escitalopram have a U.S. Food and Drug Administration (FDA) indication for the treatment of adolescent depression. As three RCTs[7–9] have demonstrated the acute efficacy of fluoxetine for depression in youth, fluoxetine is often the first choice of medications. In their meta-analysis, Bridge and colleagues[6] combined the data from all three fluoxetine RCTs for pediatric depression and found the NNT to benefit from fluoxetine was 6 (95% CI, 4–10). Bridge and colleagues[6] found the differences in response between medication and placebo were similar for children and adolescents. Likewise, Mayes and colleagues[10] combined the data from the two fluoxetine RCTs that enrolled children and found the fluoxetine response and remission rates were significantly better than placebo rates within the child subgroup (n = 134). It remains uncertain if fluoxetine is better than the other SSRIs (eg, long half-life improves adherence and outcome) or if the fluoxetine trials were better designed and conducted. For an in-depth discussion of methodologic issues please see Refs.[11,12]

Although fluoxetine is often the first choice of medication for the treatment of depression in youth given its efficacy and low cost, there are many situations when choosing a different SSRI is logical (eg, drug–drug interactions, prior lack of response to an adequate trial of fluoxetine, strong family history of therapeutic response to an alternative SSRI, or family bias).

Escitalopram

Escitalopram is another good medication choice for the treatment of adolescent depression, as two RCTs have demonstrated its efficacy in this population and the FDA has approved it for the treatment of adolescent depression. The first RCT with escitalopram compared flexible-dose medication (10–20 mg/day, mean dose 12 mg/day) and placebo for 8 weeks.[13] On the primary outcome measure, there was no significant difference between escitalopram and placebo. In a post hoc analysis of adolescents (aged 12–17 years) who completed the treatment, those who received escitalopram had significantly improved scores on all outcome measures. No difference between escitalopram and placebo was demonstrated with children (aged 6–11 years) on any of the efficacy measures. A second RCT compared flexible-dose escitalopram (10–20 mg/day, mean dose 13 mg/day) with placebo in depressed adolescents.[14] This trial found significant improvement in depressive symptoms in the escitalopram-treated group compared to the one receiving placebo on several outcome measures. Response rates, defined as 40% reduction in the total score on the Children's Depression Rating Scale-Revised, were 91% for escitalopram and 76% for placebo. Therefore, two RCTs have established the efficacy of escitalopram for the treatment of adolescent depression whereas no RCTs have shown escitalopram to be efficacious for children with MDD.

Citalopram and Sertraline

Trials with citalopram and sertraline have shown some efficacy for the treatment of depression in youth. One trial with citalopram[15] has demonstrated positive results and another[16] has shown negative results. In the positive study, children and adolescents (mean age 12.1 years) were randomized to flexible-dose citalopram (20–40 mg/day, mean dose 24 mg/day) or placebo. Response rates on the primary outcome measure were 36% for citalopram and 24% for placebo. Differences in response between child and adolescents were not examined in this trial. In the negative study, only adolescents (aged 13–18 years) received citalopram (10–40 mg/day) or placebo. Unlike in other RCTs for adolescent depression, participants in this study included both inpatients and outpatients. Some adolescents received psychotherapy or other medications including antipsychotics, benzodiazepines, anticonvulsants, hypnotics, and stimulants, or both psychotherapy and medication. Response rates on the primary outcome measure were 60% for citalopram and 61% for placebo. For sertraline, two identical multicenter randomized, double blind, placebo-controlled studies of sertraline were conducted with children and adolescents.[17] Youth received a flexible dose sertraline (50–200 mg/day, mean dose 131 mg/day) or placebo. When results from the two studies were combined, response rates were 69% for sertraline and 56% for placebo. Bridge and colleagues[6] reported the NNT to benefit from sertraline was 10 (95% CI, 6–500). Although this study was not adequately powered to detect differences between children and adolescents, a significant change in depressive symptoms between adolescents treated with sertraline and placebo was found. No significant difference in depressive symptoms between children treated with sertraline and placebo was observed. Because only one RCT supports the use of citalopram or sertraline for the treatment of adolescent depression, the FDA has not given either medication an indication for adolescent depression.

Paroxetine

The efficacy of paroxetine has been evaluated in three RCTs,[18–20] all of which were negative on the primary outcome measures. In the first trial,[20] adolescents received a flexible dose of paroxetine (20–40 mg/day, mean dose 28 mg/day) or placebo. On the two primary outcome measures, there was no significant difference between paroxetine and placebo. In contrast, four secondary measures of efficacy demonstrated significant differences between paroxetine and placebo. In the second trial,[19] adolescents were randomized to receive either a flexible dose of paroxetine (20–40 mg/day, mean dose 26 mg/day) or placebo. On the two primary outcome measures, there was no significant difference between paroxetine and placebo. In the third trial,[19] children and adolescents were randomized to flexible-dose paroxetine (10–50 mg/day, mean dose 28 mg/day) or placebo. On the primary outcome measure and all secondary efficacy measures there were no significant differences between paroxetine and placebo. In the meta-analysis of Bridge and colleagues,[6] the NNT to benefit from paroxetine was not calculated because no benefit was shown in these studies.

Factors That Influence the Outcome of RCTs for Depression in Youth

When interpreting the results of RCTs for depression in youth, caution must be exercised as several factors may influence the outcomes of these studies:

1. Industry-sponsored trials are usually conducted at more sites than studies funded by the National Institute of Mental Health. In the meta-analysis of Bridge and colleagues,[6] the number of sites was inversely associated with efficacy, suggesting a decrease in antidepressant effectiveness as the number of study sites is increased.
2. The high placebo response rate in studies of youth with MDD decreases the power of RCTs to detect differences between medication and placebo. Bridge and colleagues[11] reported that the placebo response was higher for youth with MDD (50%) than with obsessive–compulsive disorder (OCD, 32%) or other anxiety disorders (39%).
3. Characteristics of study participants (eg, age or duration of illness) can also affect the outcome of antidepressant response in RCTs. For example, younger age and longer duration of illness have been associated with poorer treatment outcomes.[6] Thus, some RCTs of SSRIs in youth with depression may have failed to show superiority of medication compared to placebo because of study design issues or participant characteristics.

Summary of Efficacy Findings of SSRIs for Depressed Youth

In summary, findings from RCTs demonstrate the acute efficacy of SSRIs for depression in youth. Evidence from more than one RCT supports the use of fluoxetine in the treatment of childhood and adolescent depression as well as escitalopram in the treatment of adolescent depression. Based on these RCTs, fluoxetine has been given an FDA indication for the treatment of MDD in youth aged 8 years and older whereas escitalopram has been given an FDA indication for the treatment of MDD in adolescents aged 12 years and older. To date, only one RCT has demonstrated the effectiveness of sertraline or citalopram for the treatment of MDD in youth. Thus, neither of these medications has received FDA approval for the treatment of MDD in youth. Only a small number of RCTs for depression have included children and none of these trials were adequately powered to detect differences in medication efficacy between children and adolescents.

CONTINUATION AND MAINTENANCE TREATMENT WITH SSRIs

Although many RCTs have assessed the efficacy of SSRIs in the acute treatment (the initial 8–12 weeks of treatment during which the main goal is symptom reduction) of MDD in youth, only a few controlled studies have examined continuation phase treatment (the 6- to 12-month treatment phase after the acute period) and no controlled studies have examined maintenance treatments (the period beyond12 months for youth with recurrent depression during which the goal is to prevent future depressive episodes). During continuation treatment, SSRIs are continued at the same dose that resulted in clinical response during acute treatment; the SSRI dose may be increased in the absence of side effects to target residual depressive symptoms. Continuation treatment with fluoxetine was shown to be more efficacious than placebo in preventing relapse of depression in youth.[21] Relapse occurred more frequently in the placebo group than in the fluoxetine group (69.2% vs. 42.0%, $P = .009$). Further, the risk of relapse is significantly higher in youth with continued depressive symptoms at the end of acute treatment compared to youth who had no residual symptoms (46.3% vs. 22.9%, $P = .014$).[21] The addition of CBT to fluoxetine treatment during continuation treatment results in a higher rate of sustained remission and lower rate of relapse than medication alone.[22]

PHARMACOKINETICS OF SSRIs IN YOUTH

Pharmacokinetic studies in children and adolescents can provide valuable information on how to best prescribe SSRIs for pediatric populations. Understanding the pharmacokinetics of SSRIs is of clinical importance because withdrawal effects (eg, irritability or sleep disturbance) caused by SSRIs with a short half-life not only can interfere with a child's functioning, but also may be confused with medication side effects or worsening symptoms of depression. For example, if a child develops sleep disturbance or irritability after starting to use an SSRI with a short half-life, the clinician may conclude the medication is causing side effects without taking into the account that these symptoms may be due to withdrawal effects. Differences in the pharmacokinetics of SSRIs in youth are also important because dosing strategies in several RCTs not only may have contributed to the failure of these studies to demonstrate a difference in efficacy between medication and placebo, but also may have influenced our understanding of the safety and tolerability of these medications.[23]

Pharmacokinetic Studies of Fluoxetine

Single-dose pharmacokinetic studies of fluoxetine have not been performed in children and adolescents; however, studies with adults have shown the elimination half-life of fluoxetine (1–4 days) and its primary metabolite, norfluoxetine (7–15 days), to be much longer than that of other SSRIs. Other pharmacokinetic properties of fluoxetine have been described in a population pharmacokinetic study of children and adolescents.[24] High intersubject variability was observed. Mean steady-state levels of fluoxetine (127 ng/mL) and norfluoxetine (151 ng/mL) were obtained after 4 weeks of treatment. Fluoxetine and norfluoxetine concentrations were two times higher in children than in adolescents. When drug concentrations were normalized to body weight, concentrations of fluoxetine and norfluoxetine were similar for children and adolescents. These data suggest that body weight (and not developmental stage) influence fluoxetine and norfluoxetine concentrations. Based on their findings, Wilens and colleagues advise that children begin fluoxetine at 10 mg/day, whereas adolescents may start at 20 mg/day.[24]

Pharmacokinetic Studies of Escitalopram, Citalopram, Sertraline

Studies with escitalopram, citalopram, and sertraline in youth show that these medications have shorter half-lives at low doses than higher doses. (S)-citalopram, marketed in the United States as escitalopram, is the therapeutically active isomer of racemic citalopram.[25] A pharmacokinetic study of a single dose of escitalopram (10 mg/day) found that the half-life of escitalopram was shorter in adolescents (19.0 hours) than in adults (28.9 hours). Another pharmacokinetic study of adolescents tested the half-life of (R)-citalopram and (S)-citalopram after a single 20-mg dose and after 2 weeks of 20 mg/day.[26] Similar to the escitalopram study, the single-dose and steady state half-life of (S)-citalopram was found to be significantly shorter than previously reported in adults. In contrast, a pharmacokinetic study of steady-state 40 mg/day citalopram found pharmacokinetic parameters were similar in adolescents (eg, half-life of 38 hours) and adults (eg, half-life of 44 hours). This same pattern of medications having shorter half-lives at low doses is also observed in pharmacokinetics studies of adolescents prescribed sertraline. The mean steady-state half-life of sertraline in adolescents is 15.3 hours at 50 mg/day, 20.4 hours at 100 to 150 mg/day, and 27.1 hours at 200 mg/day.[27,28] However, the mean steady-state half-life of sertraline at 200 mg/day was similar to that previously observed in adults. Based on their findings, the authors[28] recommended an optimal dosing plan of twice per day at doses of 50 mg/day and once daily at 200 mg/day. In summary, when prescribing escitalopram, citalopram, or sertraline in the low-dose range, twice daily dosing should be considered if withdrawal effects are reported by the child or adolescent.

Clinical Implications of Pharmacokinetic Studies

In summary, pharmacokinetics studies in youth suggest that dosing strategies of SSRIs may be different for children, adolescents, and adults. Fluoxetine may need to be started at reduced doses in low-weight children and adolescents. Clinicians should initiate treatment with escitalopram, citalopram, or sertraline at once daily dosing and monitor closely for withdrawal effects. If withdrawal effects are reported, then switching to twice daily should be considered.

INITIATION AND TITRATION OF SSRIs

It is generally recommended to start with a low dose of SSRI and increase weekly until a minimum effective dosage (eg, citalopram 20 mg, escitalopram 10 mg, fluoxetine 20 mg, sertraline 50–100 mg) is achieved. If intolerable side effects occur or moderate side effects persist for more than 1 week, the medication dose should be lowered to the highest tolerable dose. Children and adolescents should receive an adequate and tolerable dose of SSRI for a minimum of 4–6 weeks. If the child or adolescent remains symptomatic after 4–6 weeks, a dose raise should be considered.[5,29,30] Response to treatment should be reevaluated every 4 to 6 weeks. Alternative treatment options should be considered when the child or adolescent shows only minimal or partial improvement after 10 to 12 weeks.

ADVERSE EFFECTS OF SSRIs

Common Adverse Effects of SSRIs

SSRIs are generally well tolerated in acute treatment studies. Most side effects are dose dependent and usually diminish with time.[12,31,32] The common adverse effects include:

- Sleep disturbance
- Nausea

- Abdominal pain
- Diarrhea
- Change in appetite
- Headache
- Dizziness
- Vivid dreams
- Dry mouth
- Restlessness
- Akathisia
- Sexual dysfunction.

Behavioral activation, silliness, or disinhibition can be seen in 3% to 8% of youth prescribed SSRIs, especially children. This side effect is characterized by "goofiness" and restlessness after starting or changing a medication dose, and is usually mild to moderate in severity.[33] Behavioral activation can occur with various types of medications (eg, benzodiazepines, antihistamines, or tricyclic antidepressants). Symptoms quickly resolve when the medication dose is reduced or the medication is discontinued. We recommend discussing this potential side effect with parents before prescribing medication, as this adverse effect is transient and can be easily managed. It is essential for clinicians to differentiate behavioral activation from hypomania or mania.

Treatment of children and adolescents with a predisposition for bipolar disorder may result in hypomania or mania. Depression with psychosis or a family history of bipolar disorder appears to lead to an increased risk for bipolar disorder in children and adolescents; caution should be exercised when treating depressed youth with these characteristics because 20% to 40% of these youth will develop bipolar disorder.[34,35] However, beyond this, it is not clear how to distinguish depressed youth who will develop bipolar disorder from those who will not. All children and adolescents treated with an antidepressant should be monitored for symptoms of hypomania or mania. The unmasking of a primary psychiatric disorder (eg, bipolar disorder with a hypomanic/manic episode) can be differentiated from behavioral activation by the onset of symptoms, the offset of symptoms, and the intensity and quality of the symptoms. In comparison to behavioral activation, a hypomanic or manic episode has a prolonged onset and offset and moderate to severe symptomatology that includes grandiosity, decreased need for sleep, talkativeness, flight of ideas, distractibility, and excessive seeking of pleasurable activities that have a high potential for adverse consequences. We highly recommend reading the brief article by Wilens and colleagues[33] that includes thoughtful guidance on how to distinguish behavioral activation from the unmasking of a primary psychiatric disorder (eg, bipolar disorder.)

Uncommon Adverse Effects of SSRIs

Less frequent, but more severe adverse effects of SSRIs include:

- **Increased risk of bleeding** (eg, gastrointestinal bleeding and perioperative bleeding)[36,37]
- **Serotonin toxicity** Clinical features of serotonin toxicity include neuromuscular hyperactivity (eg, tremor, hyperreflexia, and clonus), autonomic hyperactivity (eg, diaphoresis, fever, tachycardia, and mydriasis), and mental status changes (eg, agitation, excitement, or confusion)[38]
- **Abnormal heart rhythms**. In August 2011, the FDA issued a Drug Safety Communication regarding abnormal heart rhythms associated with high doses of citalopram. Based on post-marketing reports of QT-interval prolongation

and torsade de pointes, the FDA concluded that citalopram causes dose-dependent QT-interval prolongation and should no longer be prescribed at doses greater than 40 mg/day. Children and adolescents with congenital long QT syndrome should not be treated with citalopram. Youth with congestive heart failure, bradyarrhythmias, or predisposition to hypokalemia or hypomagnesemia because of illness or medication are at higher risk of developing torsade de pointes and should be monitored closely if they are prescribed citalopram

- **Suicidal ideation and behavior.** In recent years, the concern about increases spontaneous reports of suicidal ideation and behavior has become the most highly publicized side effect of SSRIs in children, adolescents, and young adults. Because of these concerns, two meta-analyses have evaluated the risk of suicidal ideation and behavior in youth taking antidepressants.[6,39]

Meta-Analyses of Risk of Suicidal Ideation and Behavior in RCTs of Youth Taking Antidepressants

A collaborative project between researchers at Columbia University and the FDA assessed the impact of 9 antidepressants in 24 RCTs of depression, anxiety disorders, or attention-deficit/hyperactivity disorder in children and adolescents.[39] *Spontaneous* reports of suicidal ideation and suicidal behavior were the primary outcome measures for this meta-analysis. The collaborative team found the overall risk ratio (RR) for suicidality in all the trials was 1.95 (95% CI, 1.28–2.98). The overall RR was 1.66 (95% CI, 1.02–2.68) when analyses were limited to depression studies. These data propose that 1 to 3 out of every 100 children will experience a suicidal adverse event (defined as suicidal ideation or behavior) when treated with an antidepressant. This meta-analysis[39] also evaluated the emergence of suicidality or worsening of suicidal ideation through the use of suicide item scores on depression rating scales from 17 RCTs. These analyses did not show a significant RR for emergence of suicidality (0.93; 95% CI, 0.75–1.15) or worsening of suicidality (0.92; 95% CI, 0.76–1.1).

Another meta-analysis tested the effect of antidepressants on suicidality in 27 published and unpublished RCTs of depression and anxiety disorders in youth.[6] This meta-analysis found comparable results to the prior study. A small but significant increase in overall RR for suicidality was found for all disorders (1.9; 95% CI, 1.3–3.0) and depression (1.9; 95% CI 1.2–2.9). Because RR analysis requires that trials have at least one event and several trials had no events, Bridge and colleagues[6] also evaluated the risk difference (RD), which allows the inclusion of studies with no events. When using random-effects analysis of RD, Bridge and colleagues found a small but significant overall RD for medication compared with placebo (0.7%; 95% CI, 0.1–1.3). No significant difference was found when analyses were restricted to studies with only depression (0.9%; 95% CI, −0.1 to 1.9%), OCD (0.5%; 95% CI, −0.4 to 1.8%), or other anxiety disorders (0.7%; 95% CI, −0.4 to 1.8%).

Epidemiologic Studies of Suicide Risk for Youth Taking SSRIs

The implication of these findings for clinical practice are not entirely clear because there had been a reduction in the rate of youth suicide in the United States during this earlier time of increased prescription of SSRIs.[40] Epidemiologic studies before the FDA black box warning on SSRIs showed a positive relationship between the reduced in adolescent suicide rates and the use of SSRIs.[40–42] Since US and European regulators placed warnings on SSRIs, there has been a decrease in the number of SSRI prescriptions to children and adolescents and an increase in completed suicides in the United States and the Netherlands.[43] Therefore, epidemiologic studies demonstrate not only a correlation between increased SSRIs use and lower suicide rates, but also an association between reduced SSRI use and increased youth suicide rates.

Suicidal Risk and Treatment of Youth with SSRIs

In summary, children and adolescents treated with SSRIs more frequently report suicidal ideation or behavior than those treated with placebo. Infrequently, youth may experience a new onset or worsening in suicidal ideation or behavior after starting an SSRI. Because of these concerns, it is important to assess for the presence of suicidal risk before and after initiating treatment with an SSRI. See section on Monitoring for Adverse Effects of SSRIs.

Long-Term Impact of SSRI Use in Children and Adolescents

The long-term impact of SSRIs use in children and adolescents is not known. The effect of medication on brain development and function is often a great concern of the patients for whom medication treatment is being considered and their families. Clinicians should remind patients and families that untreated depression may result in significant morbidity and mortality. Thus, an individual risk/benefit analysis is indicated when considering medication use. Long-term study of SSRI use in children and adolescents is clearly needed to evaluate the influence of medication on human development.

Monitoring for Adverse Effects of SSRIs

After initiating treatment with an SSRI, the prescribing clinician usually schedules weekly or twice monthly appointments to monitor for adverse effects, to make dose adjustments, and to provide support. We recommend that clinicians inquire about adverse effects including new onset or worsening of suicidal ideation and medication adherence during these appointments. After the initial 2 months of treatment, the frequency of visits is often reduced. We recommend continuing to monitor for adverse effects throughout the course of treatment.

WITHDRAWAL FROM SSRIs

When the SSRIs are abruptly stopped, taken inconsistently, or rapidly metabolized, a withdrawal syndrome may occur. Somatic symptoms consist of [44]:

- Gastrointestinal upset (such as, nausea or emesis)
- Disequilibrium (such as, dizziness, ataxia, or vertigo)
- Sleep disruption (such as, insomnia or vivid dreams)
- Flulike symptoms (such as, myalgia, fatigue, or chills)
- Sensory disturbances (such as, paresthesia).

Given the resemblance of SSRI side effects and withdrawal symptoms, it is important to ask about medication adherence when difficulties with medication are reported. Withdrawal symptoms have been shown to differ among the SSRIs in studies with adults.[45,46] Baldwin and colleagues[45] found significantly fewer withdrawal symptoms with escitalopram compared to paroxetine. Tint and colleagues[46] observed fewer symptoms with fluoxetine compared to antidepressants with short half-lives (ie, citalopram, fluvoxamine, paroxetine, and venlafaxine) and reported a comparable frequency of withdrawal symptoms regardless of the duration of medication taper (3 days vs. 14 days). Thus, tapering an SSRI is generally preferable to abrupt discontinuation, and some patients may require gradual lowering over 4 to 6 weeks to reduce withdrawal.

SSRI-RESISTANT DEPRESSION

When children and adolescents fail to respond to an SSRI, identifying and managing the cause of nonresponse (eg, severe stressors, inaccurate diagnosis, medical illness, lack of treatment for comorbid psychiatric disorders, poor adherence, or inadequate medication dose or duration) is critical. Only one RCT of SSRI-resistant depression, Treatment of Resistant Depression in Adolescents (TORDIA), has been conducted. This study found that switching to either another SSRI or venlafaxine produced a response rate of approximately 48%.[47] Switching to another SSRI is preferable before a trial of venlafaxine because venlafaxine resulted in greater rates of adverse effects. The addition of CBT to either medication produced a greater improvement than medication alone.[47] Therefore, we recommend adding CBT or another evidence-based psychotherapy for patients with SSRI-resistant depression if psychotherapy is not already being utilized.

SUMMARY

RCTs have demonstrated the acute efficacy of SSRIs for depression in youth. Evidence from more than one RCT supports the use of fluoxetine in the treatment of childhood and adolescent depression as well as escitalopram in the treatment of adolescent depression. Based on these RCTs, fluoxetine has been given an FDA indication for the treatment of MDD in youth aged 8 years and older whereas escitalopram has been given an FDA indication for the treatment of MDD in adolescents 12 years and older. To date, only one RCT has demonstrated the effectiveness of sertraline or citalopram for the treatment of MDD in youth. Pharmacokinetics studies in youth suggest that dosing strategies of SSRIs may be different for children compared to adolescents, especially for children with low weight. Fluoxetine administration may need to be started at lower doses in children. If withdrawal symptoms are reported with escitalopram, citalopram, or sertraline at once daily dosing, then switching to twice daily should be considered. SSRIs are generally well tolerated by children and adolescents, but careful monitoring for adverse events during the first 2 months of treatment is recommended.

REFERENCES

1. Lewinsohn PM, Rohde P, Seeley JR. Major depressive disorder in older adolescents: prevalence, risk factors, and clinical implications. Clin Psychol Rev 1998; 18(7):765–94.
2. Birmaher B, Arbelaez C, Brent D. Course and outcome of child and adolescent major depressive disorder. Child Adolesc Psychiatr Clin North Am 2002;11(3):619–37.
3. Birmaher B, Ryan ND, Williamson DE, et al. Childhood and adolescent depression: a review of the past 10 years. Part I. J Am Acad Child Adolesc Psychiatry 1996;35(11): 1427–39.
4. Lewinsohn PM, Rohde P, Seeley JR, et al. Psychosocial functioning of young adults who have experienced and recovered from major depressive disorder during adolescence. J Abnorm Psychol 2003;112(3):353–63.
5. Birmaher B, Brent DA, Work Group on Quality I. Practice parameter for the assessment and treatment of children and adolescents with depressive disorders. J Am Acad Child Adolesc Psychiatry 2007;46(11):1503–26.
6. Bridge JA, Iyengar S, Salary CB, et al. Clinical response and risk for reported suicidal ideation and suicide attempts in pediatric antidepressant treatment: a meta-analysis of randomized controlled trials. JAMA 2007;297(15):1683–96.

7. Emslie GJ, Rush AJ, Weinberg WA, et al. A double-blind, randomized, placebo-controlled trial of fluoxetine in children and adolescents with depression. Arch Gen Psychiatry 1997;54(11):1031–7.

8. Emslie GJ, Rush AJ, Weinberg WA, et al. A double-blind, randomized, placebo-controlled trial of fluoxetine in children and adolescents with depression. Arch Gen Psychiatry 2002;54(11):1031–7.

9. March J, Silva S, Vitiello B, et al. The Treatment for Adolescents with Depression Study (TADS): methods and message at 12 weeks. J Am Acad Child Adolesc Psychiatry 2004;45(12):1393–403.

10. Mayes TL, Tao R, Rintelmann JW, et al. Do children and adolescents have differential response rates in placebo-controlled trials of fluoxetine? CNS Spectrums 2007;12(2): 147–54.

11. Bridge JA, Birmaher B, Iyengar S, et al. Placebo response in randomized controlled trials of antidepressants for pediatric major depressive disorder. Am J Psychiatry 2009;166(1):42–9.

12. Cheung AH, Emslie GJ, Mayes TL. The use of antidepressants to treat depression in children and adolescents. CMAJ Can Med Assoc J 2006;174(2):193–200.

13. Wagner KD, Jonas J, Findling RL, et al. A double-blind, randomized, placebo-controlled trial of escitalopram in the treatment of pediatric depression. J Am Acad Child Adolesc Psychiatry 2006;45(3):280–8.

14. Emslie GJ, Ventura D, Korotzer A, et al. Escitalopram in the treatment of adolescent depression: a randomized placebo-controlled multisite trial. J Am Acad Child Adolesc Psychiatry 2009 Jul;48(7):721–9.

15. Wagner KD, Robb AS, Findling RL, et al. A randomized, placebo-controlled trial of citalopram for the treatment of major depression in children and adolescents. Am J Psychiatry 2004;161(6):1079–83.

16. von Knorring AL, Olsson GI, Thomsen PH, et al. A randomized, double-blind, placebo-controlled study of citalopram in adolescents with major depressive disorder. J Clin Psychopharmacol 2006;26(3):311–5.

17. Wagner KD, Ambrosini P, Rynn M, et al. Efficacy of sertraline in the treatment of children and adolescents with major depressive disorder: two randomized controlled trials. JAMA 2003;290(8):1033–41.

18. Berard R, Fong R, Carpenter DJ, et al. An international, multicenter, placebo-controlled trial of paroxetine in adolescents with major depressive disorder. J Child Adolesc Psychopharmacol 2006;16(1–2):59–75.

19. Emslie GJ, Wagner KD, Kutcher S, et al. Paroxetine treatment in children and adolescents with major depressive disorder: a randomized, multicenter, double-blind, placebo-controlled trial. J Am Acad Child Adolesc Psychiatry 2006;45(6):709–19.

20. Keller MB, Ryan ND, Strober M, et al. Efficacy of paroxetine in the treatment of adolescent major depression: a randomized, controlled trial. J Am Acad Child Adolesc Psychiatry 2001;40(7):762–72.

21. Emslie GJ, Kennard BD, Mayes TL, et al. Fluoxetine versus placebo in preventing relapse of major depression in children and adolescents. Am J Psychiatry 2008; 165(4):459–67.

22. Kennard BD, Emslie GJ, Mayes TL, et al. Cognitive-behavioral therapy to prevent relapse in pediatric responders to pharmacotherapy for major depressive disorder. J Am Acad Child Adolesc Psychiatry 2008;47(12):1395–404.

23. Findling RL, McNamara NK, Stansbrey RJ, et al. The relevance of pharmacokinetic studies in designing efficacy trials in juvenile major depression. J Child Adolesc Psychopharmacol 2006;16(1–2):131–45.

24. Wilens TE, Cohen L, Biederman, et al. Fluoxetine pharmacokinetics in pediatric patients. J Clin Psychopharmacol 2002;22(6):568–75.
25. Hyttel J, Bogeso KP, Perregaard J, et al. The pharmacological effect of citalopram residues in the (S)-(+)-enantiomer. J Neural Transm 1992;88(2):157–60.
26. Perel JM, Axelson DA, Rudolph G, et al. Steroselective pharmacokinetic/pharmaco-dynamic (PK/PD) of ± citalopram in adolescents, comparisons with adult findings [Abstract]. Clin Pharmacol Ther 2001;69:30.
27. Alderman J, Wolkow R, Chung M, et al. Sertraline treatment of children and adolescents with obsessive-compulsive disorder or depression: pharmacokinetics, tolerability, and efficacy. J Am Acad Child Adolesc Psychiatry 1998;37(4):386–94.
28. Axelson DA, Perel JM, Birmaher B, et al. Sertraline pharmacokinetics and dynamics in adolescents. J Am Acad Child Adolesc Psychiatry 2002;41(9):1037–44.
29. Heiligenstein JH, Hoog SL, Wagner KD, et al. Fluoxetine 40–60 mg versus fluoxetine 20 mg in the treatment of children and adolescents with a less-than-complete response to nine-week treatment with fluoxetine 10–20 mg: a pilot study. J Child Adolesc Psychopharmacol 2006;16(1–2):207–17.
30. Sakolsky DJ, Perel JM, Emslie GJ, et al. Antidepressant exposure as a predictor of clinical outcomes in the Treatment of Resistant Depression In Adolescents (TORDIA) Study. J Clin Psychopharmacol 2011;31(1):92–7.
31. Emslie G, Kratochvil C, Vitiello B, et al. Treatment for Adolescents with Depression Study (TADS): safety results. J Am Acad Child Adolesc Psychiatry 2006;45(12): 1440–55.
32. Safer DJ, Zito JM. Treatment-emergent adverse events from selective serotonin reuptake inhibitors by age group: children versus adolescents. J Child Adolesc Psychopharmacol 2006;16(1–2):159–69.
33. Wilens TE, Wyatt D, Spencer TJ. Disentangling disinhibition. J Am Acad Child Adolesc Psychiatry 1998;37(11):1225–7.
34. Geller B, Fox LW, Clark KA. Rate and predictors of prepubertal bipolarity during follow-up of 6- to 12-year-old depressed children. J Am Acad Child Adolesc Psychiatry 1994;33(4):461–8.
35. Strober M, Lampert C, Schmidt S, et al. The course of major depressive disorder in adolescents: I. Recovery and risk of manic switching in a follow-up of psychotic and nonpsychotic subtypes. J Am Acad Child Adolesc Psychiatry 1993;32(1):34–42.
36. Lake MB, Birmaher B, Wassick S, et al. Bleeding and selective serotonin reuptake inhibitors in childhood and adolescence. J Child Adolesc Psychopharmacol 2000; 10(1):35–8.
37. Weinrieb RM, Auriacombe M, Lynch KG, et al. Selective serotonin re-uptake inhibitors and the risk of bleeding. Expert Opin Drug Safety 2005;4(2):337–44.
38. Gillman PK. A review of serotonin toxicity data: implications for the mechanisms of antidepressant drug action. Biol Psychiatry 2006;59(11):1046–51.
39. Hammad TA, Laughren T, Racoosin J. Suicidality in pediatric patients treated with antidepressant drugs. Arch Gen Psychiatry 2006;63(3):332–9.
40. Olfson M, Shaffer D, Marcus SC, et al. Relationship between antidepressant medication treatment and suicide in adolescents. Arch Gen Psychiatry 2003;60(10):978–82.
41. Gibbons RD, Hur K, Bhaumik DK, et al. The relationship between antidepressant prescription rates and rate of early adolescent suicide. Am J Psychiatry 2006;163(11): 1898–904.
42. Valuck RJ, Libby AM, Sills MR, et al. Antidepressant treatment and risk of suicide attempt by adolescents with major depressive disorder: a propensity-adjusted retrospective cohort study. CNS Drugs 2004;18(15):1119–32.

43. Gibbons RD, Brown CH, Hur K, et al. Early evidence on the effects of regulators' suicidality warnings on SSRI prescriptions and suicide in children and adolescents. Am J Psychiatry 2007;164(9):1356–63.

44. Schatzberg AF, Haddad P, Kaplan EM, et al. Serotonin reuptake inhibitor discontinuation syndrome: a hypothetical definition. Discontinuation Consensus panel. J Clin Psychiatry 1997;7:5–10.

45. Baldwin DS, Montgomery SA, Nil R, et al. Discontinuation symptoms in depression and anxiety disorders. Int J Neuropsychopharmacol 2007;10(1):73–84.

46. Tint A, Haddad PM, Anderson IM. The effect of rate of antidepressant tapering on the incidence of discontinuation symptoms: a randomised study. J Psychopharmacol 2008;22(3):330–2.

47. Brent D, Emslie G, Clarke G, et al. Switching to another SSRI or to venlafaxine with or without cognitive behavioral therapy for adolescents with SSRI-resistant depression: the TORDIA randomized controlled trial. JAMA 2008;299(8):901–13.

Contextual Emotion Regulation Therapy: A Developmentally Based Intervention for Pediatric Depression

Maria Kovacs, PhD[a,]*, Nestor L. Lopez-Duran, PhD[b]

KEYWORDS

• Pediatric depression • Child psychotherapy
• Emotion regulation

For this special issue about child and adolescent depression, the authors were asked to describe contextual emotion regulation therapy[1] as an example of a developmentally informed psychosocial intervention. To this end, the article begins with the authors' definition of the elements that should comprise such an intervention. A succinct summary of this contextual emotion regulation therapy is then provided, including its explanatory paradigm of depression, followed by an exposition of how it addresses the various definitional criteria of a developmentally informed intervention. The article concludes with a brief overview of the challenges of implementing a developmentally sensitive psychotherapy for depressed children and adolescents.

WHAT IS A DEVELOPMENTALLY INFORMED PSYCHOSOCIAL INTERVENTION?

As long ago as the 1980s, clarion calls already were sounded for a merger between clinicians and developmentalists to improve interventions for pediatric mental disorders.[2] More recently, Ollendick and colleagues[3] have specifically noted that developmental theory should inform decisions regarding when to intervene for children, what to target, and how treatment goals should be implemented, and suggested that a useful template is the developmentally based utilization guidelines for behavioral techniques. Barrett[4] raised similar developmentally based concerns in connection

This work was supported by grant MH081811 from the National Institute of Mental Health. The authors have nothing to disclose.

[a] Department of Psychiatry, University of Pittsburgh School of Medicine, 3811 O'Hara Street, Pittsburgh, PA 15213, USA
[b] Department of Psychology, University of Michigan, 530 Church Street, Ann Arbor, MI 48109, USA
* Corresponding author.
E-mail address: kovacs@pitt.edu

with interventions for pediatric anxiety disorders and was especially concerned that standardized interventions tend to view children as "little adults." In a subsequent publication, Kingery and colleagues[5] underscored that anxious youngsters indeed are not "little adults" and provided a detailed exposition of age-appropriate ways to engage such youths in treatment as well as ways to modify demanding therapeutic strategies (such as cognitive restructuring, exposure tasks). We have called attention to the need to render psychosocial interventions for *depressed* young patients developmentally more appropriate.[6] We have done so because the most commonly studied psychotherapies for pediatric depression (ie, cognitive behavior therapy and interpersonal psychotherapy) represent "downward" modifications of interventions that were originally designed for adults and are not particularly developmentally sensitive.

Ollendick and colleagues,[7] along with the other scholars just noted, have identified key issues that should be considered in the delivery of interventions for pediatric mental disorders. In particular, they have emphasized the lack of autonomy of child patients and the need to tailor the level of the intervention to the developmental capacities of the child. However, in designing our treatment for childhood depression, we have taken a different approach: we used the literature on normal development as one of the foundations of contextual emotion regulation therapy (CERT). Correspondingly, our view of a developmentally informed intervention differs somewhat from what has been articulated in the field.

What constitutes a developmentally informed psychosocial intervention for pediatric depression? We believe that such an intervention has to have at least *four key features*. First, the treatment's conceptual formulation (or explanatory framework) should include an explicit developmental component. In other words, the explanatory paradigm should specify *which developmental parameters or skills* are implicated in the unfolding of depression and how dysfunction in that regard paves the way to depression. Second, a developmentally informed intervention should accommodate the fact that young patients will be at *different stages of development of the targeted skills* when they enter treatment (see Ref.[8]), which will have ramifications for what the therapist can do. Further, even at a specific developmental stage or age (eg, all 7-year-olds), young patients will not be at the same skill levels and also will differ in background and contextual variables that may affect treatment. Thus, a developmentally informed intervention should be sufficiently *flexible* to accommodate multiple sources of variability across young patients and explicate how its implementation for chronologically or developmentally younger patients differs from that for older youths.

Third, a developmentally informed intervention should *account for the importance of parents (or other key caregivers) in children's lives*. From a legal and a social perspective, children and adolescents have limited rights and are entirely dependent on their parents (at least in the United States), who control access to resources. From a psychological perspective, parents play critical roles in their children's emotional and social development and provide the crucible within which developmental skills unfold. Therefore, we believe that the explanatory paradigm of a developmentally sensitive intervention should address how parents impact the skill that is being targeted *or* else account for the role of the parents in those areas of the young patient's functioning that are relevant to treatment targets.

Finally, we strongly believe that a developmentally informed intervention must address explicitly *the training and behavior of the therapists* and require that they be knowledgeable about principles of development in general and those developmental processes in particular that are most relevant to the intervention. As discussed in the text that follows, CERT meets each criterion that was just listed, albeit to varying extents.

CERT: A BRIEF DESCRIPTION

CERT is based on the proposition that sad, despondent, dysphoric mood is *the* most salient feature of clinical depression, which must be alleviated for recovery to occur.[1] It is assumed that clinical depression starts as a response to some initiating stress event or process, which elicits sadness, distress, and dysphoria. From thereon, whether or not the dysphoric emotion develops into a disorder depends in large measure on the way in which the affected youngster responds to the emotion. As Teasdale[9] has noted, individuals who are prone to clinical depression respond in ways that impede "natural recovery."

How people respond to their own emotions has come to be called *emotion regulation.*[10] Individuals are unlikely to become clinically depressed if they are able to manage (regulate) their sadness or dysphoria in a context-appropriate fashion, such that it does not get out of hand and does not interfere with functioning. However, when the skills to attenuate or modulate those emotions are lacking, are subpar, or are not effective, the emotion will progress to persistent mood, which, in turn, will initiate a downward spiral of further depression symptoms. Because CERT focuses specifically on attenuating sadness and distress, it targets regulation that has been called mood repair[11,12] or negative mood repair.[13] Mood repair refers to the fact that when a person feels sad, dysphoric, or is in a "bad mood," there is a natural inclination to behave in ways that will result in feeling better (see Ref.[14]). Thus, *mood-repair* indexes a subset of the processes and responses that comprise emotion regulation because it concerns only sadness, dysphoria, or distress, with the goal to attenuate, reduce, or shorten that experience.

According to the explanatory framework of CERT, persistent failure to attenuate sad, dysphoric mood (ie, maladaptive mood repair) is *the* mechanism that is responsible for the child's eventual depressive disorder.[15,16] Mood repair failure contributes to clinical depression in at least two ways. First, it is the mechanism that accounts for how the initial dysphoric emotion experience segues into protracted dysphoric mood and then spirals into a depressive disorder. Second, maladaptive mood repair maintains the depressive episode by contributing to the persistent sadness, distress, and irritability that are central to clinical depression. Therefore, while acknowledging the full range of depressive symptoms, the CERT formulation of depression focuses the therapist's attention on the young patient's affective complaints and the regulatory responses that maintain them. The objectives of CERT are to help the child recover from depression and to prevent recurrence primarily by (1) reinforcing the use of responses that attenuate or modulate dysphoria (adaptive responses) and (2) reducing the child's use of responses that maintain or exacerbate dysphoria (maladaptive responses).

CERT is *developmentally based* because its target, namely mood repair, is a developmentally mediated construct. More specifically, mood repair skills, along with all emotion regulation skills, unfold as part of normal development starting as early as infancy.[17,18] Thus, the persistent mood repair failure that predates and also is evident in clinical depression is a function of some atypical feature of the given child's emotion regulatory development. That atypical aspect of mood repair, which has rendered the child particularly vulnerable to the effects of depressogenic triggers, needs to be identified and remediated. Consequently, CERT emphasizes the adaptive (and age-appropriate) self-regulation of dysphoria as the primary road to recovery from clinical depression. Adaptive regulation of dysphoria means that the child is not disabled or incapacitated by his or her mood and is in a better position to manage the broader context of his or her difficulties.

How is the explanatory, developmentally based framework of CERT translated into practice? In other words, what are the developmental skills implicated by CERT? And how does the developmental basis of CERT inform and affect the behavior of the therapist? Because a developmental perspective also implies an emphasis on individual differences, how is that construct handled in CERT? These questions are the targets of the next section and are explicated in detail in the CERT treatment manual.[15,16] Although the manual focuses on intervening with depressed 7- to 12-year-olds, CERT should be readily usable with somewhat older youngsters as well.

THE IMPACT OF DEVELOPMENTALLY MEDIATED SKILLS AND INDIVIDUAL DIFFERENCES ON THE IMPLEMENTATION OF CERT

Mood repair responding is the specific developmentally mediated skill that is targeted by CERT. However, as one considers the variety of ways in which people (including youngsters) respond to their own emotions in general, and dysphoria in particular, it is clear that mood repair is a meta-skill that is dependent on a broad array of basic skills (eg, goal-directed behavior, language, cognition, executive functions). Thus, the question is: How is CERT delivered in a way that takes into consideration (1) the *developmental unfolding of mood repair responses,* (2) *developmental trajectories* of the underlying basic skills, and (3) additional *individual differences* across young patients?

To deliver CERT appropriately requires that the therapist be fully familiar with the relevant empirical literature, including the literature on the normative development of emotion regulatory responses, the unfolding of basic skills and processes that support mood repair, and findings on the phenomenology of pediatric depression. Familiarity with the developmental literature is particularly important for the therapist to be able to tailor the focus and content of each session to the developmental phase and needs of the given young patient. More specifically, knowledge of the developmental literature frames the therapist's expectations of the type and quality of mood repair responses for a given child of a particular age; helps the therapist to identify atypical mood repair response features or developmental delay in a given child; and ensures that the therapist remains mindful of the fact that mood repair competence depends in large measure on a wide array of basic skills.

The Developmental Unfolding of Mood Repair Responses (and Related Skills) and CERT

It is known that competent emotion self-regulation and mood repair emerge as part of normal development starting around 6–8 months of age (see Ref.[17–19]). It is also known that the social environment is the crucible in which these processes unfold, with parents (or other caregivers) having the greatest developmental impact (see Ref.[20]). Further, as children mature, their own mood repair attempts become more effective in part because they are increasingly able to tailor their responses to the context of the emotion.[21,22] The increasing effectiveness of mood repair with age partly mirrors developmental trends of the various skills that subserve and support it.

Mood repair responses across childhood
Studies have identified several specific developmental trends in the acquisition of mood repair responses across infancy, toddlerhood, and early to middle childhood. One important developmental trend is the shift from *extrinsic* to mostly *intrinsic* modes of regulation.[23,24] In other words, whereas regulatory responding of infants

and very young children is typically initiated and maintained by caregivers, older children become increasingly able to *self-initiate mood repair.*[25] This developmental shift occurs around *age 3 to 4* in Western societies. Consequently, while it may not be unusual for a 6- or 7-year-old to occasionally rely on externally initiated mood repair, frequent or *persistent* failure to self-initiate mood repair in a school-age child is a cause for concern and represents a CERT target.

Another developmental imperative is to acquire mostly adaptive or helpful mood repair responses along with a few maladaptive or unhelpful responses. Adaptive responses[26] are those that help children to "lower the level of distress."[27(p.314)] Responses that diminish, attenuate, or terminate dysphoria also are defined in CERT as *adaptive, but with a caveat*: the response's adaptive value has to be evident both in the short and the long run. Attempts that prolong or exacerbate distress or dysphoria are typically regarded as countereffective or *maladaptive* both in the literature (see Refs.[27,28]) and in CERT.[16] Although laboratory studies of young children have shown that adaptive ways of responding to distress typically outnumber maladaptive responses (see Refs.[26,29]), it is not known whether the ratio of adaptive to maladaptive responses changes as a function of development. However, preliminary findings from our own research suggests that, by about the age of 7 years, the adaptive to maladaptive mood repair response ratio in typical school children is about 2:1 or 3:1, and that depressed children have an excess of maladaptive responses, rather than an absence of adaptive ways of managing distress (Kovacs, unpublished data, March 2011). Consequently, although a depressed child's presenting problem will include many examples of maladaptive mood repair, the CERT therapist knows that the child also must have adaptive ways of managing distress. The therapist therefore focuses on identifying and reinforcing the young patient's adaptive mood repair responses while minimizing the use of maladaptive responses.

Development also is believed to signal a *growing repertoire* of regulatory responses (see Refs.[24,30]), but there are scant supporting data.[25] Thus, we do not know for sure how the size and scope of the mood repair repertoires of 6-year-olds, for example, differ from those of 12-year-olds. However, children must be acquiring new responses as they mature because, by adulthood, there are hundreds of self-regulatory responses to distress,[31–34] making it necessary to have some way of categorizing them. CERT categories were based on the *types of responses* that emerge in rapid succession during the first year and a half of life: somatic–sensory, cognitive, interpersonal, and behavioral responses.[35] These response categories mirror the functional domains through which changes in affect seem to be eventuated (or the areas of functioning put to use in the service of mood repair). Based on pilot experiences, a threefold grouping of responses was created[16]: the *cognitive response domain* (involving thinking, perception, and the strategic use of attention), the *behavioral response domain* (involving action oriented and instrumental behaviors and self-focused, body-oriented behaviors not involving others), and the *interpersonal response domain* (involving the use of interpersonal processes and other people to feel better).

Preliminary findings from our own research with 7- to 14-year-old school children suggest that by 7 or 8 years of age, children have acquired the bulk of their adaptive mood repair strategies: Although there is developmental expansion of the repertoire size after that age, its magnitude is quite modest (Kovacs, unpublished data, March 2011). Further, the behavioral response domain appears to show the most notable development across the age span from 7 to 14 years. Consequently, although it is reasonable to expect a 12-year-old to have a somewhat larger overall adaptive mood repair repertoire than a 7-year-old, for example (which may make it easier to work with the older child), the CERT therapist's default position is to start with the child's existing mood repair repertoire and to resolve how it can be utilized more effectively. Toward that aim, the therapist has to identify which domain is favored by (or best fits) the given child, and enumerate the adaptive (and maladaptive) responses that comprise it. If a young patient has the propensity to learn a new way of managing dysphoria while in treatment, the developmental findings suggest that it is most likely to be a regulatory strategy in the *behavioral response domain*.

Another developmental trajectory is the gradual *shift from "rudimentary" to more complex or sophisticated* ways of responding to dysphoria. For example, whereas a 3-year-old may dissolve in helpless tears when facing a distressing stimulus and attempt to visually reference the caregiver, a school-aged child is likely to use language to communicate distress and request the intervention of the parent. Whereas a 5-year-old's response to distress may entail exploring the environment for whatever distracting activity may be available, a 10-year-old's response is likely to be more strategic, such as occupying himself by fixing a broken train set. There also are some mood repair responses that simply manifest in more age-appropriate ways across development. For example, when toddlers are put into a distressing situation, one common response is to crawl away, which has been called "leaving the scene."[17,29] Versions of "leaving the scene" in older children include barging out of a distressing situation; in adults, it includes going for a drive or taking a walk.[34] Thus, if a dysphoric youngster of any age reacts to increasing upset by running out of the room, he or she is displaying a developmentally rudimentary emotion regulatory response.

Although any mood repair response is likely to have its specific developmental trajectory, that is, the ways in which its rudimentary form evolves into a more complex version, only a few responses have been studied in sufficient detail and at different ages. For example, refocusing attention is a cognitive process that underlies various mood repair responses and can also be a specific response on its own (see Refs.[17,36–38]). The developmentally earliest version of this response is "gaze aversion."[17] When infants are presented with distressing visual stimuli (such as a still and unexpressive face), they catch on that by looking away, they are no longer subjected to the unwanted stimulus (see Ref.[39]). Partly as a function of brain maturation,[40,41] gaze aversion segues into the ability to respond to visual distracters, which does relieve distress in infancy.[42] That, in turn is transformed into the selective use of attention for distress relief (see Refs.[28,43,44]). As another example, recruiting others for distress relief is an adaptive mood repair response in the interpersonal response domain, whose developmental trajectory also has been documented. Its earliest example, around the age of 6 months, is caregiver-directed distress vocalization.[17] With maturation, mood repair via the help of others progresses from the use of nonverbal responses (eg, caregiver directed crying and visual referencing) to simple verbal requests for help, and then to more complex use of language and interpersonal discourse.[30,43–45] Turning to others to feel better is a stable component of mood repair repertoires across the life span (see Refs.[32–34]), probably reflecting the many ways in which one person can intervene in the affective experience of another.

Recognition that the extent of sophistication of mood repair responses and chronological age are related to one another can help the CERT therapist to pinpoint if a child's regulatory problems reflect age-inappropriate responding. For example, a 9-year-old girl whose mood repair response includes sucking her fingers or chewing on her hair is displaying a developmentally infantile form of self-soothing. A 12-year-old who can be soothed very effectively through getting a long hug or embrace from a parent but not via verbal parental emotional reassurance is showing some developmental delay in that response domain. Likewise, a 7-year-old who responds to distress by becoming destructive is displaying a strategy characteristic of a much younger child. Given the overall context of the child's difficulties, CERT targets may include assisting the child to deploy a more age-appropriate version of an apparently favored mood repair response.

The automaticity of mood repair responses

A further developmental dimension of note concerns the process whereby a response is implemented. Implicit in the developmental literature is the fact that regardless of whether a given regulatory response first emerges as a reflex-like behavior, a consequence of operant or classical conditioning, or a result of role-modeling, most responses seem to be deployed *automatically and without planning or deliberation.* This is particularly evident during the first few years of life. However, researchers have argued that shifting from reactive to voluntary, internal, and "effortful" or deliberate control of emotions is an important developmental trend across childhood.[23,24] Although this is likely to be the case, we propose that even "effortful" as well as "mental" mood repair responses eventually become automatic as a function of practice and experience (also noted by Davidson and colleagues[46]), which can be conscious or non-conscious. Indeed, various scholars have commented on the automaticity of much of emotion regulation (see Refs.[46,47]), although this area has been generally ignored by researchers.[47]

We believe that the automaticity of mood repair is a very important issue in treatment. In fact, one of the basic tenets of CERT is that adaptive and maladaptive mood repair responses *both are typically automatic* and that deliberate mood repair responses tend to be deployed if the automatic "default" response failed to lift the person's mood. Therefore, one of the tasks of the CERT therapist is to help parent and child identify the child's mood repair responses and to make the "unknown" "known."

The context of the unfolding of mood repair responses

An explicit developmental trend in children's mood repair concerns the changing context of their lives. Scholars agree that the family in general (and caregivers in particular) have the greatest impact early on and probably up until adolescence.[20,24] However, it also is widely believed that with the transition into preschool or school, youngsters are exposed to new role models (eg, peers, teachers) whose regulatory behavior they may emulate, who may be called upon to reduce distress, or conversely, who may become new sources of distress. Unfortunately, this developmental aspect of emotion regulation and mood repair has received scant research attention. Nonetheless, the CERT therapist is cognizant of the changing context of a given child's life and takes into consideration how specific contexts can either enable or constrain successful mood repair.[15]

The skills that support mood repair responses

As previously noted, there is no question that mood repair is a type of *meta-skill,* dependent on a broad array of *basic* developmental and maturational processes. These developmental processes include the use of language for communication, the various attention skills, executive function skills (particularly response inhibition and resistance to distraction), cognitive–information processing skills, social skills, as well as emotion-specific skills (eg, emotion naming and emotion self-monitoring). Overall, such skills are at rudimentary levels during infancy, show very rapid development during early and middle childhood, and (with some exceptions) more gradual increments after late childhood.[48–50] Importantly, these various basic skills have their own age-related trajectories.

For example, auditory attention matures quite early, with impressive gains by age 7, whereas visual attention continues to develop into early adolescence.[50] Executive attention (which involves working memory and the ability to prevent attention capture by distracting stimuli) becomes evident around age 3 and continues to develop across the adolescent years.[38,48,51] In fact, working memory and attention shifting do not fully mature until mid to late adolescence or somewhat later.[52,53] These developmental trajectories reflect in great measure the process of brain maturation. Namely, brain regions that subserve motor and sensory functions mature the earliest, whereas the prefrontal cortex, which subserves executive function skills and abstract thinking, continues to mature up to young adulthood.[40,41,54–56]

All in all, successful mood repair depends on the ability to utilize sensory, motor, perceptual, cognitive, linguistic, and social skills *in the service of mood repair* and in a context-appropriate fashion. Thus, the CERT therapist is cognizant of the fact that a child's mood repair problems may reflect developmental delay in one or more basic skills. Similarly, the therapist's decision as to which adaptive mood repair response to reinforce for a given child is informed by recognizing the various skills that are needed to deploy the target response and that child's level of command of those skills.

Development and CERT: a summary

CERT for depression is guided by the understanding that this treatment targets adaptive mood repair, which is a developmentally mediated skill; that different mood repair response types have varying developmental trajectories; that most responses are acquired early in development and become automatic; and that mood repair competence partly reflects the developmental phases of component skills. Thus, for example, the CERT therapist recognizes that school-age children (the targets of CERT) should be able to deploy responses from each of the three mood repair response domains, but that developmental stage mediates the level and sophistication of available responses. This means that the therapist *does not have the same mood repair expectations* of a 12-year-old and a 7-year-old. For example, although refocusing of attention, an adaptive mood repair strategy, can be used effectively by middle-school-age children to reduce dysphoria,[57,58] cognitive responses that require abstract thinking (eg, reframing the significance of a depressogenic situation) are infrequent and of questionable effectiveness during that age period.[16] As another example, we can expect that a distressed 12-year-old can be soothed effectively through verbal emotional reassurance from a parent, whereas a 7-year-old is much more likely to obtain emotional relief through getting a long hug or embrace.

The CERT therapist also recognizes that the mood repair problems of some depressed children do not derive from a lack of adaptive responses, or an abundance of maladaptive responses, but reflect that a preferred response is deployed in a *developmentally inappropriate* manner. For example, if a 10-year-old girl, whose mood repair relies heavily on interpersonal regulators, responds to distress with a bout of crying, drops to the floor, and waits for the parent to initiate mood repair, her method of trying to recruit the parent as regulator is characteristic of a much younger child (and is not likely to be effective). Further, the CERT therapist recognizes that suboptimal mood repair responding may reflect developmental delay in one or more of the basic skills that support the self-regulation of distress, rather than being a problem more closely related to emotional development. For example, language skills play a critical role in mood repair because they support many cognitive and interpersonal regulatory responses. Therefore, it is not surprising that 6- to 13-year-old children with language impairment have been found to have more difficulties in containing or regulating negative emotion than have typically developing peers.[59]

Individual Differences and CERT

In addition to being developmentally based, an individually tailored approach to depressed youngsters is at the heart of CERT. This means that, although CERT sets the same *overall* goals for all depressed children (symptom elimination and mood repair competence), the ways in which those goals are defined and achieved will differ across patients even of the *same age and same developmental level*. It also means that CERT accommodates the fact that certain personal characteristics as well as contextual and cultural differences affect the availability and utilization of particular mood repair responses.

CERT easily accommodates individual differences in mood repair repertoires because it does *not* assume that one mood regulatory domain is better or more desirable than is another, but instead focuses on the functional domain which is "the best fit" for the particular child. Thus, CERT easily deals with the fact that for one child, tender hugs from the parent along with reassuring words may be a guaranteed path to feeling better; for another distressed child of the same age and developmental level, listening to hip-hop music to counter dysphoria may work magic; yet another child may need to be engaged in some absorbing task to attenuate distress. Further, for one child, the therapist may need to spend some effort on modifying key contextual features in the home (eg, parental affect-related behavior), while for another child, the challenge may be to assist the parent in securing mood repair relevant material resources (eg, access to a basketball court). The flexibility inherent in CERT is reflected by the basic tenets that youths of the same age and developmental stage vary in their inclinations to deploy responses from the behavioral, cognitive, and interpersonal response domains; that some mood repair responses that "work" for some youths may not work for other youths; and that there are individual differences in the skill sets that underlie effective mood repair.

The individually tailored approach of CERT also acknowledges that there are additional personal factors that can hinder or facilitate a given child's mood repair attempts.[16] Among these factors, the child's temperament or "inborn wiring" is particularly important because it can affect both the threshold at which the child responds to affect provocation and the ease with which the arousal can be modulated.[24] Another important personal variable is the child's attachment history because the attachment behavioral system is closely related to affect regulation (see Ref.[60]). Children's early attachment experiences are believed to set the tone for (or against) turning to others to regulate emotion in later years (see Refs.[19,60,61]). Thus, a child with a suboptimal early attachment history is unlikely to develop adaptive interpersonal mood repair responses. Although addressing these issues is likely to be beyond the scope of the initial treatment contract that targets the child's depression, awareness of them should inform the therapist's decision making about what are (or are not) feasible treatment goals for a given child.

Intervention Strategies and CERT

The central goal of CERT is to help young patients recover from their depression and remain symptom free. This is accomplished primarily (but not solely) by targeting affective symptoms and remediating the problematic mood repair responses that maintain them. To achieve its goals, CERT takes an eclectic stance in regard to therapeutic strategies. That is, the therapist can select from the wide array of goal-oriented and problem-focused intervention strategies that have been documented in the literature, in order to discourage or interrupt dysfunctional mood repair responses, to strengthen or introduce adaptive ways of responding to distress, and to reduce other depression symptoms.[16]

For example, initial homework assignments typically include mood monitoring for prescribed amounts of time. For this task, younger children are provided with a page that has a variety of facial emotion expressions (along with verbal labels) and are asked to indicate their affect at a specified point in time by circling the faces "which best fit" how they feel. Depending on their verbal and writing skills, older children are asked to write down the name of the emotion at specific points in time. Another typical homework assignment includes practicing a particular adaptive mood repair sequence: for example, if the child has an upsurge of distress, he or she may be asked to approach the parent, "use words" to verbalize the affect and then receive a parental hug for at least 30 seconds. Within the CERT session itself, the therapist also may employ role-playing, modeling, and didactics to implement a particular treatment goal.

Owing to developmental considerations, CERT favors simple intervention strategies over complex ones, behavioral techniques over cognitive techniques, and action over words. For example, moderate physical activity is a well documented adaptive mood repair response. If a child is visibly dysphoric or distressed in a session, the CERT therapist will orchestrate for all participants (child, parent, and therapist together) several minutes of physical activity, such as jumping jacks, right in the treatment room. This inevitably brings the child some degree of emotional relief, demonstrates, in vivo, the association between exercise and feeling better, and accomplishes the goal of making a potential mood repair response explicit and conscious.

CERT also uses cognitive or "mental" techniques to accomplish treatment goals. In the traditional cognitive therapies for depression, cognitive techniques (eg, correcting misperceptions, questioning the evidence) serve to correct negatively biased abstract information processing. Because this use of cognitive techniques usually requires abstract operational thinking, we believe that it is developmentally inappropriate for school-age children. Instead, the CERT therapist uses (or teaches) mental or cognitive techniques (eg, mental imagery, thought interruption) in order to deter the deployment of maladaptive cognitive responses to distress and to reinforce the use of adaptive responses. For example, some depressed youngsters ruminate when they experience an upsurge in distress and thereby exacerbate their negative mood. To counter depressive rumination, such children may be taught to visualize a large, red stop sign. Rumination also can be interrupted by having young patients count backwards from a predefined number. As these strategies succeed, they are then supplemented with further adaptive response that the given child may favor.

CERT AND THE IMPORTANCE OF PARENTS IN THEIR CHILDREN'S LIVES

It seems self-evident that a child-focused intervention should engage the parents and account for their importance in their offspring's lives. After all, most psychotherapists who work with children reportedly involve the parents on some level.[62,63] Parental involvement has long been considered indispensable in the treatment of conduct problems (for a meta-analysis, see Ref.[64]) Yet, most treatment studies of depressed children and adolescents have not involved parents or involved them in separate parent groups (see Ref.[65]).

In contrast to other currently popular interventions for pediatric depression, CERT requires the active involvement of the parent (or primary adult caregiver). Indeed, the focus of CERT on mood repair explicitly calls for parental involvement because they play key roles in the developmental unfolding of children's regulatory strategies.

Parents facilitate their children's acquisition of regulatory responses across time by selectively reinforcing some responses but not others, and by serving as role models that can be emulated (for an overview, see Ref.[20]). In addition, when parents (caregivers) themselves respond to a child's distress, they function as *interpersonal regulatory agents.* The fact that parents remain the most important interpersonal regulators of a child's distress, at least up to mid-adolescence, further underscores the need for their participation in CERT.

Another reason for active parental involvement concerns the importance of reestablishing reasonable parent–child interactions. As any parent will testify, the ability of a child to respond positively to nurturing and caregiving parental behavior is part of the glue of the parent–child relationship. However, depressed children often are unaffectionate and unresponsive.[65] In addition, if the parent is depressed, which is not an infrequent occurrence,[66] a recursive pattern of negative parent–child interactions may result. By the time the family of a depressed child seeks help, it is not unusual for the original psychosocial stressor to have lost its salience and be replaced by negative parent–child interactions as part of the presenting problem. The active involvement of the parent affords the therapist the opportunity to fulfill an important (although implicit) goal of CERT, the normalization of parent–child interactions, particularly around affect-related topics.

CERT relies on a sport analogy to provide a framework for *how* the parent is expected to be involved (and how the child is expected to contribute): *the therapist is the "coach," the parent is the "assistant coach," while the child is the special team "player."* The coach and assistant coach roles make it explicit that the two adults share the goal of helping the child *and* that the child is the focus of their interactions. One consequence of this formulation is that, as assistant coach, the parent is expected to make objective observations of the child's behavior and becomes an information source for the therapist. As assistant coach, the parent also is expected to work with the child around homework assignments and facilitate the deployment of adaptive mood repair responses.

By defining the roles (and responsibilities) of the assistant coach and player in the presence of the young patient, the sport analogy also serves as a vehicle for transparency: the child knows that the parent will have to report observations (and thus information is not being conveyed behind his/her back). The parent's role as an assistant coach also underscores that the young patient (not the parent) is the treatment focus. It is important to note, however, that while the parent plays a key role in CERT, the final responsibility for the content and format of treatment rests with the therapist.

During each CERT session, the therapist engages the parent as much as possible as the assistant coach: this is often prompted by addressing the parent along the lines of *"can you now put on your coaching hat?"* Further, by identifying *coaching opportunities* for the parent outside the session, the CERT therapist provides the parent–child pair with the framework for new ways of interacting. By definition, coaching opportunities are intrinsic to homework assignments, but they also can be linked more broadly to the child's displays of adaptive (or maladaptive) mood repair responding. Importantly, coaching interactions between parent and child are guided by *rules,* which specify the needed behaviors and attitudes. There are six rules for coaches (eg, a good coach "Focuses on the player's abilities and strengths," "Hangs in there and works with the player even if the coach had a bad day"), and six rules for the child player (eg, a team player "Doesn't mind trying new ways to do things," "Uses words to tell the coaches how he or she feels"). The rules are introduced in the first CERT session, are prominently displayed as posters in the treatment room, and also are noted in the parents manual for CERT. Because coaching opportunities provide the parent–child pair with an interactional framework that is different from their usual daily interactions, their successful use signals the possibility of positive change.

CERT AND THE TRAINING OF THERAPISTS

We strongly believe that a developmentally informed intervention for youngsters must pay attention to the therapeutic skills and the empirical and conceptual knowledge of the therapists. Although one would expect that professionals trained in "child" programs possess the needed qualifications, this is not necessarily the case. Indeed, it is not uncommon to see pediatric mental health practitioners either responding to children as if they were miniature adults (a stance also bemoaned by Barrett[4]), or else modifying their behaviors in somewhat theatrical ways (eg, by altering the tempo and quality of their voice). With regard to CERT, we identified three developmentally relevant training needs.

First, it is critical that the therapist know how to establish a therapeutic relationship with children and parents. At the very least, this involves the therapist being fully aware of his or her own verbal and nonverbal behavior and communication. It is not uncommon for young therapists with excellent exposure to cognitive–behavioral interventions to have limited understanding of the dynamics of the therapeutic relationship and how their own behavior contributes to (or detracts from) actualizing that goal. A related issue is the level of oral communication with youngsters and parents. We have been surprised by the extent to which therapists fail to monitor how they use language in treatment. The vocabulary level often is far higher than that of a high school graduate, with frequent use of highly abstract concepts and terms.

One aspect of establishing a positive therapist–patient relationship is to know how to engage younger or inattentive depressed children in a goal-oriented intervention such as CERT. A withdrawn depressed child makes this task even more difficult. Therapists with limited exposure to pediatric depression frequently have difficulties in this regard. For example, it was necessary on occasion to tell therapists to get up from their chair, kneel or bend down near the child, and figuratively "get into the child's face" and visual field to capture the child's attention. The painstaking details of how to engage anxious children in treatment offered by Kingery and colleagues[5] suggest that our training experiences are not that unusual.

CERT requires that therapists have a broad knowledge base about general developmental trends of various basic skills, emotion regulation, and mood repair responding. For example, to work with a depressed child effectively, the therapist should know that attention is a multifaceted phenomenon; that is, visual attention and auditory attention are not the same and have different developmental trajectories, and further, that there is a distinction between stimulus-driven and goal-directed attention skills. The latter point is exemplified by the difference between asking a depressed boy to listen to his favorite upbeat music versus to make a list of all the things he will need for the new school year, as a way to respond to acute dysphoria. Although a comprehensive textbook of developmental psychology may provide important initial chunks of the needed knowledge about basic skills, it is harder to acquire the knowledge base about the development of emotion regulation and mood repair. This is partly because the developmental literature on the unfolding of emotion regulation, in general, and mood repair in particular, is discontinuous and uneven: most empirical work has addressed infants, toddlers, and very young children, with relatively few studies of older children, and almost none of young adolescents (eg, 11–12 years of age). Further, the few studies of older adolescents that exist have focused almost exclusively on cognitive mood repair responses. Thus, the developmental lacunae have to be filled based on literature reviews that also contain case narratives, descriptions based on clinical experience, and by extrapolating from research findings with college students. One way we addressed this issue is to include in the CERT treatment manual a summary of the findings of developmental studies, and also to require therapists to become familiar with major reviews of the field (see Refs.[17,20,23,24,30]). Unfortunately, with the exception of the article by Morris and coworkers,[20] reviews typically focus on emotion regulation in younger ages.

THE CHALLENGES OF DELIVERING A DEVELOPMENTALLY BASED TREATMENT

We end by noting some of the challenges that we have encountered in delivering CERT. Possibly the largest issue has been the lack of psychometric tools to assess children's developmental level on the key construct of interest, that is, mood repair. Owing to a lack of assessment tools, there are no standardized and age specific guidelines about what mood repair "looks like" at the various ages across childhood and adolescence. Because we lack a quantified index of *mood repair developmental stage*, the therapist must rely on qualitative information about a young patient, along with clinical experience (and knowledge of the literature), to estimate whether that young patient handles distress in age-appropriate ways. This state of affairs adds an extra layer of challenge to any training initiative.

A related issue has been that mood repair (or emotion regulation) is a meta-skill that recruits a wide array of basic skills. Thus, ideally, if one wanted to establish a child's developmental level vis-à-vis mood repair, one should assess not only the meta-skill, but also the developmental stages of the various aspects of language skills, attention skills, executive function skills, social skills, and motor skills, which subserve emotion regulation. It may be conceivable under some circumstances to use standard neuropsychological tests to assess key skill domains. For example, there are reliable and valid assessment batteries that target areas of executive function (eg, The Delis Kaplan Executive Function System[67]), domains of attention (eg, The Integrated Visual and Auditory Continuous Performance Test[68]), visual–motor skills (eg, The Developmental Test of Visual Motor Integration[69]), and aspects of language skills (eg, Test of Language Development[70]). However, the usual community- or university-based treatment setting is unlikely to accommodate full assessment of all the necessary skills. The administration and interpretation of many of these tests require specialized training, are costly, and also are very time consuming. Further, such tests typically have not been used for case conceptualization in psychotherapy.

Another challenge has concerned therapists' qualifications. There is no formal way to assess the development-specific therapeutic skills of new therapists or their knowledge of the related empirical literature. This renders training efforts less efficient than one would like. Requiring therapists to work conjointly with parent and child at the same time, and in the same room, also posed some unexpected problems. Specifically, although therapists could easily focus on the child (and thereby not attend to the parent), or focus on the parent (and thereby ignore the child), focusing on the child *while actively engaging the parent* proved to be a far more difficult undertaking. Thus, it had become necessary to dedicate parts of CERT training to some areas of basic therapeutic skills.

In summary, the two major challenges of delivering a clearly articulated, developmentally based intervention for pediatric depression include the assessment of young patients' developmental stages on the skills of interest and the training of therapists. Research attention to these dimensions should help to pave the way for innovative solutions, which, in turn, could help in further treatment-development efforts for depressed youngsters. In the meanwhile, based on the positive results of a pilot study with chronically depressed youngsters,[1] CERT is currently being tested with 7- to 12-year-old, depressed young patients and their parents. This randomized, clinical trial includes Rogerian, client-centered therapy as the comparison condition, and both treatments entail 22 sessions delivered across a 6-month period. The study also includes 6- and 12-month follow up evaluations. Initial results should be available by late 2013.

REFERENCES

1. Kovacs M, Sherrill J, George CJ, et al. Contextual emotion-regulation therapy for childhood depression. J Am Acad Child Adolesc Psychiatry 2006;45(8):892–903.
2. Kendall PC, Lerner RM, Craighead WE. Human development and intervention in childhood psychopathology. Child Dev 1984;55(1):71–82.
3. Ollendick TH, Grills AE, King NJ. Applying developmental theory to the assessment and treatment of childhood disorders: does it make a difference? Clin Psychol Psychother 2001;8(5):304–14.
4. Barrett PM. Treatment of childhood anxiety: developmental aspects. Clin Psychol Rev 2000;20(4):479–94.
5. Kingery JN, Roblek TL, Suveg C, et al. They're not just "little adults": developmental considerations for implementing cognitive-behavioral therapy with anxious youth. J Cogn Psychother 2006;20(3):263–73.
6. Kovacs M, Sherrill JT. The psychotherapeutic management of major depressive and dysthymic disorders in childhood and adolescence: issues and prospects. In: Goodyer IM, editor. The depressed child and adolescent. 2nd edition. New York: Cambridge University Press; 2001. p. 325–52.
7. Ollendick T, King N. Empirically supported treatments for children with phobic and anxiety disorders: current status. J Clin Child Adolesc Psychol 1998;27(2):156–67.
8. Cicchetti D, Toth SL. Developmental psychopathology and preventive intervention. In: Damon W, Lerner RM, editors. Handbook of child psychology. 6th edition. New York: John Wiley; 2006.
9. Teasdale JD. Cognitive vulnerability to persistent depression. Cogn Emot 1988;2(3):247–74.
10. Gross JJ. The emerging field of emotion regulation: an integrative review. Rev Gen Psychol 1998;2(3):271–99.
11. Isen AM. Asymmetry of happiness and sadness in effects on memory in normal college students: Comment on Hasher, Rose, Zacks, Sanft, and Doren. J Exp Psychol Gen 1985;114(3):388–91.
12. Josephson BR. Mood regulation and memory: repairing sad moods with happy memories. Cogn Emot 1996;10(4):437–44.
13. Parrott WG. Beyond hedonism: motives for inhibiting good moods and for maintaining bad moods. In: Wegner DM, Pennebaker JW, editors. Handbook of mental control. Century psychology series. Englewood Cliffs (NJ): Prentice-Hall; 1993.
14. Morris WN, Reilly NP. Toward the self-regulation of mood: theory and research. Motiv Emot 1987;11(3):215–49.
15. Kovacs M. Depression in childhood and its treatment by contextual emotion regulation therapy. New York: Guilford Press; 2012, in press.
16. Kovacs M. Manual of contextual emotion regulation therapy for depression in childhood-revised (CERT-CR). Pittsburgh (PA): University of Pittsburgh School of Medicine, Department of Psychiatry, WPIC; 2009.

17. Kopp CB. Regulation of distress and negative emotions: a developmental view. Dev Psychol 1989;25(3):343–54.
18. Thompson R. Emotional regulation: a theme in search of definition, the development of emotion regulation. Educ Psychol Rev 1994;58:25.
19. Hofer MA. Hidden regulators in attachment, separation, and loss. Monogr Soc Res Child Dev 1994;59(2–3):192–207.
20. Morris AS, Silk JS, Steinberg L, et al. The role of the family context in the development of emotion regulation. Social Dev 2007;16(2):361–88.
21. Davis EL, Levine LJ, Lench HC, et al. Metacognitive emotion regulation: children's awareness that changing thoughts and goals can alleviate negative emotions. Emotion 2010;10(4):498–510.
22. Garber J, Braafladt N, Weiss B. Affect regulation in depressed and nondepressed children and young adolescents. Dev Psychopathol 1995;7(01):93.
23. Eisenberg N, Morris AS. Children's emotion-related regulation. In: Kail RV, editor. Advances in child development and behavior, vol. 30. Amsterdam: Academic Press; 2002. p. 189–229. Available at: http://www.sciencedirect.com/science/article/pii/S0065240702800428. Accessed August 16, 2011.
24. Fox NA, Calkins SD. The development of self-control of emotion: intrinsic and extrinsic influences. Motiv Emot 2003;27(1):7–26.
25. Grolnick WS, McMenamy JM, Kurowski CO. Emotional self-regulation in infancy and toddlerhood. In: Balter L, Tamis-LeMonda CS, editors. Child psychology: a handbook of contemporary issues. New York: Psychology Press; 2006. p. 3–25.
26. Calkins SD, Johnson MC. Toddler regulation of distress to frustrating events: temperamental and maternal correlates. Infant Behav Dev 1998;21(3):379–95.
27. Calkins SD, Gill KL, Johnson MC, et al. Emotional reactivity and emotional regulation strategies as predictors of social behavior with peers during toddlerhood. Social Dev 1999;8(3):310–34.
28. Silk JS, Shaw DS, Skuban EM, et al. Emotion regulation strategies in offspring of childhood-onset depressed mothers. J Child Psychol Psychiatry 2006;47(1):69–78.
29. Diener ML, Mangelsdorf SC, McHale JL, et al. Infants' behavioral strategies for emotion regulation with fathers and mothers: associations with emotional expressions and attachment quality. Infancy 2002;3(2):153–74.
30. Thompson RA. Emotional regulation and emotional development. Educ Psychol Rev 1991;3(4):269–307.
31. Koole SL. The psychology of emotion regulation: an integrative review. Cogn Emot 2009;23(1):4–41.
32. Parkinson B, Totterdell P. Classifying affect-regulation strategies. PCEM 1999;13(3):277–303.
33. Rippere V. "What's the thing to do when you're feeling depressed?" — a pilot study. Behav Res Ther 1977;15(2):185–91.
34. Thayer RE, Newman JR, McClain TM. Self-regulation of mood: strategies for changing a bad mood, raising energy, and reducing tension. J Pers Soc Psychol 1994;67(5):910–25.
35. Kovacs M, Joormann J, Gotlib IH. Emotion (dys)regulation and links to depressive disorders. Child Dev Perspect 2008;2(3):149–55.
36. Eisenberg N, Fabes RA, Guthrie IK, et al. Dispositional emotionality and regulation: their role in predicting quality of social functioning. J Pers Soc Psychol 2000;78(1):136–57.
37. Mangelsdorf SC, Shapiro JR, Marzolf D. Developmental and temperamental differences in emotion regulation in infancy. Child Dev 1995;66(6):1817–28.

38. Posner MI, Rothbart MK. Developing mechanisms of self-regulation. Dev Psychopathol 2000;12(03):427–41.
39. Peláez-Nogueras M, Field TM, Hossain Z, et al. Depressed mothers' touching increases infants' positive affect and attention in still-face interactions. Child Dev 1996;67(4):1780–92.
40. Sowell ER, Thompson PM, Toga AW. Mapping changes in the human cortex throughout the span of life. Neuroscientist 2004;10(4):372–92.
41. Toga AW, Thompson PM, Sowell ER. Mapping brain maturation. Trends Neurosci 2006;29(3):148–59.
42. Harman C, Rothbart MK, Posner MI. Distress and attention interactions in early infancy. Motiv Emot 1997;21(1):27–44.
43. Diener ML, Mangelsdorf SC. Behavioral strategies for emotion regulation in toddlers: associations with maternal involvement and emotional expressions. Infant Behav Dev 1999;22(4):569–83.
44. Grolnick WS, Bridges LJ, Connell JP. Emotion regulation in two-year-olds: strategies and emotional expression in four contexts. Child Dev 1996;67(3):928–41.
45. Braungart JM, Stifter CA. Regulation of negative reactivity during the strange situation: temperament and attachment in 12-month-old infants. Infant Behav Dev 1991;14(3):349–64.
46. Davidson RJ, Jackson DC, Kalin NH. Emotion, plasticity, context, and regulation: perspectives from affective neuroscience. Psychol Bull 2000;126(6):890–909.
47. Mauss IB, Bunge SA, Gross JJ. Automatic emotion regulation. Social Pers Psychol Compass 2007;1(1):146–67.
48. Anderson V, Anderson P, Northam E, et al. Development of executive functions through late childhood and adolescence in an Australian sample. Dev Neuropsychol 2001;20(1):385–406.
49. Klenberg L, Korkman M, Lahti-Nuuttila P. Differential development of attention and executive functions in 3- to 12-year-old Finnish children. Dev Neuropsychol 2001;20(1):407–28.
50. Korkman M, Kemp S, Kirk U. Effects of age on neurocognitive measures of children ages 5 to 12: a cross-sectional study on 800 children from the United States. Dev Neuropsychol 2001;20(1):331–54.
51. Zelazo PD, Argitis G. The development of executive function in early childhood. Monogr Soc Res Child Dev 2003;68(3):1–27.
52. Huizinga M, Dolan CV, van der Molen MW. Age-related change in executive function: developmental trends and a latent variable analysis. Neuropsychologia 2006;44(11):2017–36.
53. Swanson HL. What develops in working memory? A life span perspective. Dev Psychol 1999;35(4):986–1000.
54. Casey BJ, Giedd JN, Thomas KM. Structural and functional brain development and its relation to cognitive development. Biol Psychol 2000;54(1–3):241–57.
55. Durston S, Hulshoff Pol HE, Casey BJ, et al. Anatomical MRI of the developing human brain: what have we learned? J Am Acad Child Adolesc Psychiatry 2001;40(9):1012–20.
56. Kane MJ, Engle RW. The role of prefrontal cortex in working-memory capacity, executive attention, and general fluid intelligence: an individual-differences perspective. Psychon Bull Rev 2002;9(4):637–71.
57. Morris AS, Silk JS, Steinberg L, et al. Concurrent and longitudinal links between children's externalizing behavior in school and observed anger regulation in the mother–child dyad. J Psychopathol Behav Assess 2010;32(1):48–56.

58. Reijntjes A, Stegge H, Terwogt MM, et al. Children's coping with in vivo peer rejection: an experimental investigation. J Abnorm Child Psychol 2006;34(6):873–85.
59. Fujiki M, Brinton B, Clarke D. Emotion regulation in children with specific language impairment. Lang Speech Hear Serv Sch 2002;33(2):102–11.
60. Mikulincer M, Shaver PR, Pereg D. Attachment theory and affect regulation: the dynamics, development, and cognitive consequences of attachment-related strategies. Motiv Emot 2003;27(2):77–102.
61. Kobak RR, Sceery A. Attachment in late adolescence: working models, affect regulation, and representations of self and others. Child Dev 1988;59:135–46.
62. Fauber RL, Long N. Children in context: the role of the family in child psychotherapy. J Consult Clin Psychol 1991;59(6):813–20.
63. Koocher GP, Pedulla BM. Current practices in child psychotherapy. Prof Psychol 1977;8(3):275–87.
64. Woolfenden SR, Williams K, Peat JK. Family and parenting interventions for conduct disorder and delinquency: a meta-analysis of randomised controlled trials. Arch Dis Child 2002;86(4):251–6.
65. Kovacs M, Bastiaens JT. The psychotherapeutic management of major depressive and dysthymic disorders in childhood and adolescence: issues and prospects. In: Goodyer IM, editor. The depressed child and adolescent. 1st edition. New York: Cambridge University Press; 1995.
66. Hammen C, Rudolph K, Weisz J, et al. The context of depression in clinic-referred youth: neglected areas in treatment. J Am Acad Child Adolesc Psychiatry 1999;38(1): 64–71.
67. Delis DC, Kaplan E, Kramer JH. The Delis-Kaplan executive function system: examiner's manual. San Antonio (TX): The Psychological Corporation; 2001.
68. Sandford JA, Turner A. Integrated visual and auditory continuous performance test manual. Richmond (VA): BrainTrain; 2002.
69. Beery KE. The Beery-Buktenica VMI: Developmental test of visual-motor integration with supplemental developmental tests of visual perception and motor coordination: administration, scoring, and teaching manual. Parsippany (NJ): Modern Curriculum Press; 1997.
70. Hammill DD, Newcomer P. Test of language development, primary. 4th edition. San Antonio (TX): The Psychological Corporation; 1999.

Enhancing the Developmental Appropriateness of Treatment for Depression in Youth: Integrating the Family in Treatment

Martha C. Tompson, PhD[a],*, Kathryn Dingman Boger, PhD[b,c],
Joan R. Asarnow, PhD[d]

KEYWORDS

- Youth depression • Psychosocial treatment • Family
- Developmental factors • Treatment Models
- Randomized clinical trials

Youth depression is an impairing and frequently recurrent and persistent disorder that impacts current and later development, resulting in high social and economic costs. Depression and interpersonal stress are frequently transactional, with depression powerfully negatively impacting relationships and relationship stress negatively impacting the course and outcome of depression. In this context, treatment models for youth depression that emphasize interpersonal functioning, particularly family relationships, may be particularly promising. This article has three objectives. It first reviews the current state of knowledge on the efficacy of psychosocial treatments for depression in youth, with an emphasis on the role of family involvement in treatment. Second, it discusses developmental factors that may impact the

---

This work was partially supported by NIMH grants R01 MH082856 and R01MH82856 from the National Institute of Mental Health and by a grant from the American Foundation for Suicide Prevention. We might want to also thank the many youths and families that have shared their experiences with us. Dr Asarnow reports receiving honoraria from Hathaways-Sycamores, Casa Pacifica, the California Institute of Mental Health, and the Melissa Institute.

[a] Department of Psychology, Boston University, 648 Beacon Street, Boston, MA 02215, USA
[b] McLean Hospital, 115 Mill Street, Belmont, MA 02478, USA
[c] Harvard Medical School, 25 Shattuck Street, Boston, MA 02115, USA
[d] UCLA Semel Institute for Neuroscience and Human Behavior, 760 Westwood Plaza, Los Angeles, CA 90095, USA
* Corresponding author.
E-mail address: mtompson@bu.edu

Child Adolesc Psychiatric Clin N Am 21 (2012) 345–384
doi:10.1016/j.chc.2012.01.003
1056-4993/12/$ – see front matter © 2012 Elsevier Inc. All rights reserved.

applicability and structure of family-focused treatment models for preadolescent and adolescent youth. Third, two family-based treatment models that are currently being evaluated in randomized clinical trials are described: one focusing on preadolescent depressed youth and the other on adolescents who have made a recent suicide attempt.

TREATMENT FOR YOUTH WITH DEPRESSIVE DISORDERS: CURRENT STATE OF THE FIELD

Pharmacologic treatments for depressive disorders in youth have been evaluated in numerous trials in recent years, with selective serotonin reuptake inhibitors (SSRIs) demonstrating efficacy for both adolescent and preadolescent youth (for review see Maalouf and Brent article in this issue). Several factors, in conjunction with data on the negative sequelae of youth depression, underscore the crucial need to continue to develop and evaluate psychosocial treatments:

1. Practice parameters and guidelines for youth depression emphasize an initial trial of psychosocial treatment before commencing medication intervention.[1]
2. Clinical observation and recent data indicate reluctance among adolescents and their parents to pursue medication treatments for depression and a preference for psychosocial modalities,[2,3] and this reluctance is likely to be greater among younger children.
3. Evidence of possible suicidal risk associated with SSRIs in the treatment of youth depression has led to a U.S. Food and Drug Administration (FDA) "black box" warning on all antidepressant medications, which has precipitated a reduction in prescription rates.[4,5]

Tables 1 and **2** summarize findings of current clinical trials examining psychosocial treatments for depressive disorders in youth. **Table 1** focuses on studies conducted primarily with adolescents and **Table 2** focuses on studies completed with preadolescent youth. Although a number of studies have evaluated preventive interventions for youth at risk for depression (for more details please see the article by Beardslee and colleagues elsewhere in this issue), this review is limited to those examining treatments for youth currently suffering from depression.

As evidenced in **Table 1**, recent years have witnessed significant advances in the treatment of adolescent depression. Results from large multisite trials and smaller single-site trials document the efficacy of some psychosocial and medication treatments, as well as combined treatments.[6-15] Examination of findings from these studies highlights the efficacy of cognitive–behavioral and interpersonal strategies in both reducing symptoms and enhancing functioning. Further, recent effectiveness trials have demonstrated improved depression, quality-of-life, and functioning outcomes when these evidence-based depression treatments are provided to adolescents in usual care settings.[2,7,16,17] Although most clinicians agree on the importance of family involvement in comprehensive intervention for youth depression, research has not provided clear answers regarding the optimal nature and extent of family involvement. Some family treatment sessions have been included in many of the large trials evaluating depression cognitive–behavioral therapy (CBT) for adolescents (eg, Treatment for Adolescents with Depression Study [TADS], Treatment of SSRI-Resistant Depression in Adolescents [TORDIA]), and this may have contributed to the efficacy of the CBT. Underscoring the importance accorded family involvement, Brent and colleagues,[6] in a large clinical trial comparing cognitive–behavioral, supportive, and family systemic therapies, included a few family psychoeducational sessions to enhance therapeutic engagement for all participants. However, the more extensive

Table 1
Randomized clinical intervention trials for adolescents with depression

References	Subjects	Diagnostic/Risk Assessment	Format(s)	Intervention Type(s)	Degree of Family Involvement	Post-Treatment Assessment	Impact of Treatment
Asarnow et al[2]	Ages 13–21 (n = 418)	Either: 1. Endorsed "stem items" for MDD or DD from the CIDI-12, 1 week or more of past-month depressive symptoms, and a total CES-D score >16, or 2. CES-D score ≥24	Individual	1. 6-month quality improvement intervention 2. Usual care	Parent consultation offered	Immediate	Intervention patients, compared with usual care patients, reported significantly higher mental health care utilization, fewer depressive symptoms, higher mental health-related quality of life, and greater satisfaction with mental health care.
Brent et al[6], Birmaher et al[95]	Ages 13–18 (n = 107)	Diagnosis of MDD based on K-SADS Interview and BDI ≥13	Family; Individual	1. SBFT 2. CBT 3. Supportive therapy	Extensive family involvement only in the SBFT group	Immediate; 2 years[95]	The CBT group had faster response, less diagnosable MDD at the end of the treatment, a lower number of depressive symptoms, and were more likely to be remitted. No differences in depression between treatment groups at 2-year follow-up.
Brent et al[96]	Ages 12–18 (n = 334)	Diagnosis of MDD based on K-SADS-PL, CDRS ≥40, resistant to "adequate trial" of SSRIs (equivalent to 40 mg fluoxetine)	Individual	1. CBT + medication change 2. Medication change alone	Family education plus additional family sessions, focusing on decreasing conflict and improving family communication and problem solving (mean = 1; range, 0–7 family sessions)	Immediate 24 weeks 48 weeks 72 weeks	Combined CBT + medication was associated with a significantly higher rate of clinical response/improvement at the end of the acute treatment phase (12 weeks) as compared to a medication switch alone.

(continued on next page)

Table 1
(continued)

References	Subjects	Diagnostic/Risk Assessment	Format(s)	Intervention Type(s)	Degree of Family Involvement	Post-Treatment Assessment	Impact of Treatment
Clarke et al[8]	Ages 14–18 (n = 123)	Diagnosis of MDD or DD based on the K-SADS interview	Group	1. CWD-A 2. CWD-A with nine-session parent group 3. WLC	Concurrent parent sessions plus two joint parent–adolescent groups in CWD-A plus parent group; none in other groups	Immediate; 12 months; 24 months	CBT was associated with higher depression recovery rates (66.7% vs 48.1% in wait list condition) and greater reduction in depressive symptoms. Addition of parent group had no significant effect. Booster sessions accelerated recovery among youth still depressed at the end of acute treatment but did not reduce recurrence.
Clarke et al[97]	Ages 13–18 (n = 88)	Diagnosis of DSM-III-R MDD and/or DD based on the K-SADS interview	Group	1. Usual care plus group CBT program (CWD-A) 2. Usual care	A few parent psychoeducation sessions	Immediate; 12 months; 24 months	No significant differences between CBT and usual care, either for depression diagnoses, continuous depression measures, nonaffective mental health measures, or functioning outcomes.
Clarke et al[7]	Ages 12–18 (n = 152)	Diagnoses of DSM-IV MDD based on the K-SADS-PL interview	Individual	1. Brief CBT plus treatment as usual (primarily SSRI) 2. Treatment as usual	Monthly informational parent meetings offered	Immediate; 26 weeks; 52 weeks	CBT program showed advantages on the Short-Form-12 Mental Component Scale and reductions in treatment as usual outpatient visits and days' supply of all medications. No effects were detected for MDD episodes; a nonsignificant trend favoring CBT was detected on the CES-D.

Study	Age/Sample	Inclusion Criteria	Modality	Treatment Conditions	Family Involvement	Timing	Outcomes
Diamond et al[18]	Ages 13–17 (n = 32)	Diagnoses of DSM-III-R MDD based on the K-SADS	Family	1. ABFT 2. Minimal-contact, WLC group	Extensive family involvement in ABFT	Immediate; 6 months	At post-treatment, 81% treated no longer met criteria for MDD vs 47% of patients in the waitlist group. The ABFT patients showed greater reduction in depressive and anxiety symptoms and family conflict. At follow-up, 87% of the ABFT patients continued to not meet criteria for MDD.
Diamond et al[19]	Ages 12–17 (n = 66)	Endorsement of suicidal ideation in primary care, BDI >20, and SIQ-JR >31	Family	1. ABFT 2. EUC	Extensive family involvement in ABFT	Immediate; 6 months	87% of those who participated in ABFT met criteria for clinical recovery in terms of suicidal ideation as compared to 52% receiving EUC.
Fine et al[98]	Ages 13–17 (n = 66) 83% female	Diagnosis of MDD or DD based on K-SADS interview	Group	1. TSG vs 2. SSG	None	Immediate; 9 months	At post-test both groups improved; TSG significantly more effective than SSG in reducing depression on K-SADS with more subjects in non-clinical range. Group differences disappeared at follow-up.
Goodyer et al[94]	Ages 11–17 (n = 208)	Referred to clinical care; MDD diagnosis; failure to respond to initial brief psychosocial intervention	Individual	1. SSRI + routine care 2. SSRI + routine care + CBT	Inclusion of parents at end of CBT session; no more than three family sessions	12 weeks 28 weeks	No differences between the treatment groups on Health of the Nation Outcome for children and adolescents, CDRS-R, GAF, or Clinical Global Improvement scale.

(continued on next page)

Table 1
(continued)

References	Subjects	Diagnostic/Risk Assessment	Format(s)	Intervention Type(s)	Degree of Family Involvement	Post-Treatment Assessment	Impact of Treatment
Kennard et al[99]	Ages 12–18 (n = 334)	Diagnosis of MDD on K-SADS interview, CDRS-R ≥40, CGI-S ≥4, and nonresponsive to SSRI treatment for at least 6 weeks	Individual	1. Medication switch 2. Medication switch and CBT	Family sessions offered	Immediate	Participants who had more than nine CBT sessions were 2.5 times more likely to have adequate treatment response than those with 9 sessions or fewer.
Lewinsohn et al[9]	Ages 14–18 (n = 59)	Diagnosis of major, minor, or intermittent depression based on K-SADS interview with mother and adolescent	Group; Family	1. Adolescent-only CBT training group 2. Adolescent-parent CBT training groups 3. WLC	Extensive parent involvement in the adolescent-parent CBT groups only	Immediate; 1 month; 6 months; 12 months; 24 months	Significantly fewer youths in the treatment groups met criteria for depressive disorders after treatment and at follow-up. Significantly improved on self-reported depression, anxiety, number of pleasant activities, and depressogenic thoughts. Trend for adolescent-parent condition to outperform adolescent only group.
Melvin et al[11]	Ages 12–18 (n = 73)	Diagnosis of DSM-IV MDD, DD, or DDNOS based on the K-SADS	Individual	1. CBT 2. Antidepressant medication (Sertraline) 3. Combined CBT and medication	Concurrent parent sessions plus two family sessions	Immediate; 6 months	All groups showed significant improvement on outcome measures and this was maintained at follow-up. Combined group was not superior to monotherapy. CBT alone was superior to medication alone.

Study	Age (n)	Diagnosis	Format	Conditions	Family involvement	Follow-up	Results
Mufson et al[12]	Ages 12–18 (n = 48)	Clinician diagnosis of MDD based on the HRSD	Individual	1. IPT-A 2. Clinician monitoring	None	Immediate	IPT-A patients reported greater decrease in depressive symptoms, improved social functioning, and improved problem-solving skills compared to controls. In the IPT-A condition 74% recovered compared to 46% in the control condition.
Mufson et al[16]	Ages 12–18 (n = 63)	DSM-IV diagnosis of MDD, DD, adjustment disorder with depressed mood, or DDNOS and HRSD ≥10 and a C-GAS score ≤65	Individual	1. IPT-A 2. Treatment as usual	None in IPT-A group; several family/parent sessions for some participants in the TAU group	Immediate	IPT-A associated with fewer clinician-reported depression symptoms on the HRSD, better functioning on the C-GAS, better overall social functioning on the Social Adjustment Scale-Self-Report, greater clinical improvement, and greater decreases in clinical severity on the Clinical Global Impressions scale.
Reed[100]	Ages 14–19 (n = 18)	Clinician diagnosis of MDD or DD	Group	1. Social skills training 2. Attention placebo control	None	Immediate; 6–8 weeks	Skills group participants scored significantly higher than control group on clinicians' rating of improvement. Male subjects improved, but female subjects deteriorated.

(continued on next page)

Table 1
(continued)

References	Subjects	Diagnostic/Risk Assessment	Format(s)	Intervention Type(s)	Degree of Family Involvement	Post-Treatment Assessment	Impact of Treatment
Rohde et al[13]	Ages 13–17 (n = 91)	DSM-IV diagnoses of MDD and Conduct Disorder based on the K-SADS-E-5	Group	1. CWD-A 2. Life skills tutoring/control	Two informational sessions offered to parents	Immediate; 6 months; 12 months	Post-treatment MDD recovery rates better in CWD-A group (36%), compared to ife skills/ tutoring (19%). CWD-A participants reported reductions in BDI-II and HDRS scores and improved social functioning post-treatment. Group differences in MDD recovery rates at follow-up were nonsignificant.
Rosselló and Bernal[14]	Ages 13–18 (n = 71)	Diagnosis of MDD, DD, or both	Individual	1. CBT 2. IPT 3. WLC	Parent consultations offered on an as-needed basis	Immediate; 3 months	Both active treatments were associated with significant reductions in depression when compared to wait list. IPT was superior to CBT in enhancing social functioning and self-esteem.
Roaselló et al[15]	Ages 12–18 (n = 112)	DSM-III-R criteria for MDD, deemed by clinical interviewer to be impaired, or CDI ≥13	Individual; Group	1. Individual CBT 2. Group CBT 3. Individual IPT 4. Group IPT	Three to five parent consultation sessions offered	Immediate	CBT produced greater decreases in depressive symptoms and improved self-concept as compared to IPT.

Study	Age (n)	Diagnosis	Format	Treatment	Family component	Follow-up	Results
TADS Team[10]	Ages 12–17 (n = 439)	DSM-IV diagnosis of MDD based on the K-SADS-PL	Individual	Twelve weeks of: 1. Fluoxetine alone 2. CBT alone 3. CBT with fluoxetine 4. Placebo	Two psychoeducation sessions for parents and one to three family sessions	Immediate	There were significant differences between combination treatment and placebo on the CDRS-R. Combined treatment was superior when compared with fluoxetine alone and CBT alone. Fluoxetine alone was superior to CBT alone.
Vostanis et al[20]	Ages 8–17 (n = 56)	Diagnosis of MDD, DD, or minor depression based on K-SADS	Individual	1. Depression treatment program 2. Attention placebo	None	Immediate; 9 months	No difference in remission rates; remission rates were high in both groups.
Wood et al[21]	Ages 9–17 (n = 48)	Diagnosis of MDD or RDC minor depression based on K-SADS interview with both parent and child	Individual	1. CBT 2. Relaxation training	None	Immediate; 6 months	Post-test revealed greater reductions in depressive symptoms and an advantage in overall outcome in the CBT group. At follow-up, group differences were attenuated.

Abbreviations: ABFT, Attachment-Based Family Therapy; BDI, Beck Depression Inventory; CBT, cognitive–behavioral therapy; CDI, Children's Depression Inventory; CDRS-R, Revised Children's Depression Rating Scale; CES-D, Center for Epidemiologic Studies – Depression Scale; CGI-S, Clinical Global Impression Severity Scale; CWD-A, Adolescent Coping with Depression Course; DD, dysthymic disorder; DDNOS, depressive disorder not otherwise specified; EUC, enhanced usual care; GAF, Global Assessment of Functioning Scale; HRSD, Hamilton Rating Scale for Depression; IPT-A, interpersonal psychotherapy for depressed adolescents; K-SADS, Schedule for Affective Disorders and Schizophrenia for School-Aged Children; MDD, major depressive disorder; SBFT, Systematic Behavior Family Therapy; SIQ-JR, Suicidal Ideation Questionnaire; SSG, social skills group; TAU, treatment as usual; TSG, therapeutic support group; WLC, waitlist control.

Table 2
Randomized clinical intervention trials for preadolescents with depression

References	Subjects	Diagnostic/Risk Assessment	Format(s)	Intervention Type(s)	Degree of Family Involvement	Post-Intervention Assessment	Impact of Treatment
Asarnow et al[27]	4th–6th graders (n = 23)	School screening; CDI ≥8	Group	1. CBT and family education 2. WLC	One psychoeducation session	Immediate	Children in the intervention group were more likely to show reductions in depressive symptoms, negative cognitions, and internalizing coping.
Butler et al[101]	5th–6th graders (n = 56)	Teacher referral; high scores on CDI	Group	1. Role play problem solving 2. Cognitive restructuring 3. Attention control	None	Immediate	Role play group showed significant reduction on CDI and improved classroom functioning. One of two groups in cognitive restructuring showed significant reductions on CDI.
De Cuyper et al[102]	Ages 10–12 (n = 20)	CDI score ≥11 and/or T score ≥23 on CBCL Internalizing and Anxious/Depressed subscale; at least one MDD criterion but without other apparent Axis-I	Group	1. CBT program ("Taking Action") 2. WLC group	None	Immediate; 4 months; 12 months	Four-month follow-up comparisons with baseline measures, showed significant improvement on the CDI and the Self-Perception Profile only for CBT group. At the 12-month follow-up, CBT group showed further improvement and significant decreases on the CDI, STAI, and CBCL.

| Fristad et al[29] | Ages 8–12 (n = 165) | DSM-IV diagnosis of MDD, DD, or bipolar disorder type I, type II, or mood disorder NOS | Family | Group | 1. MF-PEP + TAU 2. WLC + TAU | Extensive family involvement in the MF-PEP group | 6 months; 12 months; 18 months | MF-PEP +TAU was associated with lower MSI scores at follow-up in intent-to-treat analyses compared with WLC + TAU. The WLC group also showed a similar decrease in MSI scores 1 year later, after their treatment. |
| Jaycox et al[103], Gillham et al[104] | Ages 10–13 (n = 143) | Z-scores on CDI + Child Perception Questionnaire > 0.50 | Group | | 1. Cognitive 2. Social problem solving 3. Combined (both above treatments) 4. WLC 5. No participation control | None | Immediate; 6 months; 12 months; 18 months; 24 months | No differences between the treated groups. Treated groups had fewer depressive symptoms at post-test and at follow-up and improved classroom behavior (teacher report) than untreated groups. Effects more pronounced among children from high conflict homes. Follow-up revealed even greater group differences in depressive symptoms over time. |

(continued on next page)

Table 2
(continued)

References	Subjects	Diagnostic/Risk Assessment	Format(s)	Intervention Type(s)	Degree of Family Involvement	Post-Intervention Assessment	Impact of Treatment
Kahn et al[105]	Ages 10–14 (n = 68)	Multistage Gating. Stage 1: CDI >14; RADS >71. Stage 2: Reassessment 1 month later with CDI and RADS. Stage 3: Interview, BDI >19. No other depression treatment	Group	1. Cognitive-behavioral 2. Relaxation training 3. Self-modeling 4. WLC	None	Immediate; 1 month	All three active treatment groups showed significant improvement in depression compared to control. Most children in both CBT and relaxation groups went from dysfunctional to functional range on depressive symptoms; self-modeling group less improved than other active treatment groups.
King and Kirschenbaum[28]	Grades KG–4 (n = 135)	Children who scored above a cutoff on the Activity Mood screening questionnaire	Group	1. Social skills training plus consultation with parents and teachers 2. Consultation only	Parent consultations offered	Immediate	Combined program showed reduced depression based on interview data as compared to consultation only. Multidimensional ratings of behavior and skills improved across both groups.
Liddle and Spence[106]	Ages 7–11 (n = 31)	CDI ≥19 CDRS-R ≥40	Group	1. Social competence training 2. Attention placebo control 3. WLC	None	Immediate; 3 months	No group differences at pretest, post-test, or follow-up. All groups declined on CDI scores and increased on teacher's reports of problem behavior.

| Stark et al[107] | 4th–5th graders (n = 29) | CDI scores >12 on 2 administrations | Group | 1. Behavioral problem solving 2. Self-control 3. WLC | None | Immediate; 8 weeks | Both active treatment groups showed significant reductions in depressive symptoms; however, in Behavioral Problem Solving both mothers and children reported differences, whereas in self-control only children reported differences. |
| Stark et al[30] | Ages 9–13; all female (n = 159) | Clinical level scores on the CDI and symptom interview and a depressive disorder dx on the KSADS DSM-IV-TR | Group | 1. CBT 2. CBT + PT 3. Minimal contact control | Extensive parent involvement in the CBT + PT group | Immediate; 1 year | ACTION treatment with and without PT was more effective than the minimal contact control but the two active treatments did not differ significantly. After treatment, 80% of the girls in the active treatments no longer met criteria for a depressive disorder dx versus 47% in the control group. Treatment gains were maintained for majority of girls 1 year post treatment. Girls in the CBT+PT group reported better family communication and cohesiveness. |

(continued on next page)

Table 2
(continued)

References	Subjects	Diagnostic/Risk Assessment	Format(s)	Intervention Type(s)	Degree of Family Involvement	Post-Intervention Assessment	Impact of Treatment
Weisz et al[108]	3rd–6th graders (n = 48)	CDI ≥10 or identified by teachers/counselor as depressed; and CDRS-R interview score ≥34	Group	1. Primary and secondary control enhancement training 2. No treatment control	None	Immediate; 9 months	At post-test, treated group showed significantly greater reductions on both CDI and CDRS-R. At follow-up (60% available), group differences remained.

Abbreviations: BDI, Beck Depression Inventory; CDI, Children's Depression Inventory; CDRS-R, Revised Children's Depression Rating Scale; CES-D, Center for Epidemiologic Studies – Depression Scale; DD, dysthymic disorder; DDNOS, depressive disorder not otherwise specified; GAF, Global Assessment of Functioning Scale; K-SADS, Schedule for Affective Disorders and Schizophrenia for School-Aged Children; MDD, major depressive disorder; MF-PEP, multifamily psychoeducational psychotherapy; MSI, Mood Severity Index; PT, parent training; TAU, treatment as usual; WLC, waitlist control.

family systemic therapy had a remission rate of approximately 38%, similar to that of nondirective supportive treatment (39%) and significantly lower than that of CBT (60%). In other clinical trials examining CBT for adolescent depression, augmentation of a parent group did not add significantly to the adolescent-only treatment.[8] However, more recently, Diamond and colleagues have examined a family-based treatment model focused on repairing and enhancing the attachment between the youth and his or her parents. In their initial clinical trial with depressed adolescents,[18] 81% of those who participated in this attached-based family therapy (ABFT) showed remission from their depression, as opposed to 47% of those on a waitlist. In a randomized controlled trial (RCT) with suicidal adolescents,[19] 87% of those who participated in ABFT met criteria for clinical recovery in terms of suicidal ideation as compared to 52% receiving enhanced usual care. Thus, although a number of issues remain in understanding the most appropriate treatments for adolescents with depression, including the role of family involvement in treatment, there are currently several efficacious strategies for this condition.

In contrast, as illustrated in **Table 2**, there are relatively few RCTs of treatments for depression in childhood. Despite the morbidity of childhood-onset depression and the emphasis in current guidelines on initial psychosocial treatment, there are currently no published RCTs of psychosocial interventions exclusively for preadolescent youth with diagnosed depressive disorders (see **Table 2**), although two are currently ongoing. The few published studies with preadolescent samples have focused on children with high depressive symptoms rather than those with diagnosable disorders. Two clinical trials have included children 12 years of age and younger with depressive diagnoses in their samples,[20,21] but neither included separate analyses allowing examination of treatment effects in younger children. One study included only eight prepubertal subjects,[21] and the other included six 12-year-old participants and 13 participants younger than the age of 12 years (Vostanis P, personal communication, February 2007). There have been some treatment development studies with diagnosed school-aged youth, including our own,[22–26] but RCTs are needed to evaluate treatment efficacy. In most of these treatments, parents are included in parallel sessions[27,28] or in groups.[29,30]

Despite the limitations in the literature on psychosocial treatments for childhood-onset depression, recent meta-analysis suggests similar effect sizes for child and adolescent treatment. Weisz and colleagues[31] found an average effect size of 0.34 for depression treatments across ages. Excluding trials with mixed child and adolescent samples, the effect size for studies of youth younger than age 13 was not significantly different from the effect size for treatment of adolescents (0.41 for children vs 0.33 for adolescents). However, the effect-size estimate for younger children (vs adolescents) was based on a very small number of trials (n = 7), all of which selected subjects based on depressive symptoms (as opposed to formal diagnosis as proposed here), which likely led to less severe depression in the child samples (see **Table 2**). In addition, the overall effect size for depression treatments was lower (0.34) than that for nondepressive problems, including aggression, disruptive behavior, attention-deficit/hyperactivity, and fears (0.69), and when the experimental treatment was compared to an active control condition (rather than a waitlist or no treatment condition), the effect size was even smaller (0.24). Thus, not only is there a striking absence of "gold standard" RCTs of interventions for child (vs adolescent) depressive disorders, but also relatively small effect sizes point to the need for additional treatment development and research targeted to more severe cases.

DEVELOPMENTAL FACTORS IMPACTING YOUTH DEPRESSION AND DEPRESSION TREATMENT

As emphasized in multiple papers throughout this issue, depression is associated with a host of negative correlates and sequelae. Depressed adolescents are at increased risk for suicidal behavior,[32] substance use,[33] academic failure,[34] and depression in adulthood.[35–39] Adolescent depression is frequently accompanied by high levels of family conflict, control,[40] negative interactional patterns,[41] major life stressors,[42] daily hassles,[43] bullying, and negative peer interactions.[44] Depressed adolescents often report low levels of social support[45] and low family cohesion.[46] Recent conceptualizations of depression generally and adolescent depression specifically[47] emphasize the role of the interpersonal context in the perpetuation of symptoms. In a bidirectional fashion, stressful events and interpersonal interactions may contribute to the development and maintenance of depression, and depressive symptoms may contribute to an increase in interpersonal stress—a process referred to as stress generation.[48] Hence, targeting the interpersonal context in the treatment of depression may be particularly germane in adolescence.

Although rarer than adolescent depression, childhood-onset depression is associated with significant morbidity, high risk of relapse, and high levels of dysfunction due to its early onset and interference with negotiation of developmental tasks. The research literature indicates that depression in children is frequently chronic and severe,[49–51] associated with the risk of high relapse and continuing impairment[49,50,52–54] as well as bipolar outcome.[53] Child depression also correlates with increased risk of drug and alcohol abuse, suicide, and other significant public health problems[55–57] and is accompanied by substantial social impairments, both during and after resolution of depressive episodes.[58,59] When untreated or ineffectively treated, child depression is predictive of chronic problems during adolescence as well as adult depression.[39,60,61]

Although depression occurs in both adolescent and preadolescent youth, there are a number of important differences:

First, **depression is more common in adolescents**. Epidemiologic studies suggest that depression may impact up to 20% of adolescents by age 18,[1,62] whereas extant data indicate 1% to 2% of school-aged youth suffer from major depressive disorder (MDD) and another 0.6% to 1.7% from dysthymic disorder (DD).[1]

Second**, different risk models may underlie adolescent and preadolescent forms of depression**. For example, the cognitive vulnerability model of depression[63] may apply more readily to adolescent youth because, before adolescence, youth may not have well-developed negative schema for processing stress-relevant information.[64]

Although forms of depression may differ across development, there are also clear differences in the developmental context and tasks between adolescent and preadolescent youth. Adolescents are developing autonomy from parents and expanding their social worlds, while still needing to maintain adaptive parent–adolescent relationships. Successful relationship functioning in adolescence includes maintaining ongoing connectedness and yet increasing independence in family relationships, establishing strong and dependable friendships with similar-age peers, and managing emerging romantic desires and experiences. In contrast, during middle to late childhood, there is greater dependence on parents and other adult figures for negotiating social interactions as children focus on developing social abilities and academic skills. Compared to adults and adolescents, preadolescents are strongly embedded in their family context. Parents provide support and feedback throughout this period, and children are more dependent on their parents' abilities to interface with the community, support their development, and model/teach coping and other key life skills than are older adolescents or adults. In addition, the rapidly changing cognitive capacity during this developmental phase makes it unlikely that adult treatments can simply be extended downward.

These differences in both depression and developmental tasks point to a need for developmentally informed treatments during both childhood and adolescence. As a result, family-focused interventions, in which parents can help provide support, model new behavior, and help generalize skills to the home and other context, are likely to be particularly beneficial during childhood. In contrast, traditional cognitive therapies, which rest on the assumption that negative/maladaptive ways of attending to, processing, and remembering render an individual vulnerable to depression, eg,[65,66] may be a better fit for adolescents. Interventions need to be designed with development in mind and should be tailored to address the different cognitive levels and psychosocial contexts of adolescent and preadolescent youth.

DESIGNING FAMILY-CENTERED INTERVENTIONS FOR YOUTH DEPRESSION

Data documenting the efficacy of family-based interventions for adults with mood disorders and showing promise with adolescents, in conjunction with treatment development work and data suggesting the important role of family factors in childhood depression, indicate that family approaches may be a particularly promising modality for depression both in children and adolescents (for review,[67,68]). Specifically, a family-focused approach has potential for addressing depression across multiple family members. The high rate of depressive disorders found among parents of depressed youth underscores the fact that both depressed children and adolescents are likely to be living with depressed parents, particularly mothers.[69] For instance, in our data, the lifetime rate of major depression in mothers and fathers of children with depressive disorders (MDD or DD) was 0.63 and 0.33 respectively.[69] A family-based intervention, which can address disorders in multiple family members and enhance family functioning, may decrease risk of depressive episodes in the family as a whole. This is particularly important because depressions tend to be temporally linked across family members, with depressions in one family member seeming to be triggered by stress associated with another family member's depression.[70]

A family-focused approach can also target specific family processes and stresses that are associated with poor depression outcomes (for review, see Ref.[71]). In our prior work, for example, parental expressed emotion (EE), an index of criticism and emotional overinvolvement in the home, was a strong predictor of outcome for 7- to 14-year old child psychiatric inpatients with MDD or DD.[72] Whereas 100% of children returning to homes with high-EE parents relapsed or showed continuing depression 1 year after hospital discharge, only 20% of children discharged to low-EE homes showed continuing depression or relapsed within that first year. Among a wide range of clinical and demographic variables, only two additional factors were found to be negatively associated with outcome: presence of a comorbid disruptive behavior disorder (attention deficit/hyperactivity, conduct, and oppositional disorders) and chronicity (>1 year of previous illness). However, even after controlling for these factors, EE remained a potent predictor of outcome. With this in mind, we developed a family-based treatment designed to specifically address the developmental needs of school-aged children and their parents through an emphasis on fostering positive and supportive parent–child interactions that scaffold the development of a positive self. This treatment appreciates the multidimensional nature of depression and addresses it systemically by helping parents provide their child additional positive feedback on his or her developmentally appropriate achievements and enhancing family and child coping.

Another advantage of family interventions is that they have greater potential, as compared to individual approaches, for addressing the range of comorbid problems typical in depressed youth. Depressed children often present with comorbid conditions, particularly anxiety and disruptive behavioral disorders.[73] Although family interventions may be depression focused, enhanced family coping, support, and problem solving may have broad effects on child psychopathology more generally.

Family psychoeducational approaches have been used in the treatment of mood disorders in youtheg,[27,74–76] and in adults (for review, see Ref.[67]). These psychoeducational approaches combine education about the disorder with skills enhancement to augment coping. In this article, we describe two intervention approaches as examples of how a family-centered approach can be used to support youth recovery: Family-Focused Treatment for Childhood Depression (FFT-CD) is a developmentally informed treatment specifically designed for preadolescent youth with depression and their families.[26] SAFETY is an intensive 12-week intervention designed to decrease suicide and suicide attempt risk among with a recent history of suicidal behavior.

FFT-CD

Our FFT (formerly referred to as FFI[26]) has roots in family psychoeducational approaches, family-focused treatments developed for adults and adolescents, and cognitive–behavioral interventions. It has also been strongly influenced by interpersonal theories of depression,[77] which emphasize the role of interpersonal stress and functioning as both risk and maintaining factors. Indeed, recent research underscores the bidirectional association between depression and stress, particularly increased interpersonal conflicts and stressors; it emphasizes how depression leads to "stress-generating" interpersonal interactions that then further fuel depression. Thus, the FFT approach conceptualizes depression in youth as a biopsychosocial phenomenon. Biological and environmental factors contribute to depression onset, and cognitive, behavioral, emotional, and biological processes as well as stress impact course and outcome, leading to a downward spiral of escalating symptoms, interactions, and stressors.[78] FFT is designed to reverse the downward spiral of depression and negative interpersonal interactions and provide enhanced support in combating feelings and maladaptive cognitive, behavioral, and emotion regulation processes that are associated with depression.

In creating a family-centered approach that would address the unique developmental needs of depressed preadolescent children, we integrated family systems and cognitive–behavioral models to provide expanded psychoeducation and skills-building within a family context. Specific FFT interventions focus on understanding the family's unique interactional processes while increasing adaptive and decreasing maladaptive interactional sequences. Using the concept of emotional spirals, families are introduced to the idea that interpersonal processes are related to mood states, providing a rationale for intervening in these processes. Two individual sessions, one with the parent(s) and one with the child, are conducted at the outset to facilitate the alliance, address questions, and provide psychoeducation at an appropriate developmental level. All other sessions are conducted with the child and parent(s) together, with siblings and others (eg, grandparents) incorporated as judged to be appropriate.

The FFT consists of five modules:

1. Rapport-building and education about depression, including introduction of an interpersonal model
2. Communication training

3. Fun activities scheduling
4. Problem solving
5. Termination.

This treatment was designed to be flexible in the face of the diverse challenges families bring to treatment. Although modules typically proceed in order, modules 2 through 4 are sometimes reordered depending on the needs of particular families.

Careful attention was paid to constructing a developmentally appropriate and informed intervention that could support durable behavioral change and generalization across multiple settings. Four specific features of the intervention are noted in this regard.

First, because school-aged youths may be uncomfortable talking about family problems, ideas are presented slowly. Handouts are used to describe concepts, and families are provided with numerous hypothetical examples; once they become comfortable with the concepts, they are asked to come up with examples from their own family.

Second, exercises are presented as "games" initially to make them more palatable to school-aged youth, increase the likelihood that these "games" could become "family tools" for combating depression after treatment is over, and create a fun/engaging "behavioral activation" exercise within the session. For example, giving positive feedback is initially presented as a game in which participants draw cards with positive statements written on them from a "hat" and have to give others the (sometimes silly) feedback. In previous work implementing a cognitive behaviorally focused family intervention,[27] depressed school-aged youth preferred the behavioral aspects of CBT over its cognitive aspects, and thus we were careful to emphasize active, behavioral strategies in this family-based model.

Third, because of limits on cognitive development, school-aged children are generally more concrete than adolescents and adults. Therefore, we expanded on Rotheram-Borus and colleagues'[79] approach of using tokens to facilitate positive communication within the family. These tokens, referred to as "thanks chips," are used throughout the treatment; the therapist models using the thanks chips to express appreciation to the child and parents and to give positive feedback. In-session "thanks chips" exercises/games are also used to help youths and parents express positive feelings/appreciation and give positive feedback to one other. In addition, between sessions, "homework" is used to promote generalization and practice of positive communication patterns. Family members are each given a number of thanks chips to take home each week with the goal of "giving all of them away" to other family members before the next session.

Fourth, session handouts use simple language, and skills are broken down into small components that can be mastered in a stepwise fashion. For example, giving positive feedback consists of identifying positive behavior ("catching upward spirals") and giving feedback ("keeping upward spirals going").

Family-Focused Treatment Modules

MODULE 1 includes three psychoeducational sessions:

1. One with the child
2. One with his/her parent(s)
3. One joint session.

Parent session goals include:

1. Providing psychoeducation about depression

2. Supporting parents' roles as models and change agents for their children
3. Emphasizing the role of "stress" in perpetuating family difficulties and child problems/symptoms
4. Refocusing the problem from one of "fixing" the child to one of helping the family to cope with stress and promoting the child's recovery.

Depressed children are often coping with multiple stressors, and teaching new ways of coping with these stressors is meant to enhance parental efficacy. The first session with the parents begins by providing feedback on the diagnostic evaluation, including diagnoses, a brief case conceptualization (emphasizing the role of stress), and treatment recommendations. Although each conceptualization differs depending on life circumstances, comorbidity, and other factors, each includes a description of the symptoms that were apparent, a review of some of the stressors that might be contributing to the symptoms, and a biopsychosocial model for how the symptoms developed and how they could be ameliorated through treatment. The therapist normalizes the frustration and, often, helplessness that parents may feel. Given the fact that depression in children is frequently characterized by irritability as well as the research underscoring the negative interaction qualities of depressed children,[80] we are careful to underscore the bidirectional nature of depression and stress in families; stress can fuel depression and depression can fuel negative family interactions. For example, a child who is dysphoric in facing a negative life event (eg, losing a much loved pet) or an ongoing life stressor (eg, severe bullying at school) may become more anhedonic and negative when interacting with parents, increasing the likelihood of conflicts and impacting his or her ability to access parental support. Parents can become frustrated as their attempts to provide assistance may be unsuccessful. Therapy is presented as an opportunity to learn skills for overcoming depression and for the parents to mobilize family resources and parenting strategies to support the child's recovery.

Module 1 then proceeds to an individual session with the child, in which the therapist engages the child in a discussion of "happy," "sad," and "angry" feelings. The child is then presented a model demonstrating how the behavior of others and the behavior of self and moods are all connected. As with the parent session, the bidirectional association between moods and interpersonal relationships is emphasized. The idea of upward and downward interactional spirals is presented and the child is encouraged to provide examples. Throughout, negative interactions are normalized and their role in perpetuating depression is emphasized.

In the final Module 1 session, the therapist reviews the interactional depression model and the rationale for FFT with the parents and child together. The therapist establishes the family as the unit of treatment by reframing the problem as an interactional one in which, working together, parents and children can help combat depression and create ways of responding within the family that protect the child from some of the negative sequelae of stress. Children and their families are provided information about the ways in which family and other social interactions affect mood, using the concept of emotional spirals (illustrated on handouts). As illustrated in **Fig. 1**, in downward emotional spirals, negative interpersonal communication contributes to negative emotions that further contribute to negative communication and so on. In upward emotional spirals (**Fig. 2**), positive interpersonal interactions contribute to positive emotions that further fuel positive interpersonal interactions. Good family communication and problem solving can be used to turn downward spirals into upward spirals, and all families need to work on these skills, practicing

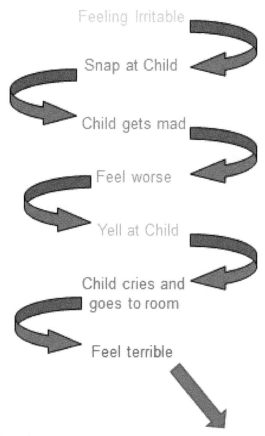

Fig. 1. Downward spiral.

ways to work together effectively. Families are shown pictorial examples of escalating cycles of both positive and negative family communication and are asked to identify similar patterns within their families. Normalizing is used to remind families that all families experience negative and positive spirals, thus disrupting the tendency to blame. The session focus is to identify the understandable patterns that families get into when someone is depressed or confronting high levels of stress and to engender hope that family members can have a positive and effective impact on the depressed individual. The rationale of the treatment is clearly laid out: "to stop downward spirals and to start upward spirals so that everyone feels better."

MODULE 2—"Families Talking to One Another"—takes three or four sessions, includes the child and parent(s), and focuses on communication training. The goals of these sessions are to:

1. Increase the child's assertiveness skills
2. Decrease depressive withdrawal and irritability
3. Engage the family members

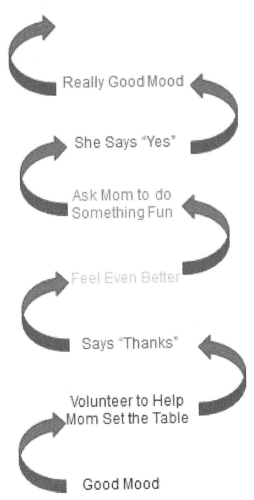

Really Good Mood

She Says "Yes"

Ask Mom to do Something Fun

Feel Even Better

Says "Thanks"

Volunteer to Help Mom Set the Table

Good Mood

Fig. 2. Upward spiral.

4. Encourage the development of empathy.

Specific skills include giving positive feedback to other family members, listening actively, making positive requests for behavioral change, and giving negative feedback. Handouts describe each of the skills to be learned. Role-playing, behavioral rehearsal, and homework assignments are used to help shape these behaviors. The therapist actively models, directs, and provides verbal reinforcement to family members during this learning process. We have created a number of games to reinforce learning. For example, in practicing active listening, players draw a card on which instructions are written for specific self-disclosure (eg, "Describe a time when you felt really afraid"). One player engages in the self-disclosure, another is the "active listener," while other family members have the job of making sure the listener is implementing all the skills listed on the active listening handout. To make it less anxiety provoking for children, this game starts with items that focus on listening for content (eg, "Describe how to make a peanut butter-and-jelly sandwich"), moves to listening for emotion about a third party (eg, "Bob just found out he failed a test, describe how he would feel"), and finally moves to listening to personal emotional self-disclosure (eg, "Describe a time when you felt really angry"). Again, normalization is frequently used, conveying to family members that although these skills are important, it is natural and understandable for all families to need to practice them.

MODULE 3—"Things we do affect how we feel"—takes two or three sessions, includes the child and parents(s), and is based on pleasant activity scheduling strategies. The goals of these sessions are to:

1. Increase positive reinforcers in the child's environment
2. Increase positive family interactions.

Each member specifies several activities that make him or her "feel better after a rough day." The therapist uses this discussion to normalize stress, to emphasize measures that can be taken to reduce its impact, and to encourage communication of needs between family members. Family members use communication exercises to ask others family members to engage in activities. Families are then encouraged to plan and implement several fun activities together as homework. Care is taken to help them select "do-able" activities that require limited resources and time (eg, walking the dog, playing a game, reading a book, or watching a family movie together).

MODULE 4—"We can solve problems together"—takes three or four sessions and includes two sections: problem identification and problem solving. These sessions include the child and parent(s), and at times also include a sibling or siblings, particularly if problems with siblings were contributing to the perpetuation of downward spirals in the family. The goals of the first section of this module, problem identification, are to:

1. Have family members develop problem identification skills
2. Practice self-monitoring of emotional states
3. Reframe problems as choices and opportunities to problem solve.

The goals of the second section of this module, problem solving, are to:

1. Practice conflict resolution skills
2. Empower the family to solve and become more flexible in approaching problems.

Children and their parents are taught to brainstorm possible solutions, to decide upon the optimal solution(s), and to effectively implement the solution(s). The therapist actively presents the family with the steps of problem solving, aids in defining the problem and evaluating the solutions, and reviews the success of the implemented solution(s). Throughout this process, therapists lower family expectations by normalizing problems, framing problem solutions as experiments to be tested, and by emphasizing the need to adjust problem solutions over time.

MODULE 5—"Saying goodbye"—takes one or two sessions. The child is given a colorful notebook including all the handouts that were used in treatment and is provided the opportunity to decorate the cover in order to more take ownership of the material. The therapist, child, and parent(s) look through the handouts together, remembering and reviewing the material. A problem-solving exercise is conducted to solve the problem of how to "keep your new skills going" after termination. The goals of these sessions are to:

1. Provide additional practice in problem solving
2. Encourage generalization of skills
3. Establish a regular family meeting time.

During these sessions, the family members are praised for their hard work, progress is acknowledged, and further work planned as necessary. See **Family-Focused Treatment Case Vignette** and **Fig. 3** for details on FFT in practice.

Family-Focused Treatment Case Vignette

"Emily" was a 9 1/2-year-old girl with dysthymic disorder. She was the middle of three children in an intact family with an older sister and a younger brother. At treatment outset she reported depressed, and frequently "grumpy" and "frustrated," mood most of the day. Emily had good school performance and relationships with peers, but tended to isolate from others when sad. Her mother and father reported intense temperament, perfectionism, and high rejection sensitivity. She had frequent verbal and sometimes physical altercations with her siblings and mother and reported feeling that she was "not part of the family." Her mother believed that Emily hated her, felt hopeless about improving the relationship, and described frequent interactions in which Emily demanded attention but seemed to reject it when it was offered.

Early Treatment

Emily and her mother attended 12 sessions of FFT, and her father joined in when his travel schedule allowed. The first two sessions focused on psychoeducation and engaging the family. Despite the mother's initial expressions of frustration and indications they she had "tried everything," she was quickly engaged. The child initially displayed limited affect, but was able to engage in role plays readily. Initial sessions focusing on enhancing positive interactions resulted in more warmth between the mother and daughter during sessions and reports of more shared enjoyment at home. Thus, positive feedback and active listening exercises and fun activities scheduling were used to strengthen the relationship between Emily and her mother, as well as to enhance the bond with her father, whose frequent travel schedule limited their time together.

Middle Phases of Treatment

The next phase of treatment focused on identifying downward spirals in the family and using communication and problem-solving exercises to address these spirals. Using the FFT model, we were quickly able to identify a downward spiral that recurred with some frequency in which Emily felt sad and wished for support from her mother; however, she did not communicate this wish. In the absence of direct communication, Emily's mother did not recognize her wish and respond as desired, leading Emily to become angry and resentful and push her mother away. This cycle fueled Emily's continuing feelings of increasing isolation, sadness, and anger. **Fig. 3** illustrates this downward spiral.

At session 5, Emily became increasingly withdrawn from treatment and expressed a desire to discontinue. With much support and active listening on the part of the therapist and her mother, she was able to articulate her concerns— the timing of sessions interfered with some valued school activities. The therapist was able to use this problem to illustrate the downward spiral in the therapy, underscore its similarity to the downward spiral that frequently occurred with

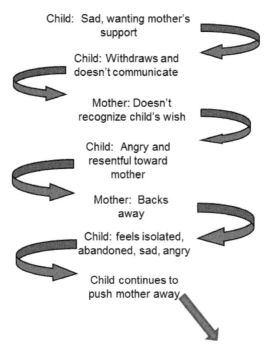

Child: Sad, wanting mother's
support

Child: Withdraws and
doesn't communicate

Mother: Doesn't
recognize child's wish

Child: Angry and
resentful toward
mother

Mother: Backs
away

Child: feels isolated,
abandoned, sad, angry

Child continues to
push mother away

Fig. 3. Emily's downward spiral.

her mother, and model the use of both direct communication and problem solving. This represented a turning point in treatment. Communication training was utilized to help Emily to express her needs and desires to her mother and help her mother to listen actively. Problem-solving training focused on ways in which Emily and her mother could work more effectively together when intense feelings were aroused.

Final Phase of Treatment

During the final treatment sessions, gains were extended and consolidated and plans were made for the future. A sibling session was conducted to identify the "downward spirals" associated with the sibling conflicts (particularly the quick escalation of teasing behavior) and to problem solve potential solutions. This session was lighthearted and Emily enjoyed seeing her siblings "on the hot seat." Problem solving led to the use of a "stop" signal that siblings could employ when teasing interactions felt overwhelming to anyone; this solution appeared to decrease downward spirals at home. The family reported frequently using their skills at home and posting the Communication Training handouts on the refrigerator as a reminder. At the final session, which occurred before the beginning of the new school year, a booklet of handouts from the treatment was provided for Emily, and she was given the opportunity to decorate the cover. The book was used with the family to review the content of the previous 11 sessions. Time was spent anticipating potential problems, including school stress, that might derail progress, and plans were made to confront this stress as a family.

Emily and both her mother and father reported improvements in her mood and in their family interactions by treatment end. These improvements were maintained at the 9-month follow-up and, indeed, continued to be reported by her mother 2 years later.

Our experience to date with FFT for depressed children demonstrates that, first, the intervention is safe, feasible, and acceptable. There were no adverse events associated with FFT; it can be effectively implemented with a wide range of families; and families are interested in such a treatment, seldom dropping out once treatment is initiated. Second, this FFT can positively impact the course of depression.[26] Finally, children report improved family functioning after treatment. Currently a two-site clinical trial (Boston University and UCLA) is being conducted to examine the efficacy of FFT compared to an individual supportive treatment modeled after usual care. In addition to evaluating efficacy, this trial will allow examination of potential moderators (parental EE, severity/chronicity of depression, externalizing comorbidity) and mediators (reduction in parental depression, reduction in family conflict) of treatment impact.

SAFETY TREATMENT FOR ADOLESCENT SUICIDE ATTEMPTERS

The SAFETY treatment was developed as a 12-week intervention designed to be incorporated in emergency mental health services for youths presenting with suicide attempts. SAFETY stands for Safe Alternatives for Teens and Youths, with the program name intended as a reminder to youths and parents that the goal of the program is to enhance SAFETY and identify safe and healthy alternatives to suicidal behavior when problems and stress appear insurmountable. Although this trial is still in progress, and results are not yet available, we offer this description as an illustration of another approach to family treatment that has been developed for adolescents versus younger children.

Our treatment development approach involved a community partnership model in which community providers and service organizations were included from the start, the approach was piloted in community settings early in the treatment development process, and feedback/discussions between the community partners and the research team helped shape the developing treatment strategy. The SAFETY treatment is rooted in cognitive–behavioral and family systems models; builds directly on our work on emergency department (ED) interventions for suicidal youths[81,82] and the "first-generation" Specialized Emergency Room intervention on which the Family Intervention for Suicide Prevention (FISP) was based[83]; and draws on strategies from CBT, dialectical behavior therapy (DBT),[84,85] and multisystemic therapy (MST).[86,87] The target age range for the SAFETY program is 12 through 18 years, primarily because suicide attempt rates are lower before adolescence. A team of two therapists delivers the treatment: one therapist identifies primarily as the child's therapist and the other primarily as the parent(s)' therapist. Sessions generally include an "individual component" with youth and parents seen by their respective therapists and a family component in which youths and parents are brought together to practice or reinforce skills emphasized in the individual session components.

Treatment is conceptualized as involving three phases, although issues addressed in one phase often reemerge in other phases.

1. Phase 1 emphasizes maximizing safety by developing an initial "cognitive–behavioral fit analysis" (CBFA; **Fig. 4**) that describes the risk and protective factors for reattempts and highlights the most important targets for intervention. This CBFA is developed collaboratively with the youth and family and forms the basis for the development of a collaborative treatment plan.
2. Phase 2 emphasizes work on specific skills or areas identified in the CBFT.

3. Phase 3 focuses on consolidation of gains/skill learning and relapse prevention.

Consistent with the MST approach, sessions and phone contacts are scheduled based on youth and parental need. Sessions generally occur on a weekly basis. At the early phases of treatment when attempt risk is high, a more frequent treatment dose is often used to promote learning and strengthen safe coping behavior. Each of these phases is described in greater detail in the text that follows.

The initial phase 1 goal of maximizing youth safety is addressed through an initial in-home session, unless the family is unwilling to have the treatment team visit the home. As in the FISP[81,82] and specialized Emergency Room intervention,[83] this session is conceptualized as a therapeutic intervention and "imminent risk assessment" that focuses on four major tasks.[83] Youths or families who cannot address these tasks are viewed as high-risk and possibly requiring more intensive evaluation and a more restrictive/intensive treatment (eg, hospitalization).

- The first task of the in-home session is to strengthen family support and healthy communication by assisting the youth and parent(s) in identifying positive attributes in the youth and the family as a whole.
- Second, an "emotional thermometer," a hierarchy of "suicide-triggering situations," is identified and youths are supported in identifying feelings, triggers, and associated physiologic signals, thoughts, and behaviors.
- Third, this information is used to develop and practice using a "safety plan" that youths can use to reduce their "emotional temperature" when it is getting too hot and risk for uncontrolled, dangerous, or suicidal behavior is elevated. Diverse coping strategies are encouraged, including behavioral, self-soothing strategies (ie, putting a cool wash cloth on the forehead, listening to comforting music, relaxation, distraction, seeking support from parents), cognitive strategies ("helpful" thoughts), and the development of a "Hope Box" or "Emergency Kit" filled with reminders of reasons for living and cues/facilitators of the safety plan (coping cards, CDs, telephone numbers of people to call for support).
- Fourth, the therapist works to obtain a commitment from the youth to use the SAFETY plan if he or she feels suicidal rather than attempting suicide and a SAFETY plan card is developed to serve as a concrete support that youth can keep and use at times of acute stress/suicide attempt risk to cue him or her to use adaptive coping strategies.

These treatment tasks can be conducted individually with the youth and parent or with the family together; therapists make this choice based on their assessments of which format will prove most effective. However, parents and youths are brought together to finalize the safety plan and share the positive characteristics they each identified in the youth and family. The safety plan always includes telling the youth and parents to page the therapist in the event of concerns about increasing risk and to call 911 or go to the nearest emergency room in a suicidal crisis. Safety plans are used in a wide range of treatments for suicidal youths. The model used here is rooted in that developed by Rotheram-Borus and colleagues[83] and emphasizes identifying specific skills and strategies that youths can use to down-regulate their emotional temperatures and decrease the risk of suicidal behavior.

The initial session also includes psychoeducation regarding the importance of continuing treatment and restricting access to dangerous suicide attempt methods. Indeed, this session is held in the home partly to evaluate potentially dangerous suicide attempt means in the home environment and to facilitate engineering of the environment to reduce suicide attempt risk. The parent therapist meets with the parent(s) individually to identify potentially dangerous suicide attempt (SA) methods in the house, lock up or remove any medications or other dangerous potential SA means, find a strategy for eliminating access to loaded guns if they are present in the home, and address any other major safety issues (eg, on home visits we have discovered balconies that could be used to jump and have arranged for doors to these upper floor balconies to be locked). A metaphor used in this work is to ask the parents to imagine that they are on a diet and their refrigerator is full of your favorite ice cream; we want to change the environment to create as many obstacles as possible to SAs just like they would not want to have the ice cream right there if they had the urge to eat ice cream. Families are taught that as time passes, the more likely it is that the "suicide attempt urge" will pass, something may interrupt the process, or some other protective factor may emerge. The youth therapist meets with the youth individually at this time and asks to see his or her room and any other key features of the environment (eg, a favorite spot in the yard). The therapist works with the youth to restrict access to potentially dangerous SA methods, create cues for using the SAFETY plan in the home (eg, arranging the location of the HOPE Box, coping resources, reminders of reasons for living), and uses any remaining time to get to know the youth better, strengthen the relationship, and reinforce the work completed in session. The therapist also introduces the mood diary as a "practice" between sessions, with youths charting their mood daily as well as any thoughts of deliberate self-injury/suicide attempts and any suicidal or self-injurious behavior. The mood diary is continued as a standard practice throughout treatment.

The second and third sessions during phase 1 focus on developing the CB fit analysis and to identify risk and protective factors at the individual, family, peer, and community level. A chain analysis of the target SA is conducted with the youth and parent(s) in individual sessions to understand the sequence of events, feelings, thoughts, behaviors, and reactions leading up to, during, and after the SA.[84,85] This information is combined with a broader assessment of risk and protective factors to develop the CBFT and collaborative treatment plan. The concept of a SAFETY pyramid is used in the development of the treatment plan.

1. **SAFE settings** form the base of the pyramid, with the importance of restricting access to dangerous SA methods and providing protective supervision and monitoring emphasized.
2. **SAFE people** are emphasized at the next level; the importance of working to increase the likelihood that the youth will turn to the parents and other responsible adults and youths as safe people at times of SA risk is discussed. Because of the increasing focus on peer support during the adolescent years, this is challenging for many families and the structure of the SAFETY program is designed to explicitly promote and practice turning to parents/parent figures instead of self-harm behavior at times of acute risk.
3. **SAFE activities** are promoted, through an analysis of the ways in which youths spend their time, the effect of activities on mood and SA risk, and the development of strategies for increasing time spent in activities that build "a life worth living."[84]
4. **SAFE thoughts** are emphasized at this next level of the pyramid, with an emphasis on finding realistic but helpful ways of thinking that allow individuals to accept what they cannot change and to think about problems in helpful as opposed to hopeless/unhelpful ways.
5. **SAFE stress reactions** form the tip of the pyramid, with an emphasis on the need to develop strategies for managing stress without turning to SA or self-harm.

As in all phases of the intervention, the mood diary is reviewed at the start of each youth session and skills are introduced to facilitate using skills as opposed to resorting to self-harm in high-risk moments. The Hope Box, filled with reminders of reasons for living and cues/resources for using the SAFETY plan (as described earlier) and coping skills is developed and expanded on during phase 1. Because of the high rate of depression among youths attempting suicide (79% reported severe depressive symptoms in our prior study,[81] CBT strategies, such as activity scheduling and developing helpful ways of thinking, are often introduced during phase 1, in addition to the concept of reversing downward spirals into depression and hopelessness through trying different activities and ways of thinking about events. Activity monitoring also provides information regarding the youth's life situation and context, and this is helpful for developing the CBFA. In parent sessions, a safety plan is developed with the parent(s) that focuses on how the parent(s) can identify signs that the youth is moving into a "high-risk temperature zone," how they can regulate their own emotional temperature, and ways they can respond to help their child down-regulate his or her emotional temperature and cope in a safe manner (without suicidality or self-harm).

Across all treatment phases, family sessions follow a standard format and begin with a round of "thanks notes," sticky notes on which family members write something they appreciate about someone else in the family. Family members give these notes to one another to say "thank you" and express appreciation for things done during the week. This is intended to encourage family members to notice and attend to things they appreciate about each other, strengthen their tendencies to tell one another what they like and appreciate, build a more supportive home environment, and increase the likelihood that youths will turn to parents in the event that SA risk should reappear. Therapists generally join this exercise to model the skill and reinforce progress in youths and parents. To promote consolidation and generalization of the individual work to the family environment, each team (youth and parents) then presents a capsule summary of the work they did in session, designed to encourage optimism regarding the work and changes being accomplished. If appropriate, an aspect of one of the skills is introduced in the session. For instance, if the youth has done mood and activity monitoring as part of the session, he or she could introduce this to the parents and have them practice the skill during the next week. Conversely, if parents have worked on active listening during the individual session component, during the family session the parents could share that they are working on being better listeners and introduce the active listening skills and an active listening practice activity/game during the session. The session ends with a practice assignment for the next week that always includes "thanks notes," and therapists may conclude the session with another round of "thanks notes." Some families have opted to send text messages as "thanks notes," which has appeal for many youths and parents who are more technologically inclined.

Given the heterogeneity among youths who attempt suicide and their environmental circumstances, the CBFA varies across youths. However, several common themes emerge in phase 2 of treatment. As noted previously, much of the work done individually with youths focuses on CBT and DBT strategies; they are asked to monitor their moods, self-harm thoughts, and behavior between sessions using the mood diary and skills are frequently introduced as part of the card as a reminder that the goal is to use the "skills" versus self-injurious behavior to cope with stress/ "unbearable" emotions and to obtain data on the effects of skill use/practice. We have found that in almost every case we have done some work on activities, thoughts, emotion regulation, and communication/problem solving. With parents, we have found that active listening is consistently a key target, as many parents rush to problem solve or give advice when the youth is in need of understanding and validation before effective problem solving can occur. Because depression and suicidal tendencies can run in families, and having a child attempt suicide is very stressful for any parent, a focus on parental emotional needs is important; in some instances the CBFT or parent reactions to the SA and sequelae of the SA dictate a need to focus on strategies for addressing parental depression, anxiety, distress, or even suicidality, including referral for treatment (medication or individual). Regardless of the treatment plan and specific skills emphasized during phase 2 (based on the CBFT), a consistent theme across families has been to develop and practice strategies for youths to be able to turn to their parents for support at times of emerging suicidal impulses/SA-risk, and for parents to develop strategies for responding that facilitate youths down-regulating their emotional temperatures and returning to safer affective states. This frequently involves helping parents listen and support youths in using distress tolerance skills such as distraction (ie, validating the youths emotional reactions/stress and shifting the focus to activities like making cookies, taking the dog for a walk) to help youths regain a sense of emotional control so that they can get through the stressful moment and address the stressor with greater emotional strength and skill. Based on the CBFT and treatment plan, other responsible adults may be brought into the treatment or introduced as another resource to which youths can turn. This could include other relatives, providers (ie, primary care, therapists, school counselors), or adults in their school or community.

Phase 3 emphasizes relapse prevention. Strategies that have proven helpful to the youth and family over the course of treatment are reviewed and the youth is asked to engage in a relapse prevention task.[88,89] This task is introduced as an opportunity for the youth to review the chain of events leading to the index SA and to replay the events using the new skills developed during treatment. The youth is also asked to consider potential new stresses that might have previously triggered self-harm/SA impulses and how he or she could use skills to respond to these stresses in safe ways without resorting to self-harm. A guided imagery approach is used to help the youth capture the emotions associated with the initial SA chain to assess the youth's ability to reexperience intense distress, tolerate these emotions, and use skills instead of self-harm behavior/SAs. A similar approach is used with parents to help them to consolidate skills for supporting their youths in times of high SA risk. Throughout phase 3, skill practice is emphasized to further strengthen the abilities of youths to use skills instead of SA/self-harm behavior and the increase the parental ability to support youths in tolerating stress and distress and using skills to down-regulate their child's emotional response. This often involves continuing work with parents on practicing skills to down-regulate their own emotional reactions so that they can provide effective support to their children and feel more confident and less stressed. Although youths and parents know that the treatment is time limited from the start, phase 3 also emphasizes termination and links youths and families to additional treatment resources as needed. A goal of phase 3 is to have youths and families connected to other providers at the end of the SAFETY treatment for additional mental health treatment and, when needed, to primary care, school, or other services. Because of the barriers to mental health care, both real and perceived (ie, stigma and the desire of youths and parents to feel that they have developed new and effective strategies for addressing stress, intense emotions, and self-harm tendencies), we consistently emphasize primary care as a resource for mental health as well as health monitoring and care.[2,27,81]

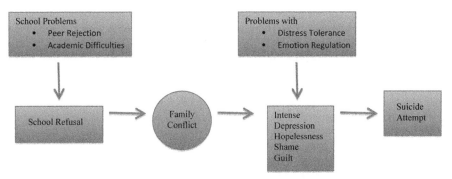

Fig. 4. Sample Cognitive-Behavioral Fit Analysis.

Safety Case Vignette

"Jane" was a 15-year-old girl who lived with her single mother. She presented to the emergency department (ED) after a suicide attempt by overdose. As illustrated in the initial cognitive–behavioral fit analysis below, Jane's suicide attempt was triggered by a conflict with her mother that developed when Jane refused to go to school and her mother insisted. At school, Jane was rejected by peers, had academic difficulties, and had few positive experiences. She disliked school, frequently faked illness to avoid going to school, and felt hopeless and helpless to change her life situation. Her mother worked hard to support them and could not stay home with Jane because of fear of losing her job. Jane was aware of that, which made her feel guilt and shame and intensified her emotional distress. When asked about what happened before the suicide attempt, Jane stated: "I couldn't stand it. Nothing helps. I hate school. I can't get along with my mother. I just wanted to die, make all of the bad feelings go away, when I saw the pills I just took all of the pills in the bottle. I was done with it." Jane had a history of one prior suicide attempt by overdose.

Phase 1 (Sessions 1–3): Development of CBFA and Intervention Plan

Session 1 was conducted in the home and represented an expansion on our ED intervention.[81,82] The session began by working with Jane to notice her strengths and positive characteristics and help Jane and her mother notice strengths and positive characteristics in their family. Using standard procedures from our ED intervention, a feeling thermometer was used to assist Jane in identifying high-risk situations for suicidal behavior and her reactions to these situations, with the goal of identifying feelings, thoughts, and physiologic and behavioral warning signs that her temperature was reaching a high-risk zone.

Based on these data, an initial SAFETY plan was developed that emphasized strategies that Jane could use to "reduce her temperature" (regulate her emotion and enhance distress tolerance), such as putting a cold cloth on her head and focusing on the way this felt, watching a funny video, reading a series of coping self-statements (eg, Just take things one step at a time), and going to her mother and asking her to engage in an activity with her without talking about anything except the activity. Jane and her mother enjoyed each other when engaged in an activity (eg, baking cookies), but unstructured conversation frequently led to escalating tension and feelings of shame and guilt. Jane appeared enthusiastic about treatment. She agreed to use the SAFETY plan if she felt her temperature rising and contracted to tell her mother if she felt she could not control a suicidal impulse. Emergency telephone numbers were given to Jane and her mother and they agreed to contact the therapist in an emergency. To restrict access to potentially dangerous suicide attempt methods, all medications, razor blades, and other potentially dangerous means of self-harm were removed/locked up (SAFE SETTINGS/ENVIRONMENT). Standard practices/homework were assigned, including the mood diary for Jane and thanks notes for Jane and her mother.

In **Session 2**, the individual work with Jane began with a check on the week's practice/mood diary and thanks notes, her safety, how the coping strategies listed in her SAFETY plan had worked, and to conduct an expanded fit analysis aimed at obtaining a chain analysis of the events leading up to the suicide attempt and consequences of the attempt. The session ended with the "hope box" task, with Jane creating a box in which she placed cues and "tools" to facilitate and cue the use of SAFE coping strategies (eg, a washcloth, favorite video, pictures of good times in her life and places she wanted to go, cookie recipes she wanted to try, and a "relaxation CD" given to her by the therapist). She called this box "Kelly," as she thought "hope box" was "weird." In addition to the mood diary, her practice for the week also involved trying out "Kelly" during the week and creating a "mini-Kelly" that she could take to school with her to help her get through the day. The session with the mother similarly involved practice review (thanks notes); review of SAFETY and incidents during the week; a chain analysis of the suicide attempt; introduction of the SAFETY pyramid; and review of risk and protective factors for suicide attempts in the family, peer, school, and community systems. The family component of the session was 15 minutes and involved a round of thanks notes, capsule summaries in which Jane presented "Kelly" and the idea of developing a "mini-Kelly" to help her get through the stress of school, as well as her mother discussing the SAFETY pyramid and how she was working on being a SAFE person for Jane and creating a SAFE environment with reduced stress.

Session 3 built on the work of the prior sessions with the standard format. The focus was on identifying SAFETY versus RISK within multiple systemic contexts (family, peers, school, community) and at the different intervention levels (SAFETY pyramid), and developing a collaborative treatment plan. Based on the CBFA, the treatment plan emphasized the importance of maintaining a SAFE home environment (SETTING) where access to suicide attempt methods was restricted and interactions between Jane and her mother were more supportive and less tense (SAFE PEOPLE). The positive behaviors and activities that they had identified through the "thanks notes" practice were used to highlight SAFE ACTIVITIES & ACTIONS. The importance of SAFE THOUGHTS versus. thoughts of hopelessness, guilt, and shame was emphasized; and the coping strategies that Jane had found most helpful were related to SAFE STRESS REACTIONS on the SAFETY pyramid and tools and reminders that Jane could keep in "Kelly" and "mini-Kelly." Treatment options were discussed, including the possibility of considering an evaluation for possible medication treatment, which neither Jane nor her mother wanted. During the family portion of the session, there was an emphasis on reinforcing progress using the "thanks notes" to communicate things that Jane and her mother appreciated in their daily interactions.

Phase 2: Intervention Plan Implementation
Based on the CBFA, the most proximal triggers of suicidal behavior appeared to be (1) hopelessness and maladaptive depressotypic thought patterns, (2)

problems with distress tolerance and emotion regulation, and (3) family tension. Therefore, building on the foundation of the initial sessions and practices that emphasized building family support (eg, family "thanks notes"), a decision was made to begin with modules designed to build hope and more hopeful and SAFE thoughts as well as teaching skills for tolerating distress and regulating intense emotions. The goal was to support Jane in using her emotion regulation and distress tolerance skills instead of engaging in non-suicidal self-injury or suicidal behavior. With the mother, the emphasis was on strengthening family support, communication, and problem solving. Because family conflict had triggered the attempt, it was viewed as critical to enhance the mother's ability to listen to and understand Jane's experiences and reactions, communication, and conflict resolution skills. Family sessions emphasized promoting "active listening," communication, and problem solving with the goal of increasing supportive interactions and the likelihood that Jane would be able to turn to her mother rather than engaging in suicidal behavior. Throughout all sessions, there was an emphasis on reinforcing the skills presented in prior sessions (eg, when addressing family communication, ways in which different thoughts could help vs impede the communication process were discussed). A plan was developed with the school to create a more supportive school environment, with some class changes, a counselor whom Jane could go to if she had a problem, and a plan for Jane to help out at the library during lunch period (a time that Jane found particularly stressful).

Phase 3: Consolidation and Relapse Prevention

During the final 3 sessions, the problems and issues that Jane and her mother brought up were addressed using strategies introduced in previous sessions. The mother was encouraged to continue to speak with the school counselor about strategies for improving Jane's school situation. Following the relapse prevention task, a relapse prevention plan was developed that emphasized noting early warning signs, seeking help through her primary care physician (whom Jane liked and confided in), seeking support at school from the school counselor, and practicing and reinforcing strategies for coping with stress. At the intervention end point, Jane had begun weekly therapy with the school counselor and a follow-up appointment had been scheduled with the primary care physician. She had not shown any suicidal behavior during the treatment period. Although she had experienced suicidal ideation at times, she had been able to manage these thoughts with her coping strategies and "Kelly," and at the treatment end-point she reported significant improvements in suicidal ideation, hopelessness, depression, and family communication and support.

DEVELOPMENTAL ISSUES

These two approaches—FFT for childhood depression and the SAFETY program for adolescent suicide prevention—highlight a number of ways in which interventions are tailored to meet the developmental levels and needs of youths. Some of these are noted below.

First, we have found that cognitive and emotional differences across development have influenced how quickly we can address issues within families. With younger children, we have found that "warm-up" activities, like games and practice focused on problems not specific to the child, are often helpful in engaging the child in a nonblaming atmosphere. Thus, in working with families of younger children, we take a slow approach, gradually addressing family-specific problems as children gain skills and become more comfortable in the family therapy setting. In contrast, when working with adolescents, we continue to use "games" to practice skills and begin with examples that are not likely to trigger intense emotions, yet we are able to move to emotionally charged issues more quickly and focus communication and problem-solving exercises on issues that are specifically relevant to individual adolescents and their families (ie, curfews, tensions in the home).

Second, developmental factors influence the degree to which family members are seen in conjoint versus individual sessions and how other family members might be integrated in the treatment model. Younger children are strongly embedded within the family context and, often, dependent on parents for support in solving problems both within the family context and the larger social environment. When parents demonstrate good listening skills and support, younger children generally welcome their input in solving problems with peers, providing an opportunity for the therapist to underscore the role of parents as potential helping agents. Thus, we have found it useful to include both the child and parent in most family sessions. When individual sessions are needed, they usually are briefer, involve parents alone, and focus on implementation of behavior management techniques/strategies and or marital/family stressors that impact parenting. In addition, younger children often benefit from the inclusion of siblings in some sessions, particularly those focused on problem solving. In working with families of younger children, several specific family problems regularly emerge, including cleaning up around the house, doing homework, TV/computer time, and, regularly, conflicts with siblings. Thus, problem-solving sessions focused on developing strategies for improving sibling relationships can reduce stress for all family members. In contrast, given the tendencies for adolescents to shift their focus to peers and outside/nonfamily activities as they mature, we have found that it is often useful to have more individual time with adolescents to address issues that they may not be able to discuss with their parents present (ie, romantic breakups that are often precipitants of depression and suicidal behavior, bullying, and risky behavior or situations). Conversely, individual time with parents provides opportunities to address sensitive issues openly, without the potential of adverse youth reactions (ie, parent depression, marital tensions, parental concerns about youth friends or behavior). By combining the individual time with youths and parents, we have found that we are able to effectively address individual issues, gain information that would not emerge in family sessions, prepare youths and parents to come together in "new ways," disrupt negative family interactional sequences/scripts, enhance skills for working together as a family to reduce SA risk in the youth, and promote healthy functioning. This approach is similar to those employed by Beardslee and colleagues[90] in their preventive interventions and Diamond and colleagues[91] in attachment-based family therapy.

SUMMARY

In sum, brief family psychoeduction has been used to improve treatment engagement[74] and is considered a standard of care.[1] Evidence is emerging that more intensive family interventions may be efficacious in the prevention[92,93] and treatment of youth depression[24,90] and suicidality.[19]

In this article we have reviewed the literature on family treatments for youth depression and described and illustrated two family-based treatment models that specifically incorporate developmental factors. We expect that the next few years will demonstrate more conclusively that increased inclusion of families in the treatment of depression and suicide may broaden social support, help skill generalization, and enhance treatment efficacy.

REFERENCES

1. Birmaher B, Brent D, Bernet W, et al. Practice parameter for the assessment and treatment of children and adolescents with depressive disorders. J Am Acad Child Adolesc Psychiatry 2007;46(11):1503–26.
2. Asarnow JR, Jaycox LH, Duan N. Depression and role impairment among adolescents in primary care clinics. J Adolesc Health 2005;37(6):477–83.
3. Jaycox LH, Asarnow JR, Sherbourne CD, et al. Adolescent primary care patients' preferences for depression treatment. Admin Policy Ment Health Ment Health Serv Res 2006;33(2):198–207.
4. Nemeroff CB. The burden of severe depression: a review of diagnostic challenges and treatment alternatives. J Psychiatr Res 2007;41(3):189–206.
5. Libby AM, Orton HD, Valuck RJ. Persisting decline in depression treatment after FDA warnings. Arch Gen Psychiatry 2009;66(6):633–9.
6. Brent DA, Holder D, Kolko D, et al. A clinical psychotherapy trial for adolescent depression comparing cognitive, family, and supportive therapy. Arch Gen Psychiatry 1997;54:877–85.
7. Clarke G, Debar L, Lynch F, et al. A randomized effectiveness trial of brief cognitive-behavioral therapy for depressed adolescents receiving antidepressant medication. J Am Acad Child Adolesc Psychiatry 2005;44(9):888–98.
8. Clarke GN, Rohde P, Lewinsohn PM, et al. Cognitive-behavioral treatment of adolescent depression: efficacy of acute group treatment and booster sessions. J Am Acad Child Adolesc Psychiatry 1999;38:272–9.
9. Lewinsohn PM, Clarke FN, Hops H, et al. Cognitive-behavioral treatment for depressed adolescents. Behav Ther 1990;21:385–401.
10. March J, Silva S, Petrycki S, et al; Treatment for Adolescents With Depression Study (TADS) Team. Fluoxetine, cognitive-behavioral therapy, and their combination for adolescents with depression: Treatment for Adolescents with Depression Study (TADS) randomized controlled trial. JAMA 2004;292(7):807–20.
11. Melvin GA, Tonge BJ, King NJ, et al. A comparison of cognitive-behavioral therapy, sertraline, and their combination for adolescent depression. J Am Acad Child Adolesc Psychiatry 2006;45(10):1151–61.
12. Mufson L, Weissman MM, Moreau D, et al. Efficacy of interpersonal psychotherapy for depressed adolescents. Arch Gen Psychiatry 1999;56:573–9.
13. Rohde P, Clarke GN, Mace DE, et al. An efficacy/effectiveness study of cognitive-behavioral treatment for adolescents with and without comorbid major depression and conduct disorder. J Am Acad Child Adolesc Psychiatry 2004;43:660–8.
14. Rosselló J, Bernal G. The efficacy of cognitive-behavioral and interpersonal treatments for depression in Puerto Rican adolescents. J Consult Clin Psychol 1999;67:734–45.
15. Rosselló J, Bernal G, Rivera-Medina C. Individual and group CBT and IPT for Puerto Rican adolescents with depressive symptoms. Cult Divers Ethnic Minor Psychol 2008;14:234–45.
16. Mufson L, Dorta KP, Wickramaratne P, et al. A randomized effectiveness trial of interpersonal psychotherapy for depressed adolescents. Arch Gen Psychiatry 2004;61:577–84.
17. Weersing VR, Iyengar S, Kolko DJ, et al. Effectiveness of cognitive-behavioral therapy for adolescent depression: a benchmarking investigation. Child Adolesc Psychiatr Clin North Am 2006;15(4):939–57.

18. Diamond GS, Reis BF, Diamond GM, et al. Attachment based family therapy for depressed adolescents: a treatment development study. J Am Acad Child Adolesc Psychiatry 2002;41:1190–6.

19. Diamond GS, Wintersteen MB, Brown GK, et al. J Am Acad Child Adolesc Psychiatry 2010;49(2):122–31.

20. Vostanis P, Feehan C, Grattan E, et al. A randomized controlled out-patient trial of cognitive-behavioral treatment for children and adolescents with depression: 9-month follow-up. J Affect Disord 1996;40:105–16.

21. Wood A, Harrington R, Moore A. Controlled trial of a brief cognitive-behavioral intervention in adolescent patients with depressive disorders. J Child Psychiatry Allied Disciplines 1996;37:737–46.

22. Flory V. A novel clinical intervention for severe childhood depression and anxiety. Clin Child Psychol Psychiatry 2004;9(1):9–23.

23. Kaslow NJ, Baskin ML, Wyckoff SC. A biopsychosocial treatment approach for depressed children and adolescents. In: Kaslow FW, editor. Comprehensive handbook of psychotherapy: integrative/eclectic, vol. 4. Hoboken (NJ): John Wiley & Sons; 2002. p. 31–57.

24. Kovacs M, Sherrill J, George CJ, et al. Contextual emotion-regulation therapy for childhood depression: description and pilot testing of a new intervention. J Am Acad Child Adolesc Psychiatry 2006;45(8):892–903.

25. Stark KD, Hoke J, Ballatore M, et al. Treatment of child and adolescent depressive disorders. In: Hibbs ED, Jensen PS, editors. Psychosocial treatments for child and adolescent disorders: empirically based strategies for clinical practice. 2nd edition. Washington, DC: American Psychological Association; 2005. p. 239–65.

26. Tompson MC, Pierre CB, McNeil Haber F, et al. Family-focused treatment for childhood-onset depressive disorders: results of an open trial. Clin Child Psychol Psychiatry 2007;12:403–20.

27. Asarnow JR, Scott CV, Mintz J. A combined cognitive-behavioral family education intervention for depression in children: a treatment development study. Cogn Ther Res 2002;26:221–9.

28. King CA, Kirschenbaum DS. An experimental evaluation of a school-based program for children at risk: Wisconsin Early Intervention. J Commun Psychol 1990;18:167–77.

29. Fristad MA, Verducci JS, Walters K, et al. Impact of multifamily psychoeducational psychotherapy in treating children aged 8 to 12 years with mood disorders. Arch Gen Psychiatry 2009;66(9):1013–20.

30. Stark KD, Streusand W, Krumholz LS, et al. Cognitive-behavioral therapy for depression: the ACTION treatment program for girls. In Weisz JR, Kazdin AE, editors. Evidence-based psychotherapies for children and adolescents. 2nd edition. New York: Guilford Press; 2010. p. 93–109.

31. Weisz JR, McCarty CA, Valeri SM. Effects of psychotherapy for depression in children and adolescents: a meta-analysis. Psychol Bull 2006;132(1):132–49.

32. American Academy of Child and Adolescent Psychiatry. Practice parameter for the assessment and treatment of children and adolescents with suicidal behavior. J Am Acad Child Adolesc Psychiatry 2001;40:24S–51S.

33. Lewinsohn PM, Shankman SA, Gau JM, et al. The prevalence and comorbidity of subthreshold psychiatric conditions. Psychol Med 2004;34:613–22.

34. Kessler RC, Foster CL, Saunders WB, et al. Social consequences of psychiatric disorders I: Educational attainment. Am J Psychiatry 1995;152(7):1026–32.

35. Bardone AM, Moffitt T, Caspi A, et al. Adult mental health and social outcomes of adolescent girls with depression and conduct disorder. Dev Psychopathol 1996;8(4): 811–29.

36. Fleming JE, Boyle MH, Offord DR. The outcome of adolescent depression in the Ontario Child Health Study follow-up. J Am Acad Child Adolesc Psychiatry 1993; 32(1):28–33.

37. Lewinsohn PM, Rohde P, Klein DN, et al. Natural course of adolescent depression. J Am Acad Child Adolesc Psychiatry 1999;38:56–63.

38. Pine DS, Cohen P, Gurley D, et al. The risk for early-adulthood anxiety and depressive disorders in adolescents with anxiety and depressive disorders. Arch Gen Psychiatry 1998;55(1):56–64.

39. Weissman MM, Wolk S, Wickramaratne P, et al. Children with prepubertal-onset major depressive disorder and anxiety grown up. Arch Gen Psychiatry 1999;56(9): 794–801.

40. Kashani JH, Burbach DJ, Rosenberg TK. Perception of family conflict resolution and depressive symptomatology in adolescents. J Am Acad Child Adolesc Psychiatry 1988;27(1):42–8.

41. Sheeber L, Hops H, Davis B. Family processes in adolescent depression. Clin Child Fam Psychol Rev 2001;4(1):19–35.

42. Hazel NA, Hammen C, Brennan PA, et al. Early childhood adversity and adolescent depression: the mediating role of continued stress. Psychol Med 2008;38:581–9.

43. Sim H. Relationship of daily hassles and social support to depression and antisocial behavior among early adolescents. J Youth Adolesc 2000;29:647–59.

44. Wang J, Nansel TR, Iannotti RJ. Cyber and traditional bullying: differential association with depression. J Adolesc Health 2011;48(4):415–7.

45. McFarlane AH, Bellissimo A, Norman GR, et al. Adolescent depression in a school-based community sample: preliminary findings on contributing social factors. J Youth Adolesc 1994;23(6):601–20.

46. Stein D, Williamson DE, Birmaher B, et al. Parent-child bonding and family functioning in depressed children and children at high risk and low risk for future depression. J Am Acad Child Adolesc Psychiatry 2000;39(11):1387–95.

47. Harkness KL, Stewart JG. Symptom specificity and the prospective generation of life events in adolescence. J Abnorm Psychol 2009;118:278–87.

48. Hammen C. Stress generation in depression: reflections on origins, research, and future directions. J Clin Psychol 2006;62:1065–82.

49. Birmaher B, Arbelaez C, Brent D. Course and outcome of child and adolescent major depressive disorder. Child Adolesc Psychiatr Clin North Am 2002;11(3):619–38.

50. Kovacs M, Feinberg TL, Crouse-Novak MA, et al. Depressive disorders in childhood. Arch Gen Psychiatry 1984;41:643–9.

51. McCauley E, Myers K, Mitchell J, et al. Depression in young people: initial presentation and clinical course. J Am Acad Child Adolesc Psychiatry 1993;32(4):714–22.

52. Harrington R, Fudge H, Rutter M, et al. Adult outcomes of childhood and adolescent depression. I. Psychiatric status. Arch Gen Psychiatry 1990;47(5):465–73.

53. Kovacs M. Presentation and course of major depressive disorder during childhood and later years of the life span. J Am Acad Child Adolesc Psychiatry 1996;35(6): 705–15.

54. Kovacs M, Obrosky S, Gatsonis C, et al. First-episode major depressive and dysthymic disorder in childhood: clinical and sociodemographic factors in recovery. J Am Acad Child Adolesc Psychiatry 1997;36(6):777–84.

55. Gould MS, King R, Greenwald S, et al. Psychopathology associated with suicidal ideation and attempts among children and adolescents. J Am Acad Child Adolesc Psychiatry 1998;37(9):915–23.
56. King SM, Iacono WG, McGue M. Childhood externalizing and internalizing psychopathology in the prediction of early substance use. Addiction 2004;99(12):1548–59.
57. McCauley E, Myers K. The longitudinal clinical course of depression in children and adolescents. Child Adolesc Psychiatr Clin North Am 1992;1:183–96.
58. Puig-Antich J, Lukens E, Davies M, et al. I. Psychosocial functioning in prepubertal major depressive disorders. I. Interpersonal relationships during the depressive episode. Arch Gen Psychiatry 1985;42(5):500–7.
59. Puig-Antich J, Lukens E, Davies M, et al. II. Interpersonal relationships after sustained recovery from affective episode. Arch Gen Psychiatry 1985b;42(5):511–7.
60. Garber J, Kriss MR, Koch M, et al. Recurrent depression in adolescents: a follow-up study. J Am Acad Child Adolesc Psychiatry 1988;27(1):49–54.
61. NIMH. National plan for research on child and adolescent mental disorders: a report requested by the U.S. Congress. 1990.
62. Lewinsohn PM, Hops H, Roberts RE, et al. Adolescent psychopathology: I. Prevalence and incidence of depression and other DSM-III-R disorders in high school students. J Abnorm Psychol 1993;102:133–44.
63. Alloy LB, Abramson LY. The adolescent surge in depression and emergence of gender differences: a biocognitive vulnerability-stress model in development context. In: Romer D, Walker EL, editors. Adolescent psychopathology and the developing brain. New York: Oxford University Press; 2007. p. 284–312.
64. Nolen-Hoeksema S, Girgus JS. Explanatory style and achievement, depression, and gender differences in childhood and early adolescence. In: Buchanan G, Seligman MP, editors. Explanatory style. Hillsdale (NJ): Lawrence Erlbaum Associates; 1995. p. 57–70.
65. Abramson LY, Seligman ME, Teasdale JD. Learned helplessness in humans: critique and reformulation. J Abnorm Psychol 1978;87(1):49–74.
66. Beck AT, Rush AJ, Shaw BF, et al. Cognitive therapy of depression. New York: Guilford Press; 1979.
67. Miklowitz DJ, Tompson MC. Family variables and interventions in schizophrenia. In: Sholevar G, editor. Textbook of family and couples therapy: clinical applications. Arlington (VA): American Psychiatric Publishing; 2003. p. 585–617.
68. Tompson MC, Dingman K. Treatment strategies for depression in youth. In: Matson JL, Andrasik F, Matson ML, editors. Treating childhood psychopathology and developmental disabilities. New York (NY): Springer Science & Business Media, LLC; 2008. p. 221–52. Chapter 8.
69. Asarnow JR, Woo S, Mintz J, et al. Family factors in youth depression: implications for personalized treatment. Paper presented at the Annual Meetings of the American Academy of Child and Adolescent Psychiatry. Honolulu, HI, October, 2009.
70. Hammen C, Burge K, Adrian C. Timing of mother and child depression in a longitudinal study of children at risk. J Consult Clin Psychol 1991;59:341–5.
71. Tompson MC, McKowen JW, Asarnow JR. Adolescent mood disorders and familial processes. In: Allen NB, Sheeber L, editors. Adolescent emotional development and the emergence of depressive disorders. Cambridge (UK): Cambridge University Press; 2009. p. 280–98. Chapter 15.
72. Asarnow JR, Goldstein MJ, Tompson MC, et al. One-year outcomes of depressive disorders in child psychiatric in-patients: evaluation of the prognostic power of a brief measure of expressed emotion. J Child Psychol Psychiatry 1993;34(2):129–37.

73. Birmaher B, Ryan ND, Brent DA, et al. Childhood and adolescent depression: a review of the past 10 years, Part I. J Am Acad Child Adolesc Psychiatry 1996;35:1427–39.

74. Brent DA, Poling K, McKain B, et al. A psychoeducational program for families of affectively ill children and adolescents. J Am Acad Child Adolesc Psychiatry 1993; 32(4):770–4.

75. Fristad MA, Gavazzi SM, Soldano KW. Multi-family psychoeducation groups for childhood mood disorders: a program description and preliminary efficacy data. Contemp Fam Ther 1998;20:385–402.

76. Miklowitz DJ, Biuckians A, Richards JA. Early-onset bipolar disorder: a family treatment perspective. Dev Psychopathol 2006;18(4):1247–65.

77. Joiner T, Coyne JC. The interactional nature of depression. Washington, DC: American Psychological Association Press; 1999.

78. Asarnow J, Jaycox LH, Tompson MC. Depression in youth: psychosocial interventions. J Clin Child Psychol 2001;30:33–47.

79. Rotheram-Borus M, Goldstein AM, Elkavich AS. Treatment of suicidality: a family intervention for adolescent suicide attempters. In: Hofmann SG, Tompson MC, editors. Treating chronic and severe mental disorders: a handbook of empirically supported interventions. New York: Guilford Press; 2002. p. 191–212.

80. Hamilton EB, Asarnow JR, Tompson MC. Social, academic, and behavioral competence of depressed children: relationship to diagnostic status and family interaction style. J Youth Adolesc 1997;26(1):77–87.

81. Asarnow JR, Berk M, Baraff LJ. Family intervention for suicide prevention: a specialized emergency department intervention for suicidal youth. Prof Psychol Res Pract 2009;40(2):118–25.

82. Asarnow JR, Baraff L, Berk M, et al. Effects of an emergency department mental health intervention for linking pediatric suicidal patients to follow up mental health treatment: a randomized controlled trial. Psychiatr Serv, in press.

83. Rotheram-Borus MJ, Piacentini J, Cantwell C, et al. The 18-month impact of an emergency room intervention for adolescent suicide attempters. J Consult Clin Psychol 2000;68:1081–3.

84. Linehan MM. Cognitive-behavioral treatment of borderline personality disorder. New York: Guilford Press; 1993.

85. Miller AL, Rathus JH, Linehan MM. Dialectical behavior therapy with suicidal adolescents. New York: Guilford Press; 2007.

86. Henggeler SW, Rowland MD, Halliday-Boykins C, et al. One-year follow-up of multisystemic therapy as an alternative to the hospitalization of youths in psychiatric crisis. J Am Acad Child Adolesc Psychiatry 2003;42(5):543–51.

87. Huey SJ Jr, Henggeler SW, Rowland MD, et al. Multisystemic therapy effects on attempted suicide by youths presenting psychiatric emergencies. J Am Acad Child Adolesc Psychiatry 2004;43(2):183–90.

88. Berk MS, Henriques GR, Warman DM, et al. A cognitive therapy intervention for suicide attempters: an overview of the treatment and case examples. Cognitive and Behavioral Practice 2004;11(3):265–77.

89. Brown TA, Chorpita BF, Korotitsch W, et al. Psychometric properties of the Depression Anxiety Stress Scales (DASS) in clinical samples. Behav Res Ther 1997;35:79–89.

90. Beardslee WR, Salt P, Porterfield K, et al. Comparison of preventive interventions for families with parental affective disorder. J Am Acad Child Adolesc Psychiatry 1993; 32(2):254–63.

91. Diamond GS, Levy SA, Israel P, et al. Attachment-based family therapy for depressed adolescents. In: Essau CA, editor. Treatments for adolescent depression: theory and practice. New York: Oxford University Press; 2009. p. 215–37.

92. Beardslee WR, Wright EJ, Gladstone TRG, et al. Long-term effects from a randomized trial of two public health preventive interventions for parental depression. J Fam Psychol 2007; 21(4):703–13.

93. D'Angelo EJ, Llerena-Quinn R, Shapiro R, et al. Adaptation of the Preventive Intervention Program for Depression for use with predominantly low-income Latino families. Fam Process 2009;48(2):269–91.

94. Goodyer I, Dubicka B, Wilkinson P, et al. Selective serotonin reuptake inhibitors (SSRIs) and routine specialist care with and without cognitive behaviour therapy in adolescents with major depression: randomised controlled trial. BMJ 2007;335:142.

95. Birmaher B, Brent DA, Kolko D, et al. Clinical outcome after short-term psychotherapy for adolescents with major depressive disorder. Arch Gen Psychiatry 2000;57(1):29–36.

96. Brent D, Emslie G, Clarke G, et al. Switching to another SSRI or to venlafaxine with or without cognitive behavioral therapy for adolescents with SSRI-resistant depression: The TORDIA randomized controlled trial. JAMA 2008;299(8):901–13.

97. Clarke GN, Hornbrook M, Lynch F, et al. Group cognitive-behavioral treatment for depressed adolescent offspring of depressed parents in a health maintenance organization. J Am Acad Child Adolesc Psychiatry 2002;41(3):305–13.

98. Fine S, Forth A, Gilbert M, et al. Group therapy for adolescent depressive disorder: a comparison of social skills and therapeutic support. J Am Acad Child Adolesc Psychiatry 1991;30(1):79–85.

99. Kennard BD, Clarke GN, Weersing V, et al. Effective components of TORDIA cognitive-behavioral therapy for adolescent depression: preliminary findings. J Consult Clin Psychol 2009;77(6):1033–41.

100. Reed MK. Social skills training to reduce depression in adolescents. Adolescence 1994;29:293–302.

101. Butler L, Mietzitis S, Friedman R, et al. The effect of two school-based intervention programs on depressive symptoms in preadolescents. American Educational Research Journal 1980;17(1):111–9.

102. De Cuyper S, Timbremont B, Braet C, et al. Treating depressive symptoms in schoolchildren: a pilot study. Eur Child Adolesc Psychiatry 2004;13(2):105–14.

103. Jaycox LH, Reivich KJ, Gillham JE, et al. Prevention of depressive symptoms in school children. Behav Res Ther 1994;32(8):801–16.

104. Gillham JE, Reivich KJ, Jaycox LH, et al. Prevention of depressive symptoms in schoolchildren: Two-year follow-up. Psychol Sci 1995;6(6):343–51.

105. Kahn JS, Kehle TJ, Jenson WR, et al. Comparison of cognitive-behavioral, relaxation, and self-modeling interventions for depression among middle-school students. Sch Psychol Rev 1990;19(2):196–211.

106. Liddle B, Spence SH, Cognitive-behaviour therapy with depressed primary school children: A cautionary note. Behav Psyc Ther 1990;18:85–102.

107. Stark KD, Reynolds WM, Kaslow NJ. A comparison of the relative efficacy of self-control therapy and a behavioral problem-solving therapy for depression in children. J Abnorm Child Psychol 1987;15(1):91–113.

108. Weisz JR, Thurber CA, Sweeney L, et al. Brief treatment of mild-to-moderate child depression using primary and secondary control enhancement training. J Consult Clin Psychol 1997;65(4):703–7.

The Complex Role of Sleep in Adolescent Depression

Greg Clarke, PhD[a],*, Allison G. Harvey, PhD[b]

KEYWORDS

- Sleep • Adolescents • Depression • Youth • Insomnia
- Behavioral problems

Unipolar depression is one of the most common disorders in adolescence, with point prevalence estimated at 3% to 8%, and episodes typically last 6 to 8 months.[1,2] It has a chronic, episodic course marked by frequent recurrence and considerable impairment.[3,4] An estimated 20% of adolescents will have had a depressive episode by age 18,[2] with as many as 75% experiencing a second episode within 5 years.[5,6] Depression is associated with substantial impairment in school, interpersonal relationships, and occupational adjustment; tobacco and substance abuse; suicide attempts; and a 30-fold increased risk of completed suicide.[3,7–9] The diagnostic criteria for major depression are presented in **Box 1**.

INADEQUACY OF TREATMENTS FOR YOUTH DEPRESSION

The critical need to augment traditional depression treatments is evident. Even in the largest, highly controlled clinical trial of youth depression treatment (Treatment for Adolescents With Depression Study [TADS]),[10] the maximally effective condition (cognitive behavioral therapy [CBT]+ fluoxetine) yielded a 3 month *remission* (full recovery) rate of only 37%[11] and *response* rates no greater than 71%[10] (*response* includes both recovered and partially improved youth). The need for improvement is reinforced by several recent meta-analyses and reviews[12–14] indicating only modest effects for traditional youth depression treatments such as CBT and antidepressants. Less is known about treatments for prepubertal depressed children, but similar inadequacies are generally presumed to be evident for this younger age range as well.

This project was supported by National Institute of Mental Health grant R34 MH 82034. We are grateful to Rachel Manber, Richard Booztin, Ron Dahl, and Dana McMakin for serving as consultants on this grant and to Alison Firemark, Sue Leung, and Ellie McGlinchey for serving as therapists for the duration of the R34.
The authors have nothing to disclose.

a Kaiser Permanente Center for Health Research, 3800 North Interstate Avenue, Portland, OR 97227, USA
b Department of Psychology, University of California, Berkeley, 3210 Tolman Hall #1650 Berkeley, CA 94720, USA
* Corresponding author.
E-mail address: Greg.Clarke@kpchr.org

Child Adolesc Psychiatric Clin N Am 21 (2012) 385–400
doi:10.1016/j.chc.2012.01.006   childpsych.theclinics.com
1056-4993/12/$ – see front matter © 2012 Elsevier Inc. All rights reserved.

Box 1
Diagnostic and Statistical Manual (DSM-IV) criteria for major depression

At least 5 of the 9 symptoms below for 2 weeks or longer, for most of the time almost every day, representing a change from prior functioning. One of the symptoms must be either (a) depressed mood or (b) loss of interest.

a. Depressed mood. For children and adolescents, this may be irritable mood.

b. A significantly reduced level of interest or pleasure in most or all activities.

c. Significant loss or gain of weight (5% or more change in a month when not dieting). This may also be an increase or decrease in appetite. For children, they may not gain an expected amount of weight.

d. Difficulty falling or staying asleep (insomnia) or sleeping more than usual (hypersomnia).

e. Behavior that is agitated or slowed down. Others should be able to observe this.

f. Feeling fatigued or diminished energy.

g. Thoughts of worthlessness or extreme guilt.

h. Reduced ability to think, concentrate, or make decisions.

i. Frequent thoughts of death or suicide, or a suicide attempt.

The person's symptoms must result in great distress or difficulty in functioning at home, work, or other important areas. The condition is also not caused or explained by (1) effects of drugs or medication, (2) a medical condition, or (3) bereavement.

Summarized from the Diagnostic and Statistical Manual of Mental Disorders—Fourth Edition, Text Revision.

Nonetheless, we will focus on adolescents as our research focuses on these older youth.

IMPROVING SUBOPTIMAL TEEN DEPRESSION TREATMENT OUTCOME

Given the unsatisfactory outcomes of conventional treatments for youth depression, various strategies are being pursued to improve outcomes (eg, improving the adherence-fidelity-duration of existing depression treatments; developing *novel* depression treatments; combining multiple depression-focused treatments—eg, antidepressants *and* CBT). Here, we describe the reason we are pursuing another strategy: we hypothesize that the concurrent treatment of depression *and insomnia* in depressed youth will improve both sleep and depression outcomes, even beyond the effects of traditional depression treatment. We next review the specific evidence pointing to the promise of this program of research.

SLEEP IN THE ADOLESCENT YEARS
Magnitude of Youth Insomnia Problem

Although improved depression is our primary goal, improved sleep is an important intermediary target. Researchers have increasingly identified an epidemic of sleep deprivation in youth.[15–17] An estimated 25% of adolescents have some form of sleep disturbance.[18,19] Sleep deprivation of varying severity is reported by 10% to 40% of high school youth.[20,21] This is a persistent problem for many; 12.4% of adolescents in another study reported insomnia symptoms nearly every day of the past month, with higher rates for girls and lower socioeconomic status youth.[22] Lifetime prevalence of *DSM-IV* insomnia (**Box 2** describes the diagnostic criteria) through age 18 has

---

Box 2
Research diagnostic criteria for insomnia*

A. The individual reports 1 or more of the following sleep-related complaints:

  1. Difficulty initiating sleep

  2. Difficulty maintaining sleep

  3. Waking up too early, or

  4. Sleep that is chronically nonrestorative or poor quality

B. The above sleep difficulty occurs despite adequate opportunity and circumstances for sleep.

C. At least 1 of the following forms of daytime impairment related to the nighttime sleep difficulty is reported by the individual:

  1. Fatigue/malaise

  2. Attention, concentration, or memory impairment

  3. Social/vocational dysfunction, poor school performance

  4. Mood disturbance/irritability

  5. Daytime sleepiness

  6. Motivation/energy/initiative reduction

  7. Proneness for errors/accidents at work or driving

  8. Tension headaches and/or gastrointestinal symptoms in response to sleep loss; and

  9. Concerns or worries about sleep

*From Edinger JD, Wohlgemuth WK, Radtke RA, et al. Does cognitive-behavioral insomnia therapy alter dysfunctional beliefs about sleep? Sleep 2001;24:591–9.

---

been reported as 10.7%, with an increased risk among girls after the onset of menses.[23] Community rates of adolescent *DSM-IV* insomnia have been reported as 4.7% one-month prevalence[24] and approximately 4% point prevalence.[25] Rates of insomnia are even higher in depressed adolescents,[26] our target population.

Sleep Disturbance and Behavioral Problems

Sleep deprivation has significant and severe adverse impacts. Studies suggest a strong link between sleep disturbance and behavioral problems in youth,[27] in part because sleep deprivation undermines emotion regulation the following day.[28–30] Sleep problems are similarly associated with increased risk of suicidality.[31,32] Across multiple studies conducted in various countries using different methodologies, insomnia in teens has been associated with suicidal ideation, suicide attempts, and suicide completion (the latter was established using a psychology autopsy method). Adolescent insomnia/sleep deprivation also contributes to school absenteeism and dropout.[33] Academic performance also declines,[15,34,35] along with impaired cognitive performance and attention,[36] consistent with the emerging neuroscience findings demonstrating the importance of sleep for learning and memory.[37,38]

Sleep Disturbance and Medical Problems

Persons with insomnia also have more medical problems and more physician visits, are hospitalized more often, use more medication, and have higher absenteeism, more problems at work, and more workplace accidents.[39] Sleep deprivation is associated much higher rates of accidents, particularly motor vehicle accidents (MVAs), one of the leading causes of death among young men and adolescents[40–43] All of these incur significant direct and indirect costs for individuals, families, health care delivery systems, and society.[44] The combined annual direct and indirect costs for insomnia have been estimated between $92 and $107 billion (1994 US dollars), with indirect costs (eg, medical comorbidities and care, reduced workplace productivity, motor vehicle accidents, other accidents) accounting for $77 to $92 billion.[45] Similarly, the average annual per-person direct and indirect costs were $5010 for individuals with insomnia syndrome, $1431 for individuals presenting with symptoms, and $421 for good sleepers.[46] There may be even greater, as-yet-underestimated costs associated with lower educational attainment resulting from youth sleep disorder, which may in turn reduce lifetime income.

Insomnia Versus Sleep Disorders

Our current work is focusing on youth *insomnia* rather than the broad span of all sleep disorder in youth (eg, delayed sleep phase syndrome [DSPS] and hypersomnia). Our rationale is 2-fold. First, studies suggest insomnia is the most prevalent of sleep disorders in community youth samples.[19,23–25] Hence, an insomnia treatment will have the broadest applicability. Second, CBT treatments for insomnia, including our youth program, are better established and better evaluated than treatments for other sleep disorders such as DSPS. For these reasons, we have been focusing exclusively on the youth insomnia population.

INSOMNIA AND DEPRESSION
Insomnia: A Possible Causal and/or Treatment-Interfering Role in Depression?

This line of research is also motivated by the research priorities developed at the National Institutes of Health state-of-the-science conference on insomnia[47]—that insomnia is not just a symptom or byproduct of depression but rather, in many patients, insomnia contributes to depression onset and/or maintenance, complicates and attenuates the effectiveness of depression treatment, and is the most common residual symptom when depression is incompletely remitted.[48,49] Thus, direct treatment of insomnia seems likely to improve depression outcomes or even prevent initial onset of depression.[50–52] In the sections that follow, we review the evidence for these assertions.

Insomnia is Comorbid With Depression

Sleep disturbances are frequently comorbid with depression and anxiety,[35,53,54] and there is evidence that these conditions have bidirectional, mutually maintaining influences.[55,56] In a recent study of 553 youth with major depression, 72.7% also reported a sleep disturbance, mostly insomnia; these youth (ages 7.3–14.9) were also more severely depressed.[26] While this association would be expected if insomnia were simply a symptom of depression, a recent review examined the epidemiologic, sleep-electroencephalography, neuroendocrine, and immune research and found distinct differences between depression and insomnia, suggesting these are separate but highly associated disorders with bidirectional impacts.[57] Convergent evidence from neuroimaging research with healthy individuals and with animals shows that sleep deprivation undermines emotion/mood regulation the following day[28] and, at the neural systems level, circuits involved in emotion regulation and circuits involved in sleep regulation interact in bidirectional ways.[58] The mechanisms underlying these effects are currently under investigation.

Insomnia Contributes to Depression Risk

Evidence has steadily accrued indicating that insomnia is an independent risk factor for first and recurrent episodes of depression.[59–64] A recent review estimated that patients with persistent insomnia have a 3.5-fold increased risk for depression relative to individuals without insomnia[50]; another recent meta-analysis similarly found a 2-fold risk.[65] This pattern of findings holds across the life span: in older adults,[66,67] adults in the middle years,[64,68–70] and young adults.[71,72] Insomnia may also be an independent predictor of suicidal behavior in depressed patients.[73]

Similar results are reported in adolescents. Community residing youth (N = 4500) who reported frequent trouble sleeping were more likely than normal-sleeping controls to report anxiety or depression (odds ratio, 22.7).[74] A similar study of 1014 teens found that chronologically primary insomnia significantly predicted future depression (hazard rate, 3.8) but that primary depression did not predict subsequent insomnia.[51] Insomnia symptoms also predicted subsequent depression in another large adolescent community panel[19]; elevated insomnia at Wave 1 predicted greater depression severity at Wave 2 even when controlling for Wave 2 insomnia. Insomnia has also been found to predict adolescent hospitalization for suicide attempt.[75]

Insomnia Interferes With Depression Treatment

Thase[76] found that depressed adults with polysomnogram (PSG) profiles indicative of sleep disorder had a less favorable response to depression CBT than did patients with normal sleep. Similar results have been reported in depressed youth, with decreased sleep efficiency and delayed sleep onset predicting depression recurrence following treatment.[77] Sleep abnormality may impair depression CBT response. The mechanism seems to be via increased hypothalamic-pituitary-adrenocortical (HPA) activity, which is thought to predict poor depression treatment response.[78,79]

Residual Insomnia is a Major Component of Incompletely Remitted Depression

Insomnia was the most common residual symptom among depressed youth in the TADS study[10] who had responded to treatment but had not yet progressed to full remission.[11] Similar residual insomnia has been reported in incompletely recovered depressed adults.[48,49,80–82] Persistent residual insomnia may significantly reduce the likelihood of full depression remission by 10- to 12-fold in patients with major depression or dysthmia[83] and increase the risk of depression recurrence.[84] While our current focus is on insomnia treatment simultaneous with depression treatment, other important targets are likely to include residual insomnia remaining after depression treatment, thereby converting additional youth to full depression remission status, similar to studies with adults.[85]

OUR HYPOTHESIS: IMPROVED YOUTH SLEEP WILL CONTRIBUTE TO IMPROVED YOUTH MOOD

The review in the previous section suggests that treating sleep disorder promises to improve depression outcomes. Therefore, we have hypothesized that treating youth insomnia simultaneously with depression treatment may improve both sleep and mood outcomes.

Adult Trials Treating Sleep to Improve Depression

Three studies with adults highlight the promise of the proposed research. Manber and colleagues[86] found higher rates of depression and insomnia remission (61% and 50%, respectively) when an antidepressant was combined with CBT for insomnia

(CBT-I), versus 33% depression and 7% insomnia remission rates in a control condition consisting of an antidepressant plus sleep hygiene (SH), considered a less potent sleep intervention. Fava and colleagues[87] compared an antidepressant plus placebo versus antidepressant plus the sleep agent eszopiclone in adults with both major depression and insomnia. The joint insomnia–depression treatment condition was associated with significantly more depression response (59% vs 48%) and remission (42% vs 32%). Similar advantages were observed in clinician-rated depression, improvement at work, and all major sleep outcomes. A third trial[85] found similar results for refractory insomnia in residual depression in adults, comparing behavioral treatment (BT) for insomnia and treatment as usual (TAU) versus a TAU-only control group. The BT+TAU arm demonstrated significantly improved sleep as well as depression outcomes.

Several of these adult trials examined *pharmacologic* treatments for either depression and/or insomnia. In contrast, our focus has been CBT psychotherapy for both conditions. We have elected to focus on CBT-I and CBT-Depression (CBT-D) because surveys indicate that youth and families strongly favor CBT and other psychotherapies over pharmacotherapies,[88] as do adult patients.[89,90] ADs are also concerning to many families because of increased suicidal ideation and suicide attempts risk in youth.[91,92] For sleep medications, there have been no controlled trials of these agents in youth other than exogenous melatonin,[93–96] and at present neither melatonin nor any other sleep agent has Food and Drug Administration approval for pediatric insomnia.[55,97–99] Finally, while both CBT and medications are effective short-term treatments for adult insomnia, following discontinuation of active treatment, the benefits of CBT persist while those of medication often fade quickly.[100,101]

Youth Insomnia Treatment

The *adult* insomnia CBT treatment literature is relatively well established, with numerous clinical trials conducted over the past few decades. The evidence base for CBT for adults with insomnia has been summarized in multiple meta-analyses[102–104] and 2 practice parameters papers commissioned by the American Academy of Sleep Medicine.[105,106] The clear conclusion is that CBT for insomnia produces reliable and durable changes in sleep. In contrast, outcome literature on *youth* insomnia treatment is very slim—reinforcing the necessity for treatment research in this area. Bootzin and Stevens (2005) conducted the first uncontrolled trial of a CBT insomnia treatment in a sample of sleep-disordered, substance-abusing adolescents. All 55 enrolled youth received the CBT-I protocol. Compared to noncompleters, treatment completers showed significant improvements on multiple sleep outcomes. Self-reported drug use declined for the completers at follow-up evaluations while continuing to increase for the noncompleters. Improved sleep was associated with decreased aggression.[107] Another small (N = 18) uncontrolled pilot[108] of a 6-session insomnia behavioral therapy (BT-I) found improvement in numerous sleep parameters. While both of these trials have been limited by the lack of a randomized control condition, the generally positive results encourage us to continue this line of research.

To the best of our knowledge, there are no other published randomized controlled trials (RCTs) of CBT or any other psychological treatment for youth insomnia. We have found a few small trials of melatonin supplementation for childhood insomnia,[93–96] though most of these were with children younger than the age range of interest to us, namely adolescents. Also, as noted earlier, depressed youth and their parents favor psychotherapy over pharmacotherapy,[88] and CBT appears to be superior to sleep medication in the longer term.[100,101] Reaffirming the need for more research, this near-dearth of youth insomnia treatment development and evaluation is especially surprising given the consistent recent literature on youth insomnia prevalence and associated morbidity.

THERE IS NEED FOR AN ADOLESCENT-SPECIFIC DEVELOPMENTALLY ADAPTED INSOMNIA TREATMENT

Given the adult trials cited earlier, readers might ask whether it is really necessary to test an *adolescent* insomnia intervention. Couldn't the insomnia interventions from these adult studies be directly employed with depressed, sleep-disordered youth? We believe that separate investigation of the joint treatment of youth insomnia and depression is warranted, for 2 reasons:

1. *Adult insomnia treatments may be inappropriate for use with youth, without modification.* Our experiences with youth highlights the necessity for age-appropriate adaptations of CBT and psychoeducational materials, examples, exercises, homework, and so on, geared to the unique adolescent psychosocial environment (living with parents; reduced independence; school and peer demands), and to the differing intellectual, emotional regulation, and "executive decision-making" capacities of adolescents.[27,109] As will become evident, our CBT-I intervention program, developed and pilot tested with National Institute for Mental Health funding (R34 MH82034), illustrates the type and extent of developmental adaptations we have made.

2. *While insomnia disorder in adults and youth shares several key features, it is also sufficiently different in presentation and maintaining factors that treatments must take these distinctions into account.* For example, the number of hours of normative sleep is greater for adolescents than for adults,[110–113] likely because of dramatic maturational and brain changes during adolescence, such as neuronal pruning.[114] Similar hours of sleep deprivation may therefore result in a greater deficit in adolescents compared to adults. Other developmental differences contributing to the need for a youth-specific insomnia treatment are:

   - Developmentally normative but often subclinical delayed sleep onset (going to bed later) during adolescence[115,116]
   - Cultural and peer pressures for late night socializing
   - Need to include parents to help scaffold the motivation for change[117] and adolescent independence from parents is in transition, leading to changing parental role with regard to monitoring and enforcing regular sleep habits.[118]

In summary, the need for age-appropriate intervention content, as well as the divergent nature of insomnia in the different ages, argues for a separate investigation of the joint treatment of *youth* insomnia and depression, rather than relying simply on the similar adult trials.

Effects Beyond Depression

Although our primary aim is to improve youth depression, successful treatment of youth insomnia may improve outcomes in other domains as well. These include improved educational attainment, reduced dropout rates, and improved classroom performance. Successful youth insomnia treatment might also reduce rates of sleep deprivation–induced MVAs (particularly nighttime accidents) and other accidental injuries.[40] Finally, insomnia has a possible contributing role in obesity,[119–122] metabolic syndrome or diabetes,[123–125] and immune system dysfunction.[126,127] Successful treatment of youth insomnia could ultimately be beneficial in these domains as well.

CBT-INSOMNIA FOR YOUTH

Our CBT-I approach is based on *adult* CBT-I protocols developed by Manber and colleagues,[86] Bootzin,[128] Morin and colleagues,[129] Harvey and Greenall,[130–132] as well as the *adolescent* protocol piloted by Bootzin and Stevens.[133] The core components of this CBT-I protocol are stimulus control (SC), sleep restriction (SR), and sleep-focused cognitive therapy (CT). We have also added elements of motivational enhancement therapy (MET) to improve youth therapy participation. Collectively, we refer to this therapy approach as insomnia CBT (CBT-I). While the primary focus of these techniques is directly on sleep improvement, therapists may use elements of these therapy approaches to address related problems, such as CT for anxiety that may be contributing to insomnia. Sleep hygiene, while not a core component, may be incidentally included.

Stimulus Control and Sleep Restriction to Regularize Sleep-Wake Cycle

SC and SR are the most established of all the behavioral sleep disorder interventions. We developmentally adapted existing protocols.[86,128–132] Both SC and SR aim to regularize the sleep-wake cycle and strengthen the association between the bed and sleeping by limiting sleep-incompatible behaviors in the bedroom environment (watching television, computer use), while developing a consistent sleep-wake schedule. SC involves the following:

a. Use the bed only for sleep—ie, no television watching or talking on cell phones.
b. Go to bed only when sleepy.
c. Get out of bed and go to another room when unable to fall asleep or return to sleep within approximately 15 to 20 minutes and return to bed only when sleepy again.
d. Arise in the morning at the same time each day (no later than plus 2 hours on weekends).

In terms of SR, also review the sleep diary for the past week. If sleep efficiency (percentage of time in bed spent asleep) is lower than 85%, we discuss the possibility of implementing SR therapy with the youth and his or her parent. The goal is to gradually move toward a regular schedule 7 days a week. To achieve steps (a) and (d), we use the standard SC methods,[134] which provide a rationale, set goals for bedtime and wake-time, use a daily sleep diary to monitor progress toward goals (also required for outcomes assessment), and review the diary at weekly therapy sessions. For difficulty falling asleep, we supplement the traditional SC instruction (get up out of bed) with training in imagery[135] and relaxation techniques,[134] with the goal of reducing arousal and promoting sleep onset. The goal is to lower the potential for youth to become engaged in rewarding and arousing activities (eg, using electronics) should they arise when unable to sleep.

Cognitive Therapy to Address Dysfunctional Sleep Beliefs and Bedtime Rumination

Cognitive therapy is a treatment for insomnia[130–132,134–136] as well as a well-established treatment for depression.[13,137] Difficulty getting to sleep is often related to excessive worry, rumination, and negative cognitions and dysfunctional beliefs about sleep.[138,139] Typical unhelpful beliefs about sleep include: *"There is no point going to bed earlier because I won't be able to fall asleep," "If I don't fall asleep soon I will be a wreck tomorrow,"* and *"Getting more sleep doesn't help me."* The intervention for dysfunctional beliefs involves a 4-step process:

1. Identifying dysfunctional thoughts

2. Guided discovery and Socratic questioning to challenge beliefs
3. Individualized experiments to test the validity and utility of dysfunctional beliefs and to collect data on new beliefs
4. Identification and dropping of safety behaviors that prevent disconfirmation of dysfunctional beliefs.

We teach patients to evaluate worry and rumination, diary writing, or scheduling a "worry period" to process worries several hours prior to bedtime; creating a "to-do" list prior to getting into bed to reduce worry about future plans/events; training to disengage from pre-sleep worry and redirect attention to pleasant, distracting imagery; identifying the adverse consequences of thought suppression in bed; and scheduling a pre-sleep "wind down" period prior to bedtime to promote disengagement from daytime concerns. Therapists may also use cognitive therapy to address some common comorbidities (eg, general anxiety) if these comorbidities interfere with sleep and/or depression recovery.

Motivational Enhancement

This component is critical given that youth sleep disturbance is associated with poor self-regulation,[140] which may undermine adherence to the treatment. A recent meta-analysis[141] found that motivational enhancement significantly increases client motivation. Motivational enhancement involves a straightforward review of perceived pros and cons of change,[142] recognizing that many sleep-incompatible/interfering behaviors used by youth are rewarding (eg, text messaging with friends).

SUMMARY

In this discussion, we had 2 related goals. First, it is clear that insomnia is a significant problem in adolescence. Successful treatment of insomnia is an important goal in its own right. However, *the primary goal in our recent research*, consistent with the National Institute for Mental Health's focus on mental disorders and the future research priorities from the National Institutes of Health state-of-the-science conference on insomnia,[47] has been to improve the treatment of youth depression beyond the modest effects achieved with depression-focused interventions. We hypothesize that joint treatment of sleep *and* mood disorder, with treatment elements specific to each, may increase depression response and remission rates. This approach is suggested by the high comorbidity of insomnia with depression, by the emerging indications that sleep disturbances may play a causal role in the onset of many (but not all) depressive episodes, by preliminary adult outcome trials in which treatment of insomnia also improved depression outcomes, and by other uncontrolled pilots of youth insomnia treatment. There is also evidence that insomnia interferes with patients' ability to benefit from depression-focused CBT, suggesting that insomnia CBT might enable depression CBT to be more successful. Overall, our approach is also consistent with the *primary prevention of secondary disorders* model advocated by several researchers in other clinical contexts[143–145] and specifically in the case of insomnia and mood disorder.[51,52,61]

Developmental timing may be important, too. Animal and human research suggests that puberty is a unique period for establishing future behavioral patterns and habits[146]; intervening in this developmental period may assist youth to establish healthy patterns that will serve them well into the future. If we find that this novel intervention improves outcomes across a broad range of critical and prevalent adverse outcomes for teens (eg, depression, suicidality, insomnia, educational attainment, and others), the public health implications will be large. Even perhaps more startling for public health implications, and a fascinating domain for future research, is to treat insomnia as a *prevention* for youth depression.

REFERENCES

1. Fleming JE, Offord DR. Epidemiology of childhood depressive disorders: a critical review. J Am Acad Child Adolesc Psychiatry 1990;29:571–80.
2. Lewinsohn PM, Hops H, Roberts RE, et al. Adolescent psychopathology: I. Prevalence and incidence of depression and other DSM-III-R disorders in high school students [published erratum appears in J Abnorm Psychol 1993;102(4):517]. J Abnorm Psychol 1993;102:133–44.
3. Birmaher B, Ryan ND, Williamson DE, et al. Childhood and adolescent depression: a review of the past 10 years. Part I. J Am Acad Child Adolesc Psychiatry 1996;35: 1427–39.
4. Birmaher B, Ryan ND, Williamson DE, et al. Childhood and adolescent depression: a review of the past 10 years. Part II. J Am Acad Child Adolesc Psychiatry 1996;35:1575–83.
5. Kovacs M, Feinberg TL, Crouse-Novak M, et al. Depressive disorders in childhood. II. A longitudinal study of the risk for a subsequent major depression. Arch Gen Psychiatry 1984;41:643–.
6. Kovacs M, Feinberg TL, Crouse-Novak MA, et al. Depressive disorders in childhood. I. A longitudinal prospective study of characteristics and recovery. Arch Gen Psychiatry 1984;41:229–37.
7. Brent DA, Perper JA, Goldstein CE, et al. Risk factors for adolescent suicide. A comparison of adolescent suicide victims with suicidal inpatients. Arch Gen Psychiatry 1988;45:581–8.
8. Brent DA. Depression and suicide in children and adolescents. Pediatr Rev 1993; 14:380–8.
9. Harrington R, Fudge H, Rutter M, et al. Adult outcomes of childhood and adolescent depression. I. Psychiatric status. Arch Gen Psychiatry 1990;47:465–73.
10. March J, Silva S, Petrycki S, et al. Fluoxetine, cognitive-behavioral therapy, and their combination for adolescents with depression: Treatment for Adolescents With Depression Study (TADS) randomized controlled trial. JAMA 2004;292:807–20.
11. Kennard B, Silva S, Vitiello B, et al. Remission and residual symptoms after short-term treatment in the Treatment of Adolescents With Depression Study (TADS). J Am Acad Child Adolesc Psychiatry 2006;45:1404–11.
12. Weisz JR, McCarty CA, Valeri SM. Effects of psychotherapy for depression in children and adolescents: a meta-analysis. Psychol Bull 2006;132:132–49.
13. Weersing VR, Brent DA. Cognitive behavioral therapy for depression in youth. Child Adolesc Psychiatr Clin N Am 2006;15:939–57, ix.
14. Wagner KD. Pharmacotherapy for major depression in children and adolescents. Prog Neuropsychopharmacol Biol Psychiatry 2005;29:819–26.
15. Gibson ES, Powles AC, Thabane L, et al. "Sleepiness" is serious in adolescence: two surveys of 3235 Canadian students. BMC Public Health 2006;6:116.
16. Hansen M, Janssen I, Schiff A, et al. The impact of school daily schedule on adolescent sleep. Pediatrics 2005;115:1555–61.
17. Millman RP. Excessive sleepiness in adolescents and young adults: causes, consequences, and treatment strategies. Pediatrics 2005;115:1774–86.
18. Mindell JA, Owens JA, Carskadon MA. Developmental features of sleep. Child Adolesc Psychiatr Clin N Am 1999;8:695–25.
19. Roberts RE, Roberts CR, Chen IG. Impact of insomnia on future functioning of adolescents. J Psychosom Res 2002;53:561–9.

20. Carskadon MA. Patterns of sleep and sleepiness in adolescents. Pediatrician 1990; 17:5–12.
21. Axelson DA, Bertocci MA, Lewin DS, et al. Measuring mood and complex behavior in natural environments: use of ecological momentary assessment in pediatric affective disorders. J Child Adolesc Psychopharmacol 2003;13:253–66.
22. Roberts RE, Lee ES, Hemandez M, et al. Symptoms of insomnia among adolescents in the lower Rio Grande Valley of Texas. Sleep 2004;27:751–60.
23. Johnson EO, Roth T, Schultz L, et al. Epidemiology of DSM-IV insomnia in adolescence: lifetime prevalence, chronicity, and an emergent gender difference. Pediatrics 2006;117:e247–56.
24. Roberts RE, Roberts CR, Chan W. Ethnic differences in symptoms of insomnia among adolescents. Sleep 2006;29:359–65.
25. Ohayon MM, Roberts RE, Zulley J, et al. Prevalence and patterns of problematic sleep among older adolescents. J Am Acad Child Adolesc Psychiatry 2000;39: 1549–56.
26. Liu X, Buysse D, Gentzler AL, et al. Insomnia and hypersomnia associated with depressive phenomenology and comorbidity in childhood depression. Sleep 2007; 30:83–90.
27. Dahl RE, Lewin DS. Pathways to adolescent health sleep regulation and behavior. J Adolesc Health 2002;31:175–84.
28. Pilcher JJ, Huffcutt AI. Effects of sleep deprivation on performance: a meta-analysis. Sleep 1996;19:318–26.
29. Van Dongen HP, Maislin G, Mullington JM, et al. The cumulative cost of additional wakefulness: dose-response effects on neurobehavioral functions and sleep physiology from chronic sleep restriction and total sleep deprivation. Sleep 2003;26:117–26.
30. Yoo SS, Gujar N, Hu P, et al. The human emotional brain without sleep - a prefrontal amygdala disconnect. Curr Biol 2007;17:R877–8.
31. Liu X. Sleep and adolescent suicidal behavior. Sleep 2004;27:1351–8.
32. Goldstein TR, Bridge JA, Brent DA. Sleep disturbance preceding completed suicide in adolescents. J Consult Clin Psychol 2008;76:84–91.
33. Carskadon MA, Wolfson AR, Acebo C, et al. Adolescent sleep patterns, circadian timing, and sleepiness at a transition to early school days. Sleep 1998;21:871–81.
34. Wolfson AR, Carskadon MA. Understanding adolescents' sleep patterns and school performance: a critical appraisal. Sleep Med Rev 2003;7:491–506.
35. Wolfson AR, Carskadon MA. Sleep schedules and daytime functioning in adolescents. Child Dev 1998;69:875–87.
36. Fallone G, Acebo C, Arnedt JT, et al. Effects of acute sleep restriction on behavior, sustained attention, and response inhibition in children. Percept Mot Skills 2001;93:213–29.
37. Frank MG, Issa NP, Stryker MP. Sleep enhances plasticity in the developing visual cortex. Neuron 2001;30:275–87.
38. Stickgold R, Walker MP. Memory consolidation and reconsolidation: what is the role of sleep? Trends Neurosci 2005;28:408–15.
39. Leger D, Guilleminault C, Bader G, et al. Medical and socio-professional impact of insomnia. Sleep 2002;25:625–9.
40. Aldrich MS. Automobile accidents in patients with sleep disorders. Sleep 1989;12: 487–94.
41. Pizza F, Contardi S, Antognini AB, et al. Sleep quality and motor vehicle crashes in adolescents. J Clin Sleep Med 2010;6:41–5.

42. Taylor DJ, Bramoweth AD. Patterns and consequences of inadequate sleep in college students: substance use and motor vehicle accidents. J Adolesc Health 2010;46:610–2.
43. Carskadon MA. Risks of driving while sleepy in adolescents and young adults. In: Carskadon MA, editor. Adolescent sleep patterns: Biological, social, and psychological influences. Cambridge (UK): Cambridge University Press; 2002. p. 148–58.
44. Rosekind MR, Gregory KB. Insomnia risks and costs: health, safety, and quality of life. Am J Manag Care 2010;16:617–26.
45. Stoller MK. Economic effects of insomnia. Clin Ther 1994;16:873–97.
46. Daley M, Morin CM, Leblanc M, et al. The economic burden of insomnia: direct and indirect costs for individuals with insomnia syndrome, insomnia symptoms, and good sleepers. Sleep 2009;32:55–64.
47. NIH State-of-the-Science Conference Statement on Manifestations and Management of Chronic Insomnia in Adults. NIH Consens Sci Statements. 2005; 22(2): 1–30. AHRQ Publication No. 05-E021-1.
48. Nierenberg AA, Husain MM, Trivedi MH, et al. Residual symptoms after remission of major depressive disorder with citalopram and risk of relapse: a STAR*D report. Psychol Med 2010;40:41–50.
49. Carney CE, Segal ZV, Edinger JD, et al. A comparison of rates of residual insomnia symptoms following pharmacotherapy or cognitive-behavioral therapy for major depressive disorder. J Clin Psychiatry 2007;68:254–60.
50. Perlis ML, Smith LJ, Lyness JM, et al. Insomnia as a risk factor for onset of depression in the elderly. Behav Sleep Med 2006;4:104–13.
51. Johnson EO, Roth T, Breslau N. The association of insomnia with anxiety disorders and depression: exploration of the direction of risk. J Psychiatr Res 2006;40:700–8.
52. Smith MT, Huang MI, Manber R. Cognitive behavior therapy for chronic insomnia occurring within the context of medical and psychiatric disorders. Clin Psychol Rev 2005;25:559–92.
53. Goetz RR, Puig-Antich J, Ryan N, et al. Electroencephalographic sleep of adolescents with major depression and normal controls. Arch Gen Psychiatry 1987;44:61–8.
54. Brunello N, Armitage R, Feinberg I, et al. Depression and sleep disorders: clinical relevance, economic burden and pharmacological treatment. Neuropsychobiology 2000;42:107–19.
55. Dahl RE, Harvey AG. Sleep disorders. In: Rutter ML, editor. Oxford textbook of child and adolescent psychiatry. Oxford (UK): Oxford University Press; 2007. p. 894–905.
56. Harvey AG. What about patients who can't sleep? Case formulation for insomnia. In: Tarrier N, editor. Case formulation in cognitive behaviour therapy: The treatment of challenging and complex clinical cases. New York: Brunner-Routledge; 2006.
57. Pigeon WR, Perlis ML. Insomnia and depression: birds of a feather? Int J Sleep Disord 2006;1.
58. Saper CB, Cano G, Scammell TE. Homeostatic, circadian, and emotional regulation of sleep. J Comp Neurol 2005;493:92–8.
59. Harvey AG. Insomnia: symptom or diagnosis? Clin Psychol Rev 2001;21:1037–59.
60. Riemann D, Berger M, Voderholzer U. Sleep and depression–results from psychobiological studies: an overview. Biol Psychol 2001;57:67–103.
61. Ford DE, Kamerow DB. Epidemiologic study of sleep disturbances and psychiatric disorders. An opportunity for prevention? JAMA 1989;262:1479–84.
62. Taylor DJ, Lichstein KL, Durrence HH. Insomnia as a health risk factor. Behav Sleep Med 2003;1:227–47.
63. Riemann D, Voderholzer U. Primary insomnia: a risk factor to develop depression? J Affect Disord 2003;76:255–9.

64. Ohayon MM, Roth T. Place of chronic insomnia in the course of depressive and anxiety disorders. J Psychiatr Res 2003;37:9–15.

65. Baglioni C, Battagliese G, Feige B, et al. Insomnia as a predictor of depression: A meta-analytic evaluation of longitudinal epidemiological studies. J Affect Disord 2011;135:10–9.

66. Livingston G, Blizard B, Mann A. Does sleep disturbance predict depression in elderly people? A study in inner London. Br J Gen Pract 1993;43:445–8.

67. Mallon L, Broman JE, Hetta J. Relationship between insomnia, depression, and mortality: a 12-year follow-up of older adults in the community. Int Psychogeriatr 2000;12:295–306.

68. Eaton WW, Badawi M, Melton B. Prodromes and precursors: epidemiologic data for primary prevention of disorders with slow onset. Am J Psychiatry 1995;152:967–72.

69. Dryman A, Eaton WW. Affective symptoms associated with the onset of major depression in the community: findings from the US National Institute of Mental Health Epidemiologic Catchment Area Program. Acta Psychiatr Scand 1991;84:1–5.

70. Weissman MM, Warner V, Wickramaratne P, et al. Offspring of depressed parents. 10 Years later. Arch Gen Psychiatry 1997;54:932–40.

71. Breslau N, Roth T, Rosenthal L, et al. Sleep disturbance and psychiatric disorders: a longitudinal epidemiological study of young adults. Biol Psychiatry 1996;39:411–8.

72. Chang PP, Ford DE, Mead LA, et al. Insomnia in young men and subsequent depression. The Johns Hopkins Precursors Study. Am J Epidemiol 1997;146:105–14.

73. Agargun MY, Kara H, Solmaz M. Sleep disturbances and suicidal behavior in patients with major depression. J Clin Psychiatry 1997;58:249–51.

74. Johnson EO, Breslau N, Roehrs T, et al. Insomnia in adolescence: epidemiology and associated problems. Sleep 1999;22:s22.

75. Gasquet I, Choquet M. Hospitalization in a pediatric ward of adolescent suicide attempters admitted to general hospitals. J Adolesc Health 1994;15:416–22.

76. Thase ME, Simons AD, Reynolds CF III. Abnormal electroencephalographic sleep profiles in major depression: association with response to cognitive behavior therapy. Arch Gen Psychiatry 1996;53:99–108.

77. Emslie GJ, Armitage R, Weinberg WA, et al. Sleep polysomnography as a predictor of recurrence in children and adolescents with major depressive disorder. Int J Neuropsychopharmacol 2001;4:159–68.

78. Ising M, Horstmann S, Kloiber S, et al. Combined dexamethasone/corticotropin releasing hormone test predicts treatment response in major depression: a potential biomarker? Biol Psychiatry 2006.

79. Brouwer JP, Appelhof BC, van Rossum EF, et al. Prediction of treatment response by HPA-axis and glucocorticoid receptor polymorphisms in major depression. Psychoneuroendocrinology 2006;31:1154–63.

80. Becker PM. Treatment of sleep dysfunction and psychiatric disorders. Curr Treat Options Neurol 2006;8:367–75.

81. Smith MT, Huang MI, Manber R. Cognitive behavior therapy for chronic insomnia occurring within the context of medical and psychiatric disorders. Clin Psychol Rev 2005;25:559–92.

82. McClintock SM, Husain MM, Wisniewski SR, et al. Residual symptoms in depressed outpatients who respond by 50% but do not remit to antidepressant medication. J Clin Psychopharmacol 2011;31:180–6.

83. Pigeon WR, Hegel MT, Mackenzie T. Insomnia as a risk for increased morbidity in depressed elderly subjects treated for depression: The IMPACT cohort. Sleep 2005;28:A307.

84. Dombrovski AY, Cyranowski JM, Mulsant BH, et al. Which symptoms predict recurrence of depression in women treated with maintenance interpersonal psychotherapy? Depress Anxiety 2008;25:1060–6.

85. Watanabe N, Furukawa TA, Shimodera S, et al. Brief behavioral therapy for refractory insomnia in residual depression: an assessor-blind, randomized controlled trial. J Clin Psychiatry 2011;72:1651–58.

86. Manber R, Edinger JD, Gress JL, et al. Cognitive behavioral therapy for insomnia enhances depression outcome in patients with comorbid major depressive disorder and insomnia. Sleep 2008;31:489–95.

87. Fava M, McCall WV, Krystal A, et al. Eszopiclone co-administered with fluoxetine in patients with insomnia coexisting with major depressive disorder. Biol Psychiatry 2006;59:1052–60.

88. Jaycox LH, Asarnow JR, Sherbourne CD, et al. Adolescent primary care patients' preferences for depression treatment. Adm Policy Ment Health 2006;33:198–207.

89. Morin CM, Gaulier B, Barry T, et al. Patients' acceptance of psychological and pharmacological therapies for insomnia. Sleep 1992;15:302–5.

90. Vincent N, Lionberg C. Treatment preference and patient satisfaction in chronic insomnia. Sleep 2001;24:411–7.

91. Meyer RE, Salzman C, Youngstrom EA, et al. Suicidality and risk of suicide—definition, drug safety concerns, and a necessary target for drug development: a brief report. J Clin Psychiatry 2010;71:1040–6.

92. Bridge JA, Iyengar S, Salary CB, et al. Clinical response and risk for reported suicidal ideation and suicide attempts in pediatric antidepressant treatment: a meta-analysis of randomized controlled trials. JAMA 2007;297:1683–6.

93. Weiss MD, Wasdell MB, Bomben MM, et al. Sleep hygiene and melatonin treatment for children and adolescents with ADHD and initial insomnia. J Am Acad Child Adolesc Psychiatry 2006;45:512–9.

94. Smits MG, Nagtegaal EE, van der HJ, et al. Melatonin for chronic sleep onset insomnia in children: a randomized placebo-controlled trial. J Child Neurol 2001;16:86–92.

95. Smits MG, van Stel HF, van der HK, et al. Melatonin improves health status and sleep in children with idiopathic chronic sleep-onset insomnia: a randomized placebo-controlled trial. J Am Acad Child Adolesc Psychiatry 2003;42:1286–93.

96. Coppola G, Iervolino G, Mastrosimone M, et al. Melatonin in wake-sleep disorders in children, adolescents and young adults with mental retardation with or without epilepsy: a double-blind, cross-over, placebo-controlled trial. Brain Dev 2004;26:373–6.

97. Weiss SK, Garbutt A. Pharmacotherapy in pediatric sleep disorders. Adolesc Med State Art Rev 2010;21:508.

98. Owens JA, Rosen CL, Mindell JA, et al. Use of pharmacotherapy for insomnia in child psychiatry practice: a national survey. Sleep Med 2010;11:692–700.

99. Mindell JA, Emslie G, Blumer J, et al. Pharmacologic management of insomnia in children and adolescents: consensus statement. Pediatrics 2006;117:e1223–32.

100. Morin CM, Colecchi C, Stone J, et al. Behavioral and pharmacological therapies for late-life insomnia: a randomized controlled trial. JAMA 1999;281:991–9.

101. Sivertsen B, Omvik S, Pallesen S, et al. Cognitive behavioral therapy vs zopiclone for treatment of chronic primary insomnia in older adults: a randomized controlled trial. JAMA 2006;295:2851–8.

102. Morin CM, Culbert JP, Schwartz SM. Nonpharmacological interventions for insomnia: a meta-analysis of treatment efficacy. Am J Psychiatry 1994;151:1172–80.

103. Murtagh DR, Greenwood KM. Identifying effective psychological treatments for insomnia: a meta-analysis. J Consult Clin Psychol 1995;63:79–89.

104. Smith MT, Perlis ML, Park A, et al. Comparative meta-analysis of pharmacotherapy and behavior therapy for persistent insomnia. Am J Psychiatry 2002;159:5–11.

105. Chesson AL Jr, Anderson WM, Littner M, et al. Practice parameters for the nonpharmacologic treatment of chronic insomnia. An American Academy of Sleep Medicine report. Standards of Practice Committee of the American Academy of Sleep Medicine. Sleep 1999;22:1128–33.

106. Morin CM, Bootzin RR, Buysse DJ, et al. Psychological and behavioral treatment of insomnia: update of the recent evidence (1998–2004). Sleep 2006;29:1398–414.

107. Haynes PL, Bootzin RR, Smith L, et al. Sleep and aggression in substance-abusing adolescents: results from an integrative behavioral sleep-treatment pilot program. Sleep 2006;29:512–20.

108. Schlarb AA, Liddle HA, Hautzinger M. JuSt—a multimodal program for treatment of insomnia in adolescents: a pilot study. Nat Sci Sleep 2011;3:13–20.

109. Weisz JR, Hawley KM. Developmental factors in the treatment of adolescents. J Consult Clin Psychol 2002;70:21–43.

110. Acebo C, Millman RP, Rosenberg C, et al. Sleep, breathing, and cephalometrics in older children and young adults. Part I—normative values. Chest 1996;109:664–72.

111. Ohayon MM, Carskadon MA, Guilleminault C, et al. Meta-analysis of quantitative sleep parameters from childhood to old age in healthy individuals: developing normative sleep values across the human lifespan. Sleep 2004;27:1255–73.

112. Ohayon MM, Roberts RE, Zulley J, et al. Prevalence and patterns of problematic sleep among older adolescents. J Am Acad Child Adolesc Psychiatry 2000;39: 1549–56.

113. Walsleben JA, Kapur VK, Newman AB, et al. Sleep and reported daytime sleepiness in normal subjects: the Sleep Heart Health Study. Sleep 2004;27:293–8.

114. Waylen A, Wolke D. Sex 'n' drugs 'n' rock 'n' roll: the meaning and social consequences of pubertal timing. Eur J Endocrinol 2004;151(Suppl 3):U151–9.

115. Carskadon MA, Vieira C, Acebo C. Association between puberty and delayed phase preference. Sleep 1993;16:258–62.

116. Carskadon MA, Acebo C, Jenni OG. Regulation of adolescent sleep: implications for behavior. Ann N Y Acad Sci 2004;1021:276–91.

117. Harvey AG. The adverse consequences of sleep disturbance in pediatric bipolar disorder: implications for intervention. Child Adolesc Psychiatr Clin N Am 2009;18: 321–38, viii.

118. Dahl RE. The regulation of sleep-arousal, affect, and attention in adolescence: Some questions and speculations. In: Carskadon MA, editor. Adolescent sleep patterns: Biological, social, and psychological influences. Cambridge (UK): Cambridge University Press; 2002. p. 269–84.

119. Spiegel K, Tasali E, Penev P, et al. Brief communication: Sleep curtailment in healthy young men is associated with decreased leptin levels, elevated ghrelin levels, and increased hunger and appetite. Ann Intern Med 2004;141:846–50.

120. Spiegel K, Leproult R, L'hermite-Baleriaux M, et al. Leptin levels are dependent on sleep duration: relationships with sympathovagal balance, carbohydrate regulation, cortisol, and thyrotropin. J Clin Endocrinol Metab 2004;89:5762–71.

121. Tasali E, Van Cauter E. Sleep-disordered breathing and the current epidemic of obesity: consequence or contributing factor? Am J Respir Crit Care Med 2002;165:562–3.

122. Lumeng JC, Somashekar D, Appugliese D, et al. Shorter sleep duration is associated with increased risk for being overweight at ages 9 to 12 years. Pediatrics 2007;120:1020–9.

123. Scheen AJ, Van Cauter E. The roles of time of day and sleep quality in modulating glucose regulation: clinical implications. Horm Res 1998;49:191–201.

124. Spiegel K, Leproult R, Van Cauter E. Impact of sleep debt on metabolic and endocrine function. Lancet 1999;354:1435–9.

125. Van Cauter E, Polonsky KS, Scheen AJ. Roles of circadian rhythmicity and sleep in human glucose regulation. Endocr Rev 1997;18:716–38.

126. Spiegel K, Sheridan JF, Van Cauter E. Effect of sleep deprivation on response to immunization. JAMA 2002;288:1471–2.

127. Taylor DJ, Lichstein KL, Durrence HH. Insomnia as a health risk factor. Behav Sleep Med 2003;1:227–47.

128. Bootzin RR. Stimulus control treatment for insomnia. Proc Am Psychol Assoc 1972;7:395–6.

129. Morin CM, Bootzin RR, Buysse DJ, et al. Psychological and behavioral treatment of insomnia: update of the recent evidence (1998–2004). Sleep 2006;29:1398–414.

130. Harvey AG. A cognitive theory of and therapy for chronic insomnia. J Cogn Psychother 2005;19:41–60.

131. Harvey AG, Greenall E. Catastrophic worry in primary insomnia. J Behav Ther Exp Psychiatry 2003;34:11–23.

132. Harvey AG. A cognitive model of insomnia. Behav Res Ther 2002;40:869–93.

133. Bootzin RR, Stevens SJ. Adolescents, substance abuse, and the treatment of insomnia and daytime sleepiness. Clin Psychol Rev 2005;25:629–44.

134. Morin CM, Espie CA. Insomnia: a clinical guide to assessment and treatment. New York: Kluwer Academic/Plenum Publishers; 2003.

135. Harvey AG, Payne S. The management of unwanted pre-sleep thoughts in insomnia: distraction with imagery versus general distraction. Behav Res Ther 2002;40:267–77.

136. Harvey AG, Tang NK. Cognitive behaviour therapy for primary insomnia: can we rest yet? Sleep Med Rev 2003;7:237–62.

137. Hollon SD, Shelton RC, Davis DD. Cognitive therapy for depression: conceptual issues and clinical efficacy. J Consult Clin Psychol 1993;61:270–5.

138. Edinger JD, Wohlgemuth WK, Radtke RA, et al. Does cognitive-behavioral insomnia therapy alter dysfunctional beliefs about sleep? Sleep 2001;24:591–9.

139. Morin CM, Blais F, Savard J. Are changes in beliefs and attitudes about sleep related to sleep improvements in the treatment of insomnia? Behav Res Ther 2002;40:741–52.

140. Digdon NL, Howell AJ. College students who have an eveningness preference report lower self-control and greater procrastination. Chronobiol Int 2008;25:1029–46.

141. Hettema J, Steele J, Miller WR. A meta-analysis of research on motivational interviewing treatment effectiveness. Annu Rev Clin Psychol 2005;1:91–111.

142. Miller WR, Rollnick S. Motivational interviewing: preparing people for change. 2nd edition. New York: Guilford Press; 2002.

143. Kendall PC, Kessler RC. The impact of childhood psychopathology interventions on subsequent substance abuse: policy implications, comments, and recommendations. J Consult Clin Psychol 2002;70:1303–6.

144. Kessler RC, Price RH. Primary prevention of secondary disorders: a proposal and agenda. Am J Community Psychol 1993;21:607–33.

145. Kessler RC. The epidemiology of dual diagnosis. Biol Psychiatry 2004;56:730–7.

146. Fleming AS, Corter C. Psychobiology of maternal behavior in nonhuman mammals. Hillside (NJ): Erlbaum; 1995.

Primary Care Management of Child & Adolescent Depressive Disorders

Frances J. Wren, MD[a],*, Jane Meschan Foy, MD[b],
Patricia I. Ibeziako, MD[c,d]

KEYWORDS

- Adolescent • Child • Primary health care
- Depressive disorders • Depression

Key Points

- As for adults, it has long been noted that high numbers of youth presenting to primary care meet criteria for 1 or more DSM psychiatric disorder and that the large majority go unrecognized.
- Key is how to implement effective management of depression in the patchwork of independent small to moderate sized, single specialty (pediatrics, family practice, internal medicine) group practices that deliver much of the available primary care.

Depressive disorders are a problem with profound societal impact, whether measured by prevalence, burden of disability and suffering across the life span, mortality, or financial costs for health care and for society at large. As such, they merit strategic public health intervention. The World Health Organization estimates that 120 million people live with depressive disorders, of whom fewer than 25% receive any treatment.[1] Integrating mental health services into primary care has been cited by World Health Organization as the most viable way of closing the treatment gap in mental health care.[2] With this in mind, we discuss how recent work on the primary care management of mental health and psychosocial problems might be applied to pediatric depressive disorders.

---

[a] Department of Psychiatry and Behavioral Sciences, Stanford University School of Medicine, Stanford, CA 94305, USA
[b] Department of Pediatrics, Wake Forest University School of Medicine, Medical Center Boulevard, Winston-Salem, NC 27157, USA
[c] Harvard Medical School, 300 Longwood Avenue, Boston, MA 02115, USA
[d] Psychiatry Consult Service, Children's Hospital Boston, 300 Longwood Avenue, Boston, MA 02115, USA
* Corresponding author.
E-mail address: fwren@stanford.edu

Child Adolesc Psychiatric Clin N Am 21 (2012) 401–419
doi:10.1016/j.chc.2012.01.008
1056-4993/12/$ – see front matter © 2012 Elsevier Inc. All rights reserved.

Background for our discussion comes from several decades of adult research, which have generated key principles and models, now beginning to be evaluated in forms adapted for youth. Over the past decade many US and international health care organizations, government bodies, and professional organizations have endorsed the collaborative care approaches to primary care management of depression that have emerged from the adult research.[3,4] Tools and strategies to implement collaborative care have also been developed by groups such as the McArthur Initiative on Depression in Primary Care.[5]

Although the pediatric research remains limited, the movement to endorse collaborative care approaches has included organizations focused on child and adolescent primary care or mental health.[6,7] Factors driving this development include the strength of the evidence from adults, the fact that we now know more and are more in agreement about what is effective front-line intervention for pediatric depressive disorders,[8] and, perhaps related to this progress in treatment effectiveness, a groundswell of concern about the short supply and poor distribution of specialized mental health services for youth.[9–11] Up to two thirds of US youth with mental health needs currently receive no services.[12] Without growth in the role played by primary care, there is no realistic way to substantially reduce this figure. This reality has been recognized by the American Academy of Pediatrics (AAP) in its July 2009 policy statement, *The Future of Pediatrics, Mental Health Competencies for Pediatric Primary Care*,[13] which included identification and management of depressive disorders in the recommended areas of competence for primary care pediatricians. In addition, the AAP recommended that all primary care clinicians develop competence in the systems skills necessary to support the management of mental health problems in primary care and to build the necessary community collaborations. Tools to support the development of these skills for practicing pediatricians were developed by the AAP Task Force on Mental Health (TFOMH).[7,14–16]

We first set the stage for this discussion by briefly outlining the public health challenge presented by depressive disorders and by the current realities of depression management in primary care. We then review the models emerging from intervention research and the barriers to their implementation in practice. Drawing on this background, we discuss the recent new standards for primary care management of pediatric depressive disorders along with resources that have been developed to support their achievement.

DEPRESSION AS A PUBLIC HEALTH PROBLEM

Depression is a leading cause of disability worldwide. The World Health Organization Global Burden of Disease study has found that, by 2000,[17] depressive disorders were the second leading contributor to years lived with disability, accounting for 12.4% of the global burden: Neuropsychiatric conditions in general accounted for 37% of years lived with disability. When expressed in terms of disability adjusted life years, a measure summing lost years of potential life owing to premature mortality with lost years of productive life owing to disability, depressive disorders ranked fourth, contributing 4.47% of global burden: In the 15 to 44 age group, they ranked second.[1]

Major Depressive Disorder in Children and Adolescents

During a given year, as discussed by Beardslee and colleagues elsehwere in this issue, 4% to 7% of US adolescents will experience an episode of major depressive disorder (MDD): by the age of 18, the estimated life-time prevalence is 14%. A further 6% of 18-years-olds will have experienced other disorders on the depression spectrum: Dysthymic disorder, 1 year or more of impairing depressive symptoms that do not met full criteria for MDD; or briefer episodes of minor depression, where duration or symptom count fall below the threshold for MDD. An episode of MDD is the most common mental health condition present when an adolescent dies by suicide. According to the US Centers for Disease Control and Prevention, the third most common cause of death in the 10 to 24 age group.[18]

The 1-year prevalence rates for full syndrome MDD are lower in preadolescent children, at 2%. However, if clinical and public health strategy for youth is to reflect the state of the science reviewed by Beardslee and colleagues, Weir and colleagues, Stuart Goldman, Kovacs and Lopez-Duran, elsewhere in this issue, it will take a longitudinal, developmental, family-focused perspective. Developmental epidemiology tells us that large numbers of those preadolescent children who have not yet experienced a first episode of MDD suffer from symptoms, disorders, or life circumstances that may be risk factors or true prodromes for adolescent depressive disorders. Relevant conditions include anxiety disorders (population prevalence in preadolescent children, 5.7%–12.8%[19]), minor depressions and difficulties with emotional regulation. Also important are sleep disturbances, which by adolescence affect 25% of youth, in particular insomnia disorder, with a lifetime prevalence of 10.7% by age 18 years (see discussion by Harvey and Clarke in this issue). Worldwide, 20% to 80% of children in the population have been exposed to at least 1 traumatic stress and there is evidence for a dose effect, with the risk for depression rising with number of exposures (see review[20]). Risk for the emergence of depression in adolescence is also higher among preadolescent children who live with chronic family conflict, parental depression, other family mental illness or substance abuse, and among those who have experienced physical or sexual abuse. It seems likely that genetic vulnerability and life experience each play a role. The practical public health relevance of this literature grows as suggestive[21] and in some cases specific[22] evidence emerges that intervention to address these preceding conditions might have the potential to prevent or ameliorate subsequent depressive episodes. Underlining the special challenges for pediatric primary care is the evidence that parental depression not only increases the risk of pediatric depression, but undermines the effectiveness of treatment of the child[23]: A particular challenge in healthcare systems such as the United States, where child and parent often do not have the same primary care physician. For these and other reasons, there are likely to be differences between the public health and primary care strategies that are most effective for pediatric and for adult depression.

THE REALITY: (HOW) IS PEDIATRIC DEPRESSION MANAGED IN PRIMARY CARE?

Depression is among the most common reasons for adult primary care consultations, ranking third in 1 large, UK, adult study.[24] Depression, anxiety, and alcoholism, alone or in combination, affect as many as 1 in 3 of adults seen in primary care.[25] However, in the overwhelming majority of cases the presenting complaint is physical rather than explicitly emotional; in no more than half of cases is the presence of depression recognized by the primary care clinician[3]; and for only a minority does primary care treatment meet minimal standards for adequacy.[3]

Comparable data are more limited for youth. The information that does exist suggests important similarities with adult primary care, but also several key areas where the realities differ, raising the possibility that the most effective public health strategy may also be different. As for adults, it has long been noted that high numbers of youth presenting to primary care, at least 20% to 25%, meet criteria for 1 or more DSM psychiatric disorder and that the large majority go unrecognized (eg, Costello and associates[26]). Youth with depression and anxiety are also overrepresented in primary care, particularly among frequent visitors,[27] a statement reconfirmed by recent studies of primary care attenders: Over 10% of UK adolescents had mood symptoms at levels comparable with those seen in clinically referred samples[28]; up to 17% of pediatric primary care patients in the United States met criteria for an anxiety disorder.[29] Affected youth, like adults, often present to primary care with physical symptoms. For example, among pediatric primary care attenders with recurrent abdominal pain, a common cause for recurrent consultation, rates are as high as 42% for MDD and 79% for 1 or more DSM anxiety disorders.[30]

However, there are important differences between the role played by primary care for depressed youth and depressed adults. Compared with affected adults, youth with depression are even less likely to be recognized in primary care and are much less likely to receive treatment of any kind. Clinically significant internalizing syndromes (anxiety, depressive) were diagnosed by primary care physicians in only 3.3% of 20,861 primary care attenders aged 4 to 15 years in the United States and Puerto Rico in the late 1990s.[31] Primary care clinicians recognized depression or anxiety in no more than 30% of diagnosable cases in 1 recent study[32] in a large integrated system of care. Figures obtained by a 2004 survey by the AAP suggest that pediatricians in the United States are less likely than internists or family practitioners to see managing depression as part of their role (25% endorse this view) or to report that they routinely do so (18%).[33] Although most (88%) do see it as their responsibility to identify depression and 56% report that they usually inquire,[33] few use existing standardized screening instruments or procedures.[34] In another contrast with adult services, only a minority of youth who receive any mental health services do so through primary care—9.6% over 3 years in the Great Smoky Mountain Study of the epidemiology of youth mental health. The figures for specialty mental health and education were 14.2% and 24.1%, respectively, over the same period, with the remainder receiving care through juvenile justice and child welfare.[35] More than 60% of youth who received mental health services made their initial contact through the education sector.[35] The prominence of the education sector of the service system is another reminder that it cannot be assumed that the public health strategy for child and adolescent depression will be identical to that for adults.

To further complicate the picture, rates of primary care treatment and even identification of pediatric depression have dropped from an already low base in the years after the British (2003) and US (2003–2004) review of the safety and efficacy of antidepressants for youth[36,37] and the US Food and Drug Administration black box warning of risk of emergent suicidality in youth exposed to antidepressants. An immediate drop in the rate of prescription of antidepressants to youth by nonspecialists was perhaps predictable, but the changes in practice went beyond pharmacotherapy in ways that are of great concern. Primary care clinicians became less likely to make a diagnosis of pediatric depression, a change that persisted 5 years later.[36] Furthermore, even when identified, depressed youth in the United States were less likely than in previous years to receive treatment of any type: There was no compensatory increase in the nonpharmacologic treatments known to be effective for many. Although cause has not been established,[38] there has been justifiable disquiet about the fact that the same years also saw a rise in adolescent suicide.[39] From 1990 to 2003, after a long period of increase from the 1950s to the early 1990s, the combined suicide rate for the age group 10 to 24 years declined by 28.5%.[18] However, 2003 to 2004 saw a reversal of this positive trend; the rate increased by 8.0%, the greatest single-year increase for 15 years.[18] In particular, suicide rates for girls aged 10 to 14 and 15 to 19 years and boys aged 15 to 19 years departed upward significantly from otherwise declining trends. The changes are not limited to the United States; Canada, for example, saw, in addition to a fall in antidepressant prescription to youth, a decrease in ambulatory visits for pediatric depression and anxiety along with an increase in youth suicide (annual rate per 1000 = 0.04 before and 0.15 after the warning).[37]

WHAT WORKS IN PRIMARY CARE? OVERVIEW OF INTERVENTION RESEARCH
Adult Intervention Research

The realities outlined in our introduction have produced several decades of adult research, which have demonstrated that primary care intervention for depressive disorders can be effective clinically (see selected reviews[3,4,40]). This work has also produced data on which types of intervention are more likely to be effective in decreasing the burden of depression in primary care patient populations. The most convincing and reproducible reports of benefits come from the now over 40 randomized, controlled trials (RCT) of versions of collaborative care.[4] "Collaborative care" is an umbrella term for a family of models that comprise a multisystem strategy to reorganize treatment for depression involving combinations of 3 distinct professionals, working collaboratively within the primary care setting: A case manager, a primary care practitioner, and a mental health specialist.[41,42] Collaborative care approaches in fact restructure care according to principles of chronic illness management.[3,43] Care is not only evidence based, but planned, typically along stepped care lines that offer simpler treatments first with guideline based progression to more complex interventions and more specialized care for those who do not respond adequately. The elements of the system that delivers care are actively designed:

- Provider roles;
- Decision support for clinicians;
- Procedures for screening, continuity of care, and case tracking;
- Support and resources for active patient self-management;
- Resources for collaboration, communication, and coordination, whether between disciplines, systems, levels of care, or with community resources; and
- Tailored use of information technology.

In contrast, interventions that limit their focus to treatment decisions produce more limited and inconsistent benefit, for example, clinician training, guideline-based care alone, feedback to clinicians on depression screening results, simple case identification and referral. These findings reflect the reality that many of the barriers to effective primary care of depression, as for other chronic or recurring conditions, lie in the organization and funding of care.[44,45]

Clinical Effectiveness of Collaborative Care

The general clinical effectiveness of the collaborative care approach is now viewed as established, at least compared with usual care in the integrated US health care settings, where the dominant model was developed. The research focus has moved on to improving the efficiency or effectiveness of specific elements of the models[46] and on extending to further conditions, for example, depression comorbid with chronic medical illness,[47] and other mental health conditions, such as exposure to trauma.[48] One promising emerging approach, potentially applicable to at-risk youth, is the concept of multiple risk intervention, for example, 1 recent study piloted cognitive–behavioral (CBT) approach that aimed to increase mental and physical well-being by reducing depressive symptoms, promoting smoking cessation, and increasing physical activity.[49]

Cost and Dissemination

On the important question of cost-effectiveness of collaborative care models data are mixed,[46] although 1 recent review[50] rated the evidence for health care savings as promising, particularly with more time elapsed from the initial investment.[51] There is no information on the cost-effectiveness of primary care mental health intervention for child and adolescent depression, either for health care systems and practices or for society at large. Another strand of the adult research has been to tackle barriers both to continued use of collaborative care approaches after the initial quality improvement initiative and to dissemination[52–54]: of particular importance is whether findings on feasibility and on impact—clinical or economic—hold in systems of care that are structured differently or funded differently than the relatively integrated systems in which the bulk of the extant research has taken place.[55,56] Key is how to implement effective management of depression in the patchwork of independent small to moderate sized, single specialty (pediatrics, family practice, internal medicine) group practices that deliver much of the available primary care. In these settings, implementation of the model requires initial work to develop the necessary personnel and relationships for the core collaborative care team, in particular to put in place the role of mental health specialist, work that in itself involves overcoming significant barriers. This reality has produced a large literature on models for primary care mental health ranging from colocation to telepsychiatry and including creative approaches to collaboration with mental health practitioners and agencies in the community. This essential work is beyond the scope of the current article, but is well summarized elsewhere.[5,57]

CHILD AND ADOLESCENT INTERVENTION RESEARCH

In contrast with the extensive adult literature, there exist only 2 controlled studies of primary care intervention for adolescent depressive disorders.[58–60] In addition, there exists 1 pilot study[61] of a classical collaborative care model and 1 controlled study of primary care protocol that aimed to prevent emergence of MDD.[62] There are no controlled studies of primary care intervention for depressive disorders in preadolescent children or for preadolescent anxiety disorders, the most common emotional disorder in the age group and a common precursor of adolescent depressive disorders. The findings of the existing studies are summarized below.

Intervention for Adolescent Depressive Disorder in Primary Care and Adolescent Medicine Settings

Asarnow and colleagues[60] enrolled 418 adolescent and young adult patients (13–21 years) with current depressive symptoms who presented to primary care and adolescent medicine settings in 5 health care organizations. Participants were randomized to usual care (n = 207) or a 6-month quality improvement intervention (n = 211), which included elements of collaborative care models (care managers, a multidisciplinary expert team) with improved access to psychotherapy (manualized CBT for depression delivered by care managers) and improved access to expert support for clinicians prescribing pharmacotherapy. Patients and clinicians in the intervention arm had free choice between CBT and pharmacotherapy. At 6 months, patients in the intervention arm were more likely to have received mental health care (32.1% vs 17.2%; $P<.001$) and in particular psychotherapy, reported fewer depressive symptoms on average significantly, were significantly less likely to be rated as severely depressed, and endorsed a higher mental health-related quality of life.

Longer term follow-up suggested a favorable impact on the course of depression through 12 and 18 months.[58]

Intervention for Adolescent Depressive Disorder in Primary Care Group Model HMO

Clarke and colleagues[59] conducted a study in pediatric primary care within a group model HMO to which they recruited 152 adolescents aged 12 to 18 years who had recently been prescribed a selective serotonin reuptake inhibitor (SSRI) and who met criteria for MDD: participants were randomized to primary care treatment as usual versus augmentation of SSRI treatment with brief (mean number of sessions achieved, 5.3), manualized CBT that included a focus on adherence to the medication program. Through the 1-year follow-up period, there was no more than weak evidence for added benefit from the adjunctive CBT. However, this finding is hard to interpret: In the event the study was underpowered because of the unexpected finding that 75% of adolescents in treatment as usual (principally primary care prescribed SSRI alone) experienced remission of MDD within 12 weeks. This is a strikingly higher acute phase remission rate than achieved by SSRI monotherapy in either adult primary care, where results for treatment as usual are typically poor, or in other RCTs for adolescent MDD, where rates have been as low as 23%.[63] (See the article by Sakolsky and Birmaher elsewhere in this issue.) The investigators cite previous data that clinical standards achieved for youth pharmacotherapy in the setting where the study took place are particularly high,[59] in contrast with the standards achieved under treatment as usual in most adult studies. However, this would not explain why outcomes differ from those achieved in RCTs evaluating the efficacy of pharmacotherapy for adolescent MDD: It seems probable that this primary care sample of depressed adolescents differs in response to treatment from typical samples in clinical research settings. This unexpected finding underlines the need for caution and evaluation as current treatment standards are disseminated to front-line community settings. On another note, 1 in 4 of the youth who remitted experienced relapse within 1 year, illustrating the need for a longitudinal perspective.

Collaborative Care Model Adaptation for Adolescents

Richardson and colleagues[61] piloted an adaptation for adolescents of a version of the well-studied collaborative care model developed by Katon, Unutzer and others at the University of Washington,[64] specifically the version used in the IMPACT study, which targeted older adults. Elements in the model included a depression case manager supervised by a mental health specialist, and adolescent and parent education. The sample comprised 40 youth aged 12 to 18 years meeting criteria for major or minor depression. The investigators report that the intervention was feasible over 6 months and well accepted by parents and youth. Rates of improvement similar to those reported in similar adult studies: 74% of youth had at least a 50% reduction in depressive symptoms.

Penn Resiliency Program

Gillham and colleagues[62] evaluated the effectiveness of the Penn Resiliency Program, a CBT intervention designed for the age group, in preventing depressive disorders in early adolescents who were recruited and, importantly, also treated in primary care settings: 271 children aged 11 and 12 years were randomized to either intervention or treatment as usual. Over 2 years of follow-up, both groups experienced similar overall rates of depressive disorders. Only in the subgroup with the highest level of depressive symptoms was there evidence that intervention prevented later episodes and that only when emotional disorders were combined into 1 group (depression, anxiety, and adjustment disorders).

Conclusions on Clinical Research on Primary Care Intervention for Youth Depression

The clinical research on primary care intervention for youth depression is sparse. The existing studies are largely promising. However, the findings in primary care have not always been consistent with the findings in adult primary care research or in pediatric research in other populations, underlining the need for continued research and evaluation as the field moves quickly to disseminate the approaches.

BARRIERS TO IMPLEMENTING COLLABORATIVE CARE

The barriers to implementation of collaborative care approaches fall in 3 principal domains:

1. The training of primary care clinicians and their comfort with the role;
2. Elements of the structure and financing of care; and
3. the traditional separateness of medical and mental health services.

As described, only 22% of US pediatricians see management of depression as within their role.[33] In the same survey by the AAP, pediatricians were also asked about perceived barriers to managing mental problems:

- They endorsed lack of training in treatment of mental health problems (70%) as a primary problem.
- A majority also endorsed a range of administrative and financial barriers, including
  - Lack of time (82%);
  - Lack of qualified mental health providers to whom to refer (65%); and
  - Inadequate payment for providing mental health treatment (54%).

In 2009, the AAP and the American Academy of Child and Adolescent Psychiatry published a joint "white paper" outlining the systemic (administrative and financial) issues that impede access to primary care mental health services for US youth and limit collaboration between primary care and specialty mental health: The paper proposed policy, funding, and reimbursement solutions.[44] These changes will take time. In the interim, the need is high and there have been a number of efforts to make available the resources and information that will allow willing pediatricians and practices to take on the challenge.

MAKING IT WORK IN PRACTICE: STANDARDS, SOLUTIONS AND RESOURCES
Standards of Care

Screening and identification
In March 2009, the US Preventive Services Task Force (USPSTF) recommended screening by primary care clinicians for MDD in adolescents aged 12 to 18 years when systems are in place to ensure accurate diagnosis, psychotherapy, and follow-up.[65] Although the evidence review identified no trials of primary care screening for pediatric MDD, the authors concluded that very limited available data suggested that primary care–feasible screening tools had been reasonably accurate in identifying depressed adolescents and, on the basis of the existing intervention research, that net benefit was probable. However, the report concluded that there was still insufficient evidence to recommend for or against universal screening for children 7 to 11 years old and that screening instruments performed less well in this younger age group. The USPSTF identified 2 screening tools for which there is adequate evidence to support use in primary care.

The AAP TFOMH[66] recommended using a 2-step procedure: Starting with an instrument to screen for general psychopathology as part of health maintenance visits or in situations suggesting increased risk, then 1 of the more depression-specific tools if a risk is identified. Like the USPSTF, the AAP TFOMH emphasized the importance of having referral sources in place.

Primary care management of depression

In its July 2009 policy statement, *The Future of Pediatrics, Mental Health Competencies for Pediatric Primary Care*,[13] the AAP recommended that all primary care clinicians become competent to develop a practice environment that normalizes integration of mental health and incorporates medical home principles for the care of children with mental health concerns. Specific recommendations related to depression included that primary care clinicians be able to apply DSM criteria to the diagnosis of MDD and use evidence-based interventions. More generally, the statement recommended that primary care clinicians, alone or in collaboration with mental health specialists, be able to plan diagnostic assessment of youth presenting with depressive or withdrawn behaviors or other mental health problems and to develop a care plan, recognize mental health emergencies, assist families in seeking and using the care of appropriate specialty mental health services, develop contingency or crisis plans for youth with urgent mental health problems, and monitor adverse and positive effects of nonpharmacologic and pharmacologic mental health therapy.

Necessary elements of primary care management for pediatric depression

The intervention research on pediatric depressive disorders (see the article by Maalouf and Brent elsewhere in this issue) has developed to the point that there is now unusual clarity about the first steps of treatment, at least in adolescents and at least in those with true, impairing MDD. The current US consensus on front-line treatment for pediatric MDD has been well-outlined in the *Practice Parameter for the Assessment and Treatment of Children and Adolescents With Depressive Disorders*[8] as updated by the American Academy of Child and Adolescent Psychiatry in 2007 and endorsed by the AAP. Since the publication of the practice parameter important additional data have come from the Treatment of Resistant Depression in Adolescence,[67] the first controlled study of additional treatment for adolescents who do not respond to a first SSRI.

Information from these sources can be simply adapted for implementation in primary care, such as the 3 flow sheets provided with this article (**Figs. 1–3**). In addition, there are now valuable tools and resources (summarized below) to support the development of the necessary collaborative care infrastructure. This clarity allows primary care practitioners and settings to choose, based on local realities and practitioner comfort, how far they wish to expand their roles in the management of depression. Some practices might choose to go no further than screening, assessment, and triage, but if they are to meet the standards for care, even this involves developing collaborative care systems (**Table 1**). Beyond this, there are a range of choices and models. At one end, a practice might manage all steps as far as the second SSRI trial (see **Figs. 1–3**) backed up by psychiatric consultation and with colocated psychotherapy services; other practices might choose to refer after the first SSRI trial or opt for developing close collaboration with local psychotherapists and clinics rather than for colocation. The important point is that any of these steps in the direction of more active involvement in the management of

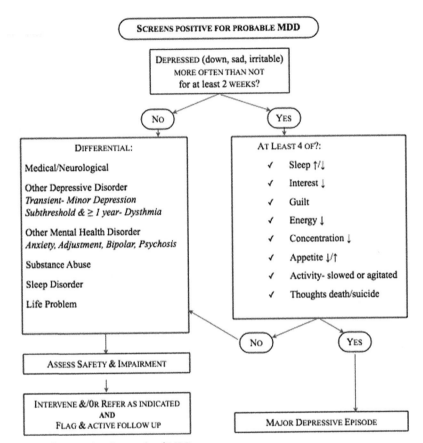

Fig. 1. Confirming the diagnosis of MDD.

depression is likely to improve access to care for the community served by the practice.

Resources to Support Primary Care Management of Pediatric Depression

American Academy of Pediatrics, Task Force on Mental Health

In 2004, the AAP convened a Task Force on Mental Health (TFOMH), charging it to assist pediatricians and other primary care clinicians in enhancing the mental health care that they provide to children and adolescents. The TFOMH acknowledged that practices taking on the challenge would need, in addition to mental health specific tools and products, strategies to produce multidisciplinary community collaboration to improve access to and coordination of care and support in the principles of producing practice change. This 6-year project generated the following products:

1. An action kit (*Strategies for System Change in Children's Mental Health: A Chapter Action Kit*) to assist AAP chapters and their organizational partners in state and regional change efforts, available for free download.[68]
2. The white paper,[44] *Improving Mental Health Services in Primary Care: Reducing Administrative and Financial Barriers to Access and Collaboration*, developed in collaboration with the American Academy of Child and Adolescent Psychiatry.

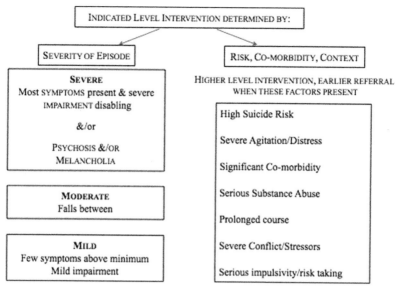

Fig. 2. Determining the indicated level of intervention for confirmed MDD. [1]For more detailed information on assessment of risk and severity see American Academy of Child and Adolescent Psychiatry: Practice parameter for the assessment and treatment of children and adolescents with depressive disorders[8] (endorsed by the American Academy of Pediatrics). Also available at http://www.aacap.org/cs/root/member_information/practice_information/ practice_parameters/practice_parameters. [2]For more detailed recommendations on management of suicide risk in primary care see the updated AAP policy statement on *Suicide and Suicide Attempts in Adolescents*[73] (available at http://aappolicy.aappublications.org/cgi/ content/full/pediatrics;105/4/871).

3. The policy statement, *The Future of Pediatrics, Mental Health Competencies for Pediatric Primary Care*.[13]
4. A special supplement to the journal *Pediatrics* in June 2010,[7] that, in addition to summarizing the work and introducing elements of the tool kit included 3 key reports: (i) Strategies for preparations for collaborative care at the community level[14] (*Enhancing Pediatric Mental Health Care: Strategies for Preparing a Community*), which includes strategies to inventory the community's mental health resources, to develop or strengthen relationships with mental health and other relevant groups including school and to develop a community protocol for managing psychiatric emergencies; (ii) a guide to change at the practice level,[15] *Enhancing Pediatric Mental Health Care: Strategies for Preparing a Primary Care Practice*, which included a Mental Health Practice Readiness Inventory to assess their practice's current capacity for effective mental health care to choose areas for targeted practice improvement; and (iii) algorithms to guide the process of integrating mental health into all facets of pediatric practice, *Enhancing Pediatric Mental Health Care: Algorithms for Primary Care*.
5. A "tool kit" (Addressing Mental Health Concerns in Primary Care: A Clinician's Toolkit)[69] designed to support the use of collaborative care/chronic illness principles in the management of child and adolescent mental health or substance abuse problems in primary care. Elements include: specific clinical materials (screening tools and protocols, intervention algorithms); materials to build practice procedures

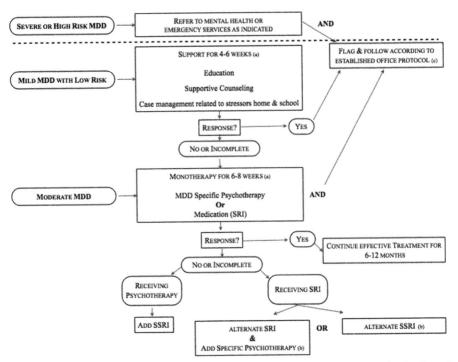

Fig. 3. Primary care treatment for confirmed MDD. For assessment of severity of episode and risk see text and **Table 1**. *Note:* At each decision point it is recommended that the clinician reassess adherence to the prescribed treatment, diagnosis, risk, severity, comorbidity, and life situation. [a]American Academy of Child and Adolescent Psychiatry: Practice parameter for the assessment and treatment of children and adolescents with depressive disorders.[8] (Endorsed by the American Academy of Pediatrics). [b]Brent and colleagues 2008.[67] [c]"Flag" typically means entering the child into a case registry which triggers relevant office protocol (see text, **Table 1**, and other resources[15,69]).

(registries, tracking protocols, information exchange, education and self-management strategies for youth/families) and primary care guidance for assessing and addressing common mental health and substance abuse symptoms (including depression), whether or not the symptoms rise to the level of a diagnosis.

6. An online educational program available through the AAP Pedialink CME program to help primary care clinicians develop the skills and knowledge to build the necessary collaborative relationships.

In addition, the TFOMH web-site is rich source of information about innovative collaborative care initiatives by practices and systems of care around the United States.[57]

TeenScreen
Technical support and resources for primary care screening programs for adolescent depressive disorders and suicidality are also available online through the TeenScreen program[70] at Columbia University. TeenScreen disseminates, free of charge, a screening package that, in addition to screening for depressive disorders, includes screening for general psychopathology and substance abuse.

Table 1
Preparing practice to screen for adolescent depressive disorders

Hierarchy of Clinical Questions	What to Know	What to Do	What the Practice Needs[a]
Is the child safe?	Imminent or high risk of harm to self or others? Of harm from others?	Do I need to act straight away by referring to emergency services and/or social services?	A protocol for accessing emergency services; procedures for flagging and following up with family and child
Is the child severely impaired?	Prolonged or highly impairing syndrome? Severe comorbidity: Severe substance abuse, risk taking, family turmoil, violence?	Do I need to get this child quickly into mental health services?	A protocol for accelerated referral of severe or at-risk cases; collaborative relationships (formal or personal) with MH clinicians and services
What is the diagnosis?	MDD or another mental health, medical, psychosocial syndrome? Emotional or behavioral symptoms that do not meet full criteria for a mental health disorder?	Which intervention or monitoring algorithm should I follow?	A protocol for differential diagnosis; algorithms for management of mental health and psychosocial conditions; procedures to flag and monitor identified youth

Abbreviation: MDD, major depressive disorder.
[a] Tools and resources to support practices in meeting these needs have been developed by the AAP Task Force on Mental Health summarized elsewhere in this paper.[7,14–16,66,69]

Screening Tools

The Patient Health Questionnaire family of screening instruments have been widely used and well-validated in primary health care for adults (PHQ; PHQ-9 item; PHQ-2 item). More recently, adolescent adapted versions have been developed (PHQ-A; PHQ-9 modified), although data on actual use in pediatric primary care are so far limited.[65] The USPSTF[65] rated the evidence for the PHQ-A as adequate to support use to screen for adolescent MDD in primary care: the PHQ-A has the advantage that, in addition to screening for mood problems, it also screens for anxiety, eating problems, and substance abuse. It has the disadvantage of being longer than other instruments and having somewhat lower sensitivity for MDD. The PHQ-9 is perhaps the instrument most widely used for screening for MDD in adult primary care; hence, it is well-known to many primary care clinicians and systems of care, an advantage. A recent study (postdating the USPSTF review) in adolescent primary care yielded a sensitivity and specificity for MDD (90/80) similar to those of adult populations but with a higher optimal screening threshold.[71] The PHQ-9 modified is a version of the PHQ-9 that has been specifically modified to screen in youth aged 12 to 18 years for MDD and suicidality; this version is included in the TeenScreen package.[70]

The USPSTF[65] also concluded that there was sufficient evidence to recommend for adolescents the use of the primary care version for Beck Depression Inventory, Primary care version, an abbreviated version of the adult Beck Depression Inventory.

Although the instruments described achieve high levels of sensitivity and specificity for the diagnosis of MDD, it remains important to conduct a brief, clinical interview to confirm the diagnosis and to screen for important somatic and psychological comorbidity (see **Figs. 1** and **2**). Equally important is determining the level of risk presented by the youth's mental health condition or life situation.

Management of youth who screen positive for probable MDD

Screening and evaluation will yield essentially 3 broad groups of youth who require attention:

1. Those with mild to moderate MDD who could safely receive front-line treatments through primary care settings that have prepared to deliver collaborative care (see **Fig. 3**);
2. Those with more severe MDD, higher levels of risk (severe suicidality, serious impulsivity/risk-taking) or more complex presentations (eg, serious comorbid substance abuse, severe family conflict) who will need early referral to mental health or, if indicated, emergency services; and
3. Those who screen positive for possible MDD, but who, on evaluation, are determined to in fact have other conditions (medical, mental health, substance abuse, life circumstances) or to have symptoms that fall below diagnostic thresholds.

Hence, an element of preparation for the practice is developing the tracking systems, protocols and collaborative relationships to support management of each of these groups (**Table 1**). Ideally, identified children in any of the groups would be flagged and entered in a manual or electronic case register, that would, in turn, trigger the relevant office management protocol, for example frequency and type of follow-up contacts with the child, family, and other professionals, and requirements for medication monitoring. Even those referred to emergency services or mental health should be flagged and followed: They are, by definition, special needs children who merit the services of a medical home and a high percentage of youth referred from primary care are seen for no or few visits in specialty mental health. The resultant case registries also can become tools for monitoring, evaluation, and improvement of the process. It is just these sorts of clinical and monitoring functions that the TFOMH tool kit was designed to support.

SUMMARY

The task of preparing primary care providers to play an effective role in the management of pediatric depressive disorders is not small. The AAP has acknowledged[7] that it represents systemic change that will take time and involve transformational changes in pediatric primary care practice, requiring new knowledge and skills, payment structures, collaborative relationships, office systems, and resources. Less overtly acknowledged is that this will involve complementary changes in child mental health practice.[6] Making these changes is a public health imperative driven by the solid data on the prevalence of adolescent depressive disorders, its risks, and the existence of effective treatments that reach few affected youth. There is now enough knowledge about first steps in treatment, at least for adolescents, and about how to house them in primary care practice to allow dedicated primary care practices, supported by the available tools, to take on the challenge.

Pediatric primary care providers have the potential to play powerful roles in reducing the burden of depression in further areas, outside the scope of this paper. We have mentioned the potential for using the longitudinal and early established relationship with the primary care clinician to identify and intervene early with conditions that are risk factors for later depressive disorders. In addition, primary care clinicians often see new mothers more than any other professional during the first year of a child's life. The data tell us that up to 12% of these mothers will be afflicted with postpartum depression,[72] usually unidentified and untreated, a current and long-term risk for their children.

It is important, however, to remember that this move to dissemination is somewhat in advance of the child- and adolescent-focused research. Even in the limited existing research, there are some flags that the clinical outcomes in pediatric primary care populations could differ from those in adult primary care settings and those in pediatric research settings.[59] There is work to be done to adapt the adult collaborative care models to the realities of clinical practice with youth, both in primary care and in specialty mental health care. These realities include working collaboratively with parents, an activity that is strongly supported both by common sense and the research literature, but poorly supported by existing funding mechanisms and the structure of care. Nor is there solid financial support for collaboration with the many other systems of care with which children and adolescents are involved. Treatment of parental mental health conditions, not captured in classic, adult-oriented models for collaborative care, can be a powerful intervention for pediatric mental health conditions, including depression. In addition, vulnerabilities and disorders are in evolution in childhood and adolescence: Evaluation of the full public health impact of intervention needs the long view. Finally, there are no data on how primary care clinicians will actually use the newly developed tools and on what impact any such changes in practice will have on the likelihood that depressed youth will receive treatment, on the types and adequacy of treatment provided and on clinical or cost outcomes. Dissemination must be accompanied by evaluation.

REFERENCES

1. World Health Organization. Disorders management: depression. Available at: http://www.who.int/mental_health/management/depression/definition/en/. Accessed November 25, 2011.

2. World Health Organization & World Organization of Family Doctors. Integrating mental health into primary care: a global perspective. Geneva: World Health Organization & World Organization of Family Doctors; 2008.

3. Katon W, Guico-Pabia CJ. Improving quality of depression care using organized systems of care: a review of the literature. Prim Care Companion CNS Disord 2011;13(1).

4. Simon G. Collaborative care for mood disorders. Curr Opin Psychiatry 2009;22:37–41.

5. McArthur Initiative on Depression in Primary Care. Available at: http://www.depression-primarycare.org/. Accessed December 22, 2011.

6. American Academy of Child and Adolescent Psychiatry: Committee on Collaboration with Mental Health Professionals. A guide to building collaborative mental health care partnerships in pediatric primary care. 2010. Available at: http://www.aacap.org/cs/systems_of_care_and_collaborative_models/collaboration_with_primary_care. Accessed January 20, 2012.

7. Foy JM, American Academy of Pediatrics Task Force on Mental Health. Enhancing pediatric mental health care: report from the American Academy of Pediatrics Task Force on Mental Health. Introduction. Pediatrics 2010;125(Suppl 3):S69–74.

8. Birmaher B, Brent D, AACAP Work Group on Quality Issues, et al. Practice parameter for the assessment and treatment of children and adolescents with depressive disorders. J Am Acad Child Adolesc Psychiatry 2007;46:1503–26.

9. Staller JA. Service delivery in child psychiatry: provider shortage isn't the only problem. Clin Child Psychol Psychiatry 2008;13:171–8.

10. Thomas CR, Holzer CE. The continuing shortage of child and adolescent psychiatrists. J Am Acad Child Adolesc Psychiatry 2006;45:1023–31.

11. Kim WJ, American Academy of Child and Adolescent Psychiatry Task Force on Workforce Needs. Child and adolescent psychiatry workforce: a critical shortage and national challenge. Acad Psychiatry 2003;27:277–82.

12. Wang PS, Sherrill J, Vitiello B. Unmet need for services and interventions among adolescents with mental disorders. Am J Psychiatry 2007;164:1–3.

13. Committee on Psychosocial Aspects of Child and Family Health and Task Force on Mental Health. Policy statement—the future of pediatrics: mental health competencies for pediatric primary care. Pediatrics 2009;124:410–21.

14. Foy JM, Perrin J, American Academy of Pediatrics Task Force on Mental Health. Enhancing pediatric mental health care: strategies for preparing a community. Pediatrics 2010;125(Suppl 3):S75–S86.

15. Foy JM, Kelleher KJ, Laraque D, American Academy of Pediatrics Task Force on Mental Health. Enhancing pediatric mental health care: strategies for preparing a primary care practice. Pediatrics 2010;125(Suppl 3):S87–108.

16. Foy JM, American Academy of Pediatrics Task Force on Mental Health. Enhancing pediatric mental health care: algorithms for primary care. Pediatrics 2010;125(Suppl 3):S109–25.

17. Ustün TB, Ayuso-Mateos JL, Chatterji S, et al. Global burden of depressive disorders in the year 2000. Br J Psychiatry 2004;184:386–92.

18. Centers for Disease Control and Prevention (CDC). Suicide trends among youths and young adults aged 10–24 years–United States, 1990–2004. MMWR Morb Mortal Wkly Rep 2007;56:905–8.

19. Ramsawh HJ, Chavira DA, Stein MB. Burden of anxiety disorders in pediatric medical settings: prevalence, phenomenology, and a research agenda. Arch Pediatr Adolesc Med 2010;164:965–72.

20. Fairbank JA, Fairbank DW. Epidemiology of child traumatic stress. Curr Psychiatry Rep 2009;11:289–95.

21. Cuijpers P, Muñoz RF, Clarke GN, et al. Psychoeducational treatment and prevention of depression: the "coping with depression" course thirty years later. Clin Psychol Rev 2009;29:449–58.
22. Garber J, Clarke GN, Weersing VR, et al. Prevention of depression in at-risk adolescents: a randomized controlled trial. JAMA 2009;301:2215–24.
23. Maalouf FT, Atwi M, Brent DA. Treatment-resistant depression in adolescents: review and updates on clinical management. Depress Anxiety 2011;28:946–54.
24. Singleton N, Bumpstead R, O'Brien M, et al. Psychiatric morbidity among adults living in private households, 2000. London: Social Survey Division of the Office for National Statistics; 2001.
25. Nordström A, Bodlund O. Every third patient in primary care suffers from depression, anxiety or alcohol problems. Nord J Psychiatry 2008;62:250–5.
26. Costello EJ, Costello AJ, Edelbrock C, et al. Psychiatric disorders in pediatric primary care. Prevalence and risk factors. Arch Gen Psychiatry 1988;45:1107–16.
27. Garralda ME, Bowman FM, Mandalia S. Children with psychiatric disorders who are frequent attenders to primary care. Eur Child Adolesc Psychiatry 1999;8:34–44.
28. Yates P, Kramer T, Garralda E. Depressive symptoms amongst adolescent primary care attenders. Levels and associations. Soc Psychiatry Psychiatr Epidemiol 2004; 39:588–94.
29. Chavira DA, Stein MB, Bailey K, et al. Child anxiety in primary care: prevalent but untreated. Depress Anxiety 2004;20:155–64.
30. Campo JV, Bridge J, Ehmann M, et al. Recurrent abdominal pain, anxiety, and depression in primary care. Pediatrics 2004;113:817–24.
31. Wren FJ, Scholle SH, Heo J, et al. Pediatric mood and anxiety syndromes in primary care: who gets identified? Int J Psychiatry Med 2003;33:1–16.
32. Richardson LP, Russo JE, Lozano P, et al. Factors associated with detection and receipt of treatment for youth with depression and anxiety disorders. Acad Pediatr 2010;10:36–40.
33. Stein RE, Horwitz SM, Storfer-Isser A, et al. Do pediatricians think they are responsible for identification and management of child mental health problems? Results of the AAP periodic survey. Ambul Pediatr 2008;8:11–7.
34. Zuckerbrot RA, Jensen PS. Improving recognition of adolescent depression in primary care. Arch Pediatr Adolesc Med 2006;160:694–704.
35. Farmer EM, Burns BJ, Phillips SD, et al. Pathways into and through mental health services for children and adolescents. Psychiatr Serv 2003;54:60–6.
36. Libby AM, Orton HD, Valuck RJ. Persisting decline in depression treatment after FDA warnings. Arch Gen Psychiatry 2009;66:633–9.
37. Katz LY, Kozyrskyj AL, Prior HJ, et al. Effect of regulatory warnings on antidepressant prescription rates, use of health services and outcomes among children, adolescents and young adults. CMAJ 2008;178:1005–11.
38. Centers for Disease Control and Prevention (CDC). Increases in age-group-specific injury mortality--United States, 1999-2004. MMWR Morb Mortal Wkly Rep 2007;56: 1281–4.
39. McCain JA. Antidepressants and suicide in adolescents and adults: a public health experiment with unintended consequences? P T 2009;34:355–78.
40. Badamgarav E, Weingarten SR, Henning JM, et al. Effectiveness of disease management programs in depression: a systematic review. Am J Psychiatry 2003;160:2080–90.
41. Gilbody S, Bower P, Whitty P. Costs and consequences of enhanced primary care for depression: systematic review of randomised economic evaluations. Br J Psychiatry 2006;189:297–308.

42. Katon W, Von Korff M, Lin E, et al. Rethinking practitioner roles in chronic illness: the specialist, primary care physician, and the practice nurse. Gen Hosp Psychiatry 2001;23:138–44.

43. Bodenheimer T, Wagner EH, Grumbach K. Improving primary care for patients with chronic illness. JAMA 2002;288:1775–9.

44. American Academy of Child and Adolescent Psychiatry Committee on Health Care Access and Economics Task Force on Mental Health. Improving mental health services in primary care: reducing administrative and financial barriers to access and collaboration. Pediatrics 2009;123:1248–51.

45. Von Korff M, Katon W, Unützer J, et al. Improving depression care: barriers, solutions, and research needs. J Fam Pract 2001;50:E1.

46. Liu CF, Rubenstein LV, Kirchner JE, et al. Organizational cost of quality improvement for depression care. Health Serv Res 2009;44:225–44.

47. Katon W, Lin EH, Von Korff M, et al. Integrating depression and chronic disease care among patients with diabetes and/or coronary heart disease: the design of the TEAMcare study. Contemp Clin Trials 2010;31:312–22.

48. Zatzick D, Rivara F, Jurkovich G, et al. Enhancing the population impact of collaborative care interventions: mixed method development and implementation of stepped care targeting posttraumatic stress disorder and related comorbidities after acute trauma. Gen Hosp Psychiatry 2011;33:123–34.

49. McClure JB, Catz SL, Ludman EJ, et al. Feasibility and acceptability of a multiple risk factor intervention: the Step Up randomized pilot trial. BMC Public Health 2011;11: 167.

50. van Steenbergen-Weijenburg KM, van der Feltz-Cornelis CM, Horn EK, et al. Cost-effectiveness of collaborative care for the treatment of major depressive disorder in primary care. A systematic review. BMC Health Serv Res 2010;10:19.

51. Unutzer J, Katon WJ, Fan MY, et al. Long-term cost effects of collaborative care for late-life depression. Am J Manag Care 2008;14:95–100.

52. Rubenstein LV, Chaney EF, Ober S, et al. Using evidence-based quality improvement methods for translating depression collaborative care research into practice. Fam Syst Health 2010;28:91–113.

53. Luck J, Hagigi F, Parker LE, et al. A social marketing approach to implementing evidence-based practice in VHA QUERI: the TIDES depression collaborative care model. Implement Sci 2009;4:64.

54. Smith JL, Williams JW, Owen RR, et al. Developing a national dissemination plan for collaborative care for depression: QUERI Series. Implement Sci 2008;3:59.

55. Katon W, Unützer J. Consultation psychiatry in the medical home and accountable care organizations: achieving the triple aim. Gen Hosp Psychiatry 2011;33:305–10.

56. Gilbody S, Bower P, Fletcher J, et al. Collaborative care for depression: a cumulative meta-analysis and review of longer-term outcomes. Arch Intern Med 2006;166: 2314–21.

57. American Academy of Pediatrics. Childrens mental health in primary care: collaborative projects. Available at: http://www2.aap.org/commpeds/dochs/mentalhealth/mh3co.html. Accessed December 22, 2011.

58. Asarnow JR, Jaycox LH, Tang L, et al. Long-term benefits of short-term quality improvement interventions for depressed youths in primary care. Am J Psychiatry 2009;166:1002–10.

59. Clarke G, Debar L, Lynch F, et al. A randomized effectiveness trial of brief cognitive-behavioral therapy for depressed adolescents receiving antidepressant medication. J Am Acad Child Adolesc Psychiatry 2005;44:888–98.

60. Asarnow JR, Jaycox LH, Duan N, et al. Effectiveness of a quality improvement intervention for adolescent depression in primary care clinics: a randomized controlled trial. JAMA 2005;293:311–9.
61. Richardson L, McCauley E, Katon W. Collaborative care for adolescent depression: a pilot study. Gen Hosp Psychiatry 2009;31:36–45.
62. Gillham JE, Hamilton J, Freres DR, et al. Preventing depression among early adolescents in the primary care setting: a randomized controlled study of the Penn Resiliency Program. J Abnorm Child Psychol 2006;34:203–19.
63. Kennard B, Silva S, Tonev S, et al. Remission and Recovery in the Treatment for Adolescents With Depression Study (TADS): acute and long-term outcomes. J Am Acad Child Adolesc Psychiatry 2009;48:186–95.
64. Katon W, Unützer J, Wells K, et al. Collaborative depression care: history, evolution and ways to enhance dissemination and sustainability. Gen Hosp Psychiatry 2010; 32:456–64.
65. Williams SB, O'Connor EA, Eder M, et al. Screening for child and adolescent depression in primary care settings: a systematic evidence review for the US Preventive Services Task Force. Pediatrics 2009;123:e716–35.
66. The Case for Routine Mental Health Screening. Pediatrics 2010;125:S133.
67. Brent D, Emslie G, Clarke G, et al. Switching to another SSRI or to venlafaxine with or without cognitive behavioral therapy for adolescents with SSRI-resistant depression: the TORDIA Randomized Controlled Trial. JAMA 2008;299:901–13.
68. American Academy of Pediatrics. Strategies for system change in children's mental health: a chapter action kit. American Academy of Pediatrics. Available at: http://www2.aap.org/commpeds/dochs/mentalhealth/mh2ch.html. Accessed January 20, 2012.
69. Foy JM, editor. Addressing mental health concerns in primary care: a clinician's toolkit. Chicago (IL): American Academy of Pediatrics; 2010.
70. National Center for Mental Health Check Ups at Columbia University. TeenScreen: Primary Care. Available at: http://www.teenscreen.org/programs/primary-care/. Accessed December 22, 2011.
71. Richardson LP, McCauley E, Grossman DC, et al. Evaluation of the Patient Health Questionnaire-9 Item for detecting major depression among adolescents. Pediatrics 2010;126:1117–23.
72. Earls MF, Committee on Psychosocial Aspects of Child and Family Health American Academy of Pediatrics. Incorporating recognition and management of perinatal and postpartum depression into pediatric practice. Pediatrics 2010;126:1032–9.
73. Shain BN. American Academy Of Pediatrics, Committee on Adolescence: Suicide and Suicide Attempts in Adolescents. Pediatrics 2007;120:3:669-76.

Education and Depression

Robert Li Kitts, MD, Stuart J. Goldman, MD*

KEYWORDS
- Depression • Education • Children • Adolescents

Primary care clinicians, including pediatricians, are often the first and only clinicians who have the opportunity to assess, diagnose, prevent, and treat child and adolescent mental health issues. They are the gatekeepers to mental health evaluations and treatment. Unfortunately, studies have shown that they warrant improvements in training around adequately evaluating depression (eg, using diagnostic criteria and ruling out medical causes), effectively recognizing suicide risk, assessing for psychiatric comorbidities, practicing evidence-based treatment with regard to depression (eg, starting antidepressant without fully meeting diagnostic criteria for major depression), and being able to establish effective relationships with mental health clinicians.[1–6]

"The identification, initial assessment, and care of mental health problems ideally take place in the child's 'medical home,' where he or she will benefit from the strengths and skills of the primary care clinician in establishing rapport with the child and family, using the primary care clinician's unique opportunities to engage children and families in mental health care without stigma," American Academy of Child and Adolescent Psychiatry in collaboration with the American Academy of Pediatrics.[7]

ELLA
Approach: Screening and Diagnostic Tools

Case: Ella is a 14-year-old Hispanic female with a strong family history of depression who seemed sad when she presented with her mother for her annual physical examination. During the examination her pediatrician asked her how she was doing, and Ella stated that she was "fine." Although concerned, her pediatrician still had to complete her examination, and she was already backed up with patients waiting.

Teaching Points

In primary care clinics, it is important that clinicians are aware of the risk factors for depression (**Box 1**) to help appropriately prioritize their time. Even though Ella stated that she was "fine," this statement should not end the screening for

The authors have nothing to disclose.
Department of Psychiatry, Children's Hospital Boston and Harvard Medical School, 300 Longwood Avenue, Boston, MA 02115, USA
* Corresponding author.
E-mail address: Stuart.goldman@childrens.harvard.edu

Child Adolesc Psychiatric Clin N Am 21 (2012) 421–446
doi:10.1016/j.chc.2012.01.007
1056-4993/12/$ – see front matter © 2012 Elsevier Inc. All rights reserved.

childpsych.theclinics.com

Box 1
Risk factors for child and adolescent depression

Biological

- Genetic predisposition, especially maternal psychopathology
- Other psychiatric condition (eg, anxiety, disruptive, eating, or substance use disorders)
- Inhibited, easily upset (negative affectivity/emotionality) and/or inflexible temperament
- Chronic medical illness
- Female gender, particularly with adolescents

Psychological

- Negative thinking pattern
- Tendency to base one's self-worth on success in interpersonal relationships
- Exposure to trauma, including neglect, sexual, physical, and emotional abuse
- Disengagement, involuntary, and emotion-focused coping (as opposed to engaged and problem-focused coping)

Social

- Childhood poverty
- Family dysfunction
- Personal disappointments, failures, and losses

Developmental

- Transition from childhood to adolescence

Data from Refs.[8–11]

---

depression, particularly if it is not consistent with her presentation along with having a strong risk factor for depression. This scenario presents a critical opportunity for a clinician to identify a highly treatable illness and make a clinical difference for the patient.

To assist busy clinicians in being more proactive and competent in the approach and management of adolescent depression, experts convened and developed the first evidence- and consensus-derived guidelines and their associated toolkit (ie, Guidelines for Adolescent Depression in Primary Care, GLAD-PC; http://www.glad-pc.org/). Educators and trainees should be encouraged to read the guidelines and use the toolkit.[6,12] Briefly, the guidelines focus on children and adolescents from 10 to 21 years old. They provide both the recommendations and the level of evidence behind each recommendation, offering clinicians the opportunity to develop their critical appraisal skills. The resources efficiently provide aids, guidelines, and/or information on early identification, screening, diagnosis, treatment, monitoring, billing, and speaking with adolescents and parents. They also provide educational materials for adolescents and parents.

In Ella's case, it would have been very useful for her busy pediatrician to have in place a systematic means (for example a waiting room questionnaire) of identifying whether Ella, or any other patient, was truly at high risk for depression, regardless of the presenting complaint. The US Preventive Services Task Force recommends screening of all adolescents between the ages of 12 and 18 years for major depressive disorder when the appropriate systems are in place.[13]

Box 2
Depressive disorders other than a major depressive disorder

- Complex grief
- Dysthymic disorder
- Substance-induced mood disorder
- Adjustment disorder with depressed mood
- Adjustment disorder with depressed mood and anxiety
- Depressive disorder not otherwise specified
- Depressive episode of a bipolar disorder

The GLAD-PC toolkit provides and reviews how to use such tools, including the Guidelines for Adolescent Preventive Services Questionnaires, Strength and Difficulties Questionnaire, Columbia Depression Scale, Kutcher Adolescent Depression Scale, and PHQ-9 modified for teens (Patient Health Questionnaire). Additionally, the Beck Depression Inventory for Youth and Children's Depression Rating Scale–Revised are both easy to administer and have good internal consistency, validity, and reliability.[11] The TeenScreen National Center (http://www.teenscreen.org/) is a potential resource for primary care clinicians that promotes screening in the community. However, these screening tools are intended to supplement and not replace the diagnostic interview, details of which are available elsewhere.[14]

Ella's pediatrician asked that her mother step out of the office and proceeded to further inquire about her mood. Upon asking Ella about how things have been going, her pediatrician discovered that Ella was not "fine." She discovered that Ella has been feeling "stupid" and "ugly" and that she has been feeling this way for almost a month. Upon direct questioning Ella also revealed feeling sadder, more tired, less interested in activities, having a decreased appetite, and acknowledging that "nothing" was "fun" anymore. She acknowledged that she did not want to tell her mother because her mother had depression and stress of her own, and therefore she did not want to upset her. Ella denied thoughts of wanting to end her life. Further questions reflected the pediatrician's understanding of the diagnostic criteria for major depression in the *Diagnostic and Statistical Manual of Mental Disorders, Fourth Edition. (DSM-IV)*,[15] and she met most of the criteria for a mild major depressive episode.

Ella's pediatrician needed to make sure that there was no underlying medical cause, because some medical disorders may mimic or exacerbate depressive disorders. These include hypothyroidism, mononucleosis, autoimmune diseases, anemia, certain neoplasms, and chronic fatigue syndrome.[8] Medications that are more often associated with depressive symptoms include cardiovascular agents, chemotherapeutic agents, corticosteroids, immunosuppressants, interferon, isotretinoin, narcotics, and oral contraceptives.[11]

A follow-up appointment was scheduled the next week to confirm a working diagnosis of major depression, rule out other depressive disorders (**Box 2**) and psychiatric comorbidities (additional psychiatric diagnosis coinciding with depression considered the rule rather than the exception[8,9]), reassess suicidal ideation, and discuss treatment recommendations. Ella's pediatrician also wanted to inquire more about their understanding of depression and to explore more in-depth factors that may be playing a role in her depression to best guide her treatment recommendations.

Box 3
Common reasons for referral or consultation with a mental health clinician

- If you have questions regarding diagnosis of depression
- Psychiatric comorbidity (eg, substance use, anxiety, disruptive behavior, or psychotic disorders)
- Concern for bipolar disorder
- More severe depression (eg, moderate to severe depression with or without psychotic features)
- Starting an antidepressant and unable to provide adequate follow-up (eg, just started an antidepressant and cannot see them for more than a week)
- Not responding to an antidepressant
- Safety concerns (eg, suicidal ideation)
- Concerns regarding adverse reaction to antidepressant
- Patient with depression and complex psychosocial issues

Although Ella was rather forthcoming upon more direct questioning, collecting information from pediatric patients can be challenging, especially when he/she is very young. Challenges include patients' limited insight and communication as a function of normal development, making them less likely to seek help from the clinician. This challenge differs from the adult patient, who is more likely to ask for treatment of his/her own self-identified and articulated depression and symptoms. Clinicians are encouraged to make the patient as comfortable as possible while assessing potentially personal and/or sensitive areas, such as feelings (eg, have parent[s] step out of the room, wait until the patient is back in her own clothes, use language that he or she can relate to). Children and adolescents have been shown to report lower levels of depressive symptoms than their parents,[16] making collateral information from parents crucial for an accurate diagnosis. Obtaining additional collateral information may also be helpful. For example, contacting a patient's teacher or guidance counselor may help clarify potential discrepancies of severity reported by two parents or between the child and parent.

Q & A

Q: When would it be appropriate to make a referral or consult with a mental health clinician?

A: The GLAD-PC toolkit outlines the referral process, provides a clinical management flowchart recommending when it is appropriate to refer, and provides tools to facilitate the process. Additionally, the American Academy of Child and Adolescent Psychiatry (AACAP) has a section that addresses this question (http://www.aacap. org/cs/root/physicians_and_allied_professionals/when_to_seek_referral_or_consultation_ with_a_child_and_adolescent_psychiatrist).

Generally speaking, any child with depression that is interfering with his or her functioning should be referred to evidence-based talking therapy. Additional common reasons for referral or consultation include those provided in **Box 3**.

Access to a mental health clinician varies based on the type of clinician (eg, fewer child and adolescent psychiatrists than licensed clinical social workers) and location (eg, metropolitan vs rural location). It is important to find out what your access is (eg, academic institution, colocation within your clinic, or telepsychiatry) and promote communication/collaboration.

Q: Does the presentation of depression vary with age and gender?

A: Yes. Child and adolescent patients are more inclined to display anxiety, irritability, temper tantrums, somatic complaints, hypersomnia, weight gain, psychomotor agitation, and poor self-esteem when compared with adults[8,17] (see discussion elsewhere in this issue). Further differences are seen when comparing children with adolescents. For example, hypersomnia, suicide attempts, melancholia, and associated psychotic symptoms are more frequently seen with depressed adolescents, whereas somatic complaints and behavioral problems are more frequently seen with depressed children.[9] Differences are also seen between genders, with depressed females more likely to report changes in appetite/weight, sleep difficulties, psychomotor retardation, increased crying, feelings of failure, guilt, and poor self-esteem, whereas males are more likely to report anhedonia, diurnal variation in mood and energy, social withdrawal, and work impairment.[9]

ALEX
Approach: Parental Depression and Prevention

Case: Alex is a 7-year-old white male who was brought in for an annual checkup by his pediatrician. His mother complained of Alex's misbehaviors at home and school. Although Alex clearly had some behavioral problems, he was appropriate in the office and did not seem sad, but his tearful mother did.

Teaching Points

Negative effects of parental depression have been documented in children ranging from infancy through adulthood.[18–23] School-aged children of depressed mothers have more school problems, are less socially competent, and have lower levels of self-esteem and higher levels of behavioral problems.[19–20] Children of depressed parents are at a significantly increased risk for developing psychopathologic conditions compared with the children of nondepressed parents, especially mothers.[18,22,23] Weissman and colleagues'[23] 20-year prospective longitudinal study revealed that offspring of depressed parents had approximately three times the risk for anxiety disorders, major depression, and substance dependence, along with increased social impairment and emerging higher rates of medical problems and mortality. Studies also support the association between improvements in children's overall functioning and in their depressive symptoms with the successful treatment of parental depression.[24–26]

Clearly, it is important for clinicians, including pediatricians, to be able to screen for parental depression and help parents get the needed support and/or treatment critical to their child's well-being. Screening for peripartum depression, such as with the Edinburgh Postnatal Depression Scale, is routinely recommended for women in primary care[26] but should continue once the postpartum period has ended. There are brief and user-friendly family-based preventive interventions, such as the Family Talk Preventive Intervention. In its five to seven sessions it aims to reduce risk and enhance protective factors by promoting positive interactions between parents and children, increasing understanding of the illness (ie, parental depression) for everyone in the family, and fostering communication between parents and children, including discussions about the effects of parental depression. It is evidence-based and has been shown to be adaptable and have positive effects among different populations, including inner-city single-parent minority families, Latino families, and outside of the United States.[27–30] Dr Beardslee's Web site, Families Preventing & Overcoming Depression (FAMPod; http://www.fampod.org/), enables clinicians to learn at no cost how to conduct this intervention by providing a downloadable manual, learning modules, and supporting videos.

Alex's pediatrician decided to call Alex's mother later in the day because she did not want to check in with her in front of Alex. The pediatrician inquired about how things have been going and said that she noticed that the mother had seemed sad during the appointment. Alex's mother responded that things have been very stressful at home because Alex's father had recently been deployed. She acknowledged that she has been more overwhelmed and less patient with Alex and his two siblings. The pediatrician decided to set up an appointment between the clinic's social worker and Alex's mother. Additionally, she referred the social worker to the Family Preventing & Overcoming Depression Web site.

An additional resource for families in the military is the Family Resiliency Training for Military Families (FOCUS; http://www.focusproject.org/) that was initiated by the Bureau of Medicine and Surgery. It is a family-centered resource focused on prevention by providing resiliency training to military children and families. It teaches practical skills to meet the challenges of deployment and reintegration, to communicate and solve problems effectively, to improve emotional regulation, and to successfully set goals together and create a shared family story.

Although there are increasing numbers of preventative interventions for depression in young people, they still lag far behind its treatment. The National Research Council and Institute of Medicine's 2009 report, Preventing Mental, Emotional, and Behavioral Disorder Among Young People, appropriately *"calls on the nation—its leaders, its mental health research and service provision agencies, its schools, its primary care medical systems, its community-based organizations, its child welfare and criminal justice systems—to make prevention of mental, emotional, and behavioral disorders and the promotion of mental health of young people a very high priority."*[26]

Q&A

Q: Are there resources adolescents can access on their own?

A: Different communities have different resources for adolescents. Being aware of what your community has to offer (eg, youth community empowerment organizations or programs) will go a long way. One additional resource is Project CATCH-IT (http://catchit-public.bsd.uchicago.edu/) a community and Internet-based project with 14 modules designed to teach coping skills to teenagers and young adults.

JEREMY
Understanding: Developmentally Informed Stressors

Case: Jeremy is an 11-year-old white male whose father called the pediatric office with concerns that his son may be depressed because he has recently seemed less happy and far less interested in school. His father acknowledged that depression runs in his family. Jeremy had been a good student who enjoys attending school. In your assessment, Jeremy did not meet criteria for major depressive disorder, but seemed sad and did not want to talk about it.

Teaching Points

Although a strong family history of depression raises concern for a major depressive disorder, it is also important to explore and educate parents for other possible reasons why their child may be sad. The understanding and insight of parents vary and are influenced by their own experiences with sadness (eg, family psychiatric history), current state (eg, currently depressed and overwhelmed), relationship with child (eg, contentious and distant), and level of involvement with child's full life (eg, actively engaged with child's school and peer group).

Helping parents understand their child's sadness and underlying stressors typically enhances their empathy, thereby strengthening their ability to support their child and potentially reduce the risk of a future depression. Universal potential sources of stress include trauma (ie, neglect, sexual, physical, or emotional), bullying, loss (especially parental), moving, divorce, or medical illness (ie, self or someone close). Other sources of stress and their impact may vary with age or developmental level and may not seem as subjectively serious to adults. Reminding parents of this fact may be helpful. For example, it may be very invalidating and frustrating for an adolescent to have his or her parent minimize the impact of the first failed romantic relationship. **Table 1** provides a list of developmentally informed sources of stress.

Exploring stressors with Jeremy's mother helped put his depression into context. His parents were about to get a divorce and he and his mother were now living in a different neighborhood. Although Jeremy was relieved that his parents were not fighting as much, he was sad over the loss of what he was so used to, his family being one unit (eg, "waking up to both of his parents in the kitchen and having breakfast together"). Although informative, his intermittent school refusal still remained unexplained.

Refusal to attend school is a serious concern. It is not only a red flag for mental health concerns, but also a risk factor for multiple poor outcomes including violence, suicide attempts, pregnancy, and substance abuse.[31] Just as the severity ranges (eg, from occasional absences to persistent daily school refusal), the underlying factors(s) may range. Depression and depressive symptoms may play a role, through reduced motivation related to anhedonia, disrupted sleep and increased fatigue, and decline in focus and attention. Anxiety disorders, somatoform disorders, and diverse medical problems may also disrupt school attendance as well as contextual factors including the home environment, parental involvement, teenage pregnancy, school climate, and peer challenges.[31] More detailed information and algorithms are available.[31–33]

Peer challenges can range from difficulties with making friends to severe bullying (eg, physical, verbal, alienation, and electronic). Violence and bullying are major concerns. A 2005 nationwide survey of 6th- to 10th-grade students reported 2-month prevalence rates of either being bullied or bullying at school at 20.8% physically, 53.6% verbally, 51.4% socially, and 13.6% electronically.[33] In a separate study, 5% of students reported not attending school on at least 1 day during the 30 days before the survey because they felt that they would be unsafe at school or on their way to or from school.[34] Longitudinal studies support the association between bullying and increased suicidal ideation and behaviors.[35,36]

According to his parents, Jeremy just started the sixth grade in a new and better school district. Neither they nor his teachers were aware of bullying, and he reportedly was making new friends. Upon further discussion, Jeremy reported that work had been more difficult, but he did not want to disappoint his parents by complaining so he just spent more time studying. In a quiet voice he says that he is smaller than many of his classmates and is wondering when he is going to hit puberty. Jeremy currently has no interest in sex or relationships, and a couple of older seventh graders have been teasing him and his friends and calling them gay.

Transitions, even positive and expected ones, can be a challenge and a source of major stress to a child or adolescent. This type of change includes transitioning from being at home to preschool, preschool to elementary school, elementary to middle school, and high school to college, military, or workforce. It includes transitioning into adolescence (ie, onset of puberty) or transitioning into a role with greater or just

Table 1
Developmentally informed sources of stress

Age Range	Self	Others/Environment	Tasks
Early Childhood (birth–5 years old)	• Sense of safety and security (eg, fear of abandonment by parent who is inconsistently present) • Feeling loved (eg, feeling less loved because of newborn sibling)	• Structure (eg, lack of daily structure provided by parents) • Predictability (eg, unpredictable parent absence due to sickness) • Ambiance of home/family environment (eg, parents getting a divorce and a lot of tension within the home)	• Developmental milestones (eg, pressure to develop skills that may signify something negative to the child)
Childhood (6–12 years old)	• Appearance (eg, being the only child with dark skin in the entire classroom) • Gender role and identity (eg, girl wanting to play sports, but being told that it is for boys)	• Caregiver validation and pressure (eg, being told by caregiver that there is nothing for the child to be upset about because he/she had it much worse) • Peer validation and pressure (eg, pressure to fit in and fear of being left out) • Ambiance of home/family environment (eg, younger sibling being treated for cancer)	• School work (eg, starting a new school that is much harder than prior school) • Extracurricular (eg, boy wanting to spend more time with father but no time because at school and over-extended with sports and music lessons)
Adolescence (12–18 years old)	• Appearance (eg, being a teenager with severe acne or overweight) • Personal identity (eg, trying to figure one's identity, but challenged by their desire conflicting with others) • Sexual identity (eg, being unsure of one's sexuality but afraid to talk to anyone because of fear of rejection)	• Caregiver validation and pressure (eg, pressure from parents to achieve) • Peer validation and pressure (eg, pressure to conform) • Ambiance of home/family environment (eg, excited about going to college but overt awareness of family's financial stress) • Sexual activity (eg, pressured by significant other to have sex) • Relationship (eg, first breakup)	• School work (eg, difficulty with adjusting to ninth grade and being told, "these grades really do count" or "these are supposed to be the best years of your life") • Extracurricular (eg, first job)

different responsibilities. Additionally, being different (eg, appearance, race, ethnicity, socioeconomic status, religion, gender role, or sexual orientation) can be a source of stress for a child or adolescent regardless of whether or not it leads to bullying. Children and adolescents who are beginning to question their sexual orientation or identify themselves as lesbian, gay, bisexual, or transgender are at increased risk for bullying, school refusal/dropping out, depression, substance use, and suicidal ideation/behaviors.[37–39] Therefore, it is important for clinicians to inquire about sexual attraction and behaviors in a developmentally appropriate manner and to educate parents on how they can be supportive.[40,41]

Regardless of the cause or severity of bullying, it is important for parents to provide a validating environment, encourage communication, and advocate against bullying. A longitudinal environmental risk study involving over a thousand twin pairs and their families identified the following factors as being associated with children's resilience to being bullied: family support, maternal warmth, sibling warmth, and atmosphere at home (eg, clean, stimulating, and happy).[42]

Q&A

Q: A patient of mine is being bullied and his parents are in need of support. Are there any resources I can provide them?

A: Stopbullying.gov (http://www.stopbullying.gov/) is an informative Web site jointly managed by the US Departments of Health and Human Services and Education and Justice. It provides children, teens, young adults, parents, and educators resources about bullying awareness, prevention, and intervention. For additional information, particularly with regard to electronic bullying, you may explore the following sites:

- Electronic Media and Youth Violence: A Centers for Disease Control and Prevention Issue Brief for Educators and Parents (http://www.cdc.gov/ViolencePrevention/pub/EA-brief.html)
- Center for Safe and Responsible Internet Use (http://www.cyberbully.org/)
- Cyberbullying Research Center (http://cyberbullying.us/)
- Internet Safety Education (http://www.isafe.org/).

Q: Parents of a patient of mine would like resources to help understand and support their daughter who recently disclosed that she was a lesbian. Are there any?

A: Certain cities and states may provide their own local resources, such as WAGLY (West Suburban Alliance of Gay and Lesbian Youth; http://www.wagly.org/) and BAGLY (Boston Alliance of Gay, Lesbian, and Transgender Youth; http://www.bagly.org/home). If they do not, you may consider exploring the following:

- Parents, Families, and Friends of Lesbians and Gays (PFLAG; http://community.pflag.org/)
- Gay, Lesbian & Straight Education Network (GLSEN)—national education organization focused on ensuring safe schools for all students (http://www.glsen.org/)
- GLBT National Help Center (http://www.glnh.org/)
- The Trevor Project—national organization focused on crisis and suicide prevention efforts among lesbian, gay, bisexual, transgender, and questioning youth (http://www.thetrevorproject.org/)
- It Gets Better Project (http://www.itgetsbetter.org/).

Box 4
Examples of impairments in child and adolescent functioning related to depression

Personal Functioning

- Decline in hygiene (eg, decreased showering)
- Room is messier than usual
- Not caring about dress as much as before
- Worsened medical adherence if he/she has a chronic medical illness

Social Functioning

- Increased isolation in room
- Preferring not to eat with the family
- Declining friends or family outings
- Friends not calling or coming over as often
- Recent breakup with significant other
- No longer engaging in extracurricular activities

Academic Functioning

- Decline in grades
- Harder to wake up and get to class
- Increased school attendance and tardiness issues

Occupational Functioning

- Fired from job (and not caring)
- No longer as interested in making money to save for particular item (eg, car, video game)

HENRY
Approach: Chronic Medical Illnesses and Hospitalizations

Case: Henry is a 13-year-old African American male who was admitted to the hospital 3 days ago for new onset of Type I diabetes mellitus. His medical team raised concerns for depression because the patient has been progressively less interactive with the medical team and recently started covering his head with the sheets when they would enter the room. Parents have noted increased irritability. The team was hoping to start him on a selective serotonin reuptake inhibitor (SSRI). A psychiatry consultation was requested.

Teaching Points

It would be important to determine whether Henry has a primary mood disorder, mood disorder secondary to a general medical condition (eg, poorly controlled diabetes), an adjustment disorder (eg, new diagnoses of diabetes), or no disorder at all. An irritable mood, rather than a depressed mood, can qualify as the predominant mood for a child or adolescent who presents with a major depressive episode. Additional criteria for such a major depressive episode would include five or more of the noted symptoms[15] for the same 2-week period along with a change from previous functioning. Examples of impairments in different types of functioning among the child and adolescent population are described in **Box 4**.

Box 5
Behaviors that may enhance therapeutic collaboration and enhance validity of an interview with a child or adolescent patient

- Showing interest in the individual and not just the disease[44]

- Actively listening

- Starting off with a friendly question as opposed to a question that the patient may be tired of hearing (eg, first ask about the movie they were watching as opposed to "have you had a bowel movement?" "how is your pain?" or "how are you doing?")

- Sitting down

- Providing good eye contact[45]

- Apologizing if you seem to be interrupting something (eg, "I'm sorry, am I interrupting your movie or lunch?")

- Asking patient what he or she prefers to be called (same with parents)

- Using developmentally appropriate language

- Explaining why you need to be doing things that may be frustrating to the patient (eg, explaining why it is important to ask about bowel movements every morning)

- Empathizing with patients when you know you are asking questions that they may not like to hear ("I'm sorry, but I have to ask this question and you may not like it when I ask it over and over again each day.")

- Giving the patient options to assist in giving them a sense of control (eg, "I need to listen to your heart, but do you prefer I do it now or in a few minutes so that you can have time to wake up?")

- Giving them time to speak when asking if they have any questions, comments, or concerns

---

Promoting cooperative collaboration with children and adolescents can be challenging, and efforts to minimize disruptive factors are crucial in promoting collaboration, information collection, and reducing clinician bias. For example, a team of physicians entering a pediatric patient's room with contact precautions, including masks, are more likely to elicit a negative response from the child,[43] and those clinicians may be more inclined to label that child as anxious, depressed, or even medically traumatized. Alternatively, the team could have displayed their faces before entering the room, smiled at the child, and limited the number entering the room. **Boxes 5** and **6** list behaviors that may enhance or worsen therapeutic collaboration with a child or adolescent patient, which is an important but understudied area.

As for Henry, the psychiatrist initially walked into the room and saw Henry watching television. He asked what he was watching and began a discussion with Henry over his favorite movies. After a couple of minutes of discussion, he asked if it was okay if they paused the movie and if he could ask Henry questions about his hospital stay and how it has been. Henry agreed, and the psychiatrist sat at his bedside and was able to engage him without difficulty for the entire assessment. Henry was pleasant with a full range of affect, but predominantly sad. He seemed quite anxious and upset when talking about his diabetes. He stated that he was tired of being in the hospital, scared by his diabetes ("If I don't take good care of my sugars, I may lose my fingers and toes!"), and frustrated with having strangers consistently coming in and waking him up to ask him the same questions.

Symptoms of depression (eg, irritability, fatigue, appetite change, challenges with concentration) and anxiety can be due to poor glucose control, making it challenging

---

Box 6
Behaviors that may worsen therapeutic collaboration and reduce the validity of an interview with a child or adolescent patient

- Entering a room with a mask on to a patient who has never seen your face
- Interviewing the patient right after an unfavorable procedure (eg, blood draw)
- Entering in large groups
- Early morning rounding when the patient is not a morning person
- Entering the room abruptly without permission (eg, knocking and not waiting for permission)
- Dismissive behaviors (eg, talking fast, standing close to the door, interrupting patient multiple times)
- Talking among medical providers as if patient is not even there or just an object
- Asking patient for permission to do something, but arguing if the patient says no (eg, "Can I listen to your heart?" "No," "But I have to")
- Monotonous behavior (eg, same tone, same questions, same responses)

---

to make a diagnosis.[46] Once Henry's glucose was under better control, the psychiatrist could determine that he met criteria for an adjustment disorder with depressed mood and anxiety.[15] According to Fritsch and colleagues,[46] approximately 30% of children develop a clinical adjustment disorder within 3 months of being diagnosed with Type 1 diabetes mellitus. This adjustment disorder often resolves within the first year, but poor adaptation in this initial phase places children at risk for later psychological difficulties.

Overall, most children and adolescents adjust to their chronic health conditions.[11] However, those who have chronic health conditions have higher levels of disorder-dependent depressive symptoms than those who are healthy.[11,16] A recent meta-analysis by Pinquart and Shen[16] found higher rates of depression in children and adolescents with cleft lip and palate, epilepsy diseases, chronic fatigue syndrome, and illnesses characterized by chronic pain (eg, migraine/tension–type headaches) among over a dozen other illnesses. However, it is important that clinicians screen for depression regardless of type of illness. Depression has often been associated with poor treatment adherence, worsened prognosis, and higher rates of adverse health risk behaviors.[11] In other words, they can transactionally worsen or improve the other. Therefore, a collaborative approach between mental health and primary care clinicians will promote the specific and overall health and well-being of patients.[6,11]

Henry's team still wanted to start him on an SSRI despite the diagnosis of adjustment disorder. His psychiatrist informed the team that this medication was not indicated. It is important for clinicians not to simply prescribe an antidepressant because the patient seems anxious and/or depressed. They need to be informed by an accurate diagnosis, treatment guidelines (eg, GLAD-PC and AACAP Practice Parameter), and the quality of evidence/studies supporting treatment recommendations. There has been increasing scrutiny with regard to industry influence on prescribing practices and the quality of influence-sponsored clinical research.[47,48] Promoting research literacy will enhance evidence-based practice.

Q&A

Q: What are some resources with regard to chronic medical illness and stress among child and adolescent patients?

A: The following are just a few Web sites that can help children and adolescents adjust to medical diagnoses and/or hospitalizations:

- The National Child Traumatic Stress Network (NCTSN) has a section devoted to medical trauma, including a Pediatric Medical Traumatic Stress Toolkit for health care providers and educational material for parents (http://www.nctsn.org/)
- The Health Care Toolbox, sponsored by NCTSN and the Children's Hospital of Philadelphia, provides tools, resources, and educational materials for parents and clinicians to help children and families cope with illness and injury (http://www.healthcaretoolbox.org/)
- The Experience Journal, sponsored by Children's Hospital Boston, provides opportunities for patients and families to read about or share their own stories, pictures, and personal experiences with illness (http://www.experiencejournal.com/)
- The National Center for School Crisis and Bereavement, sponsored by Cincinnati Children's Hospital Medical Center, provides guidance for parents and children's schools to understand and meet the needs of their children and families in times of crisis and loss (http://www.cincinnatichildrens.org/service/n/school-crisis/default/).

Thought-provoking questions: Should one treat a child who is depressed with an SSRI even if there is a direct link to a stressor (eg, having cancer and being in the hospital for a month)? How would the child interpret this approach if you are giving her a medication to treat a depression that she clearly links to a particular stressor?

SAMANTHA
Approach and Treatment: SSRIs, Psychotherapy, and Collaboration

Case: Samantha is a 16-year-old Asian female who presented to her pediatrician with a chief complaint of depression. A diagnosis of major depressive disorder was made, and her pediatrician recommended to her parents that she start on an SSRI. However, her parents refused the SSRI because when they went on the Internet, they read about the black box warning and were concerned that she might become suicidal.

Teaching Points

When approaching parents about treating depression, not all parents will respond in the same way. The responses may be influenced by the parents' past/current experience(s) with treatment, prior knowledge (whether correct or not) about the treatment, cultural background, or therapeutic relationship with the clinician. Past negative or positive experiences, whether indirect or direct, with treatments can lead to strong opinions for or against a particular treatment. For example, a father with major depression that responded quite well to an antidepressant may request that his son start one even if it was not clearly indicated. Regardless of the influence and its direction, it is often helpful to elicit the opinion of the parents before making any firm recommendation. This approach will provide the opportunity to address concerns, questions, or acquired misinformation. It may strengthen the therapeutic relationship, or at least prevent it from worsening.

Samantha's parents were immediately frustrated with the pediatrician's recommendation of the SSRI, but they kept this frustration to themselves. They were always concerned with physicians overprescribing medications, which is why they refused to have Samantha seen by a psychiatrist. They were more frustrated that the pediatrician neither asked for their opinion nor communicated with Samantha's therapist before making such a recommendation.

In 2004, the US Food and Drug Administration (FDA) came out with a black box warning for all antidepressants secondarily to an increase in suicidal thoughts and behaviors (for those who are under 25 years old). This warning was based on the finding that there was a 2% (4% vs 2% on placebo) increase in reporting of suicidal thoughts or potentially dangerous behaviors among those on antidepressants. According to Brent and colleagues,[14] across all the reviewed studies of pediatric depression, the risk of a suicidal event (ie, increased suicidal ideation, planning, or making an attempt) was approximately 1% greater in those on antidepressants than a placebo. No suicides occurred in any of these studies. Additionally, more recent studies including epidemiologic and metaanalyses indicate that the benefits of using an SSRI to treat children and adolescents with a major depressive disorder outweigh the risks.[49–54] Recommendations remain for the careful monitoring of suicidal symptoms when starting an antidepressant (ie, weekly follow-up for the first 6 weeks).

In a time-sensitive appointment, a clinician, such as Samantha's, may feel pressured into making a quick diagnosis of depression and initiate treatment with an antidepressant, even when a more careful assessment (like Ella's) would not have substantiated it. Additionally, time pressures may compromise adequately educating patients and parents on the risks, benefits, and alternatives of treatments for depression, including the black box warning, and addressing other potential concerns or questions. Not doing so makes informed consent impossible and may compromise the relationship, impairing treatment adherence. Solutions include setting up an additional appointment or making a referral to a mental health clinician who does have the time to have these important discussions and is able to provide adequate follow-up. As mentioned earlier, the GLAD-PC toolkit provides tools to aid in carrying out such education efficiently. Also, the AACAP and American Psychiatric Association, in consultation with the National Coalition of Concerned Parents, Providers, and Professional Associations, created a useful handout for patients and parents on the use of medication in treating child and adolescent depression, including information on the black box warning (http://www.parentsmedguide.org/pmg_depression.html).

Samantha's pediatrician agreed to set up a follow-up appointment in 2 weeks to provide a more thorough discussion of treatment alternatives including the use of SSRIs. It also provided him time to have a discussion with Samantha's therapist, which revealed that Samantha met criteria for mild major depression and was actually showing improvement with cognitive behavior therapy (CBT). Together they agreed that it was not essential to start an SSRI at this point in time. The pediatrician also learned that Samantha's parents were very hesitant about returning to their pediatrician for fear of Samantha being started on a medication.

CBT and interpersonal therapy (IPT) have well-established efficacy for the treatment of child and adolescent depression.[55,56] CBT is the most widely researched psychotherapeutic approach for treating depression in adolescents. It is a time-limited treatment that focuses on the relationship between how the individual thinks about the world, themselves, and the future. It is based on the belief that there is a close interrelationship between thoughts, emotions, and the body and behaviors, and that depression can be relieved by altering patterns of thinking and behavior as well as by calming the body. Common elements of CBT include mood monitoring, relaxation training, behavioral activation, cognitive restructuring, stress management, emotion regulation, distress tolerance, social skills, conflict resolution, and general problem-solving skills.[14] IPT is a time-limited treatment that approaches depression as a medical illness caused and influenced by life situations, usually a disturbing change in one's interpersonal environment, a struggle with a significant other, or some other life upheaval.[57] The task of IPT is to develop means to resolve these life situations, including improving one's interpersonal skills.

Although it may be time-consuming to obtain collateral information, ultimately it often saves time and improves care by leading to a more accurate assessment and diagnosis and subsequently a more appropriate treatment. It may help guide treatment and prevent premature initiation of a medication as with Samantha. Finally, it may provide an additional set of eyes with monitoring for improvements or worsening of symptoms.

Q&A

Q: Are there available resources on enhancing collaboration between mental health clinicians and primary care clinicians?

A: Systemically, there is a need for improved working relationships between mental health and primary care clinicians, which would include effective collaboration, communication, and coordination. Useful information on how to promote this relationship includes the following:

- AACAP's Committee on Collaboration with Medical Professionals' Guide to Building Collaborative Mental Health Care Partnerships in Pediatric Primary Care[58]
- The US Department of Health and Human Services' Strategies to Support the Integration of Mental Health into Pediatric Primary Care[59]
- American Academy of Pediatrics' Web site section Children's Mental Health in Primary Care (http://www.aap.org/commpeds/dochs/mentalhealth/).

Q: Are there resources to assist with cultural competency with regard to approach to children and adolescents with depression?

A: Please consider the following:

- The Child and Adolescent Psychiatric Clinics of North America's October 2010 edition is devoted to cultural issues in pediatric mental health.
- The American Psychiatric Association's Web site has a diversity curriculum section (http://www.psych.org/Share/OMNA/Minority-Council.aspx) that offers a few useful resources, including the following:
  ○ Diversity and cultural competency curriculum.
  ○ A 4-year model curriculum on culture, gender, LGBT (lesbian, gay, bisexual, and transgender), religion, and spirituality.
- The GLAD-PC toolkit provides a list of helpful Web sites including a site maintained by the New York City Department of Mental Health and Hygiene that provides links to a number of cultural competency resources (http://www.nyc. gov/html/doh/downloads/pdf/qi/qi-ccpriority-resources.pdf).

DENNIS
Treatment

Case: Dennis is a 16-year-old African American male who presented to his pediatrician with depression. His mother expressed concern and was hoping that Dennis could get treatment. Although the pediatrician did agree with the diagnosis of major depression, he preferred that a child and adolescent psychiatrist be the one to start him on an antidepressant. He explained this preference to the family, and he gave them the number of the intake office for the outpatient psychiatry clinic associated with his practice. A couple of weeks later, Dennis's pediatrician received a phone call from an inpatient psychiatrist informing him that Dennis was just hospitalized for attempting suicide. After the initial appointment, Dennis's mother did call the intake office but unfortunately was only able to get an appointment with a psychiatrist that was 6 weeks out.

Teaching Points

"Despite recent progress in identifying and treating children's and adolescents' mental disorders, epidemiologic studies indicate that only 20% to 35% of youth who meet full criteria for depression currently receive treatment," Stein and colleagues.[4] Barriers to treatment include stigma around mental health/treatment, lack of access to mental health clinicians (especially child and adolescent psychiatrists), insurance coverage, and primary care clinicians not feeling comfortable or responsible for treating depression. Unfortunately, although many pediatricians feel undertrained, it is a critical responsibility of the primary care clinician to appropriately identify and manage depression and suicidal ideation, particularly in those contexts in which access to a psychiatrist or another mental health clinician is limited. Given the prevalence of depression (8% of teens annually) and its impact (see discussion elsewhere in this issue), this role should be a training priority for all those who plan to work with child and adolescent patients.

Stein and colleagues[4] conducted a systematic review revealing a need for further studies on the benefits of treating adolescent depression in primary care settings and were able to identify four studies directly examining the effectiveness of primary care physicians or members of their staff in the recognition and treatment of depression in 10- to 18-year-olds. Each study had positive findings and together provided some evidence for direct efficacy of psychosocial interventions for depression management delivered in primary care.

The GLAD-PC and its accompanied toolkit were designed to make primary care clinicians more comfortable with treating and managing adolescents with depression. It fosters active monitoring (eg, providing patients and families with educational materials, recommending a peer support group, or prescribing regular exercise) and brief effective counseling (eg, empathizing with them while helping formulate clear, simple, and specific behavioral change plans). Collaborating with depressed adolescents and their families can provide the critical care and problem-solving skills they so often may be struggling with.

If Dennis's depression were more than just a mild depressive episode and his pediatrician were to start him on an antidepressant, fluoxetine would be the recommended first-choice SSRI, provided there were no contraindications (eg, drug-drug interaction). Fluoxetine and escitalopram are the only antidepressants FDA approved for use in adolescents, whereas fluoxetine is the only antidepressant approved for children (age 8). Fluoxetine has the highest number of successful trials and is advantageous because it has the longest half-life of all SSRIs, reducing the adverse withdrawal effects of poor adherence. Although not specifically FDA-approved, it is common practice to consider other SSRIs, such as sertraline, if Dennis's mother was clear that she or another immediate family member of Dennis's responded adversely to fluoxetine and/or did very well on sertraline. The GLAD-PC toolkit provides dosing and monitoring guidelines along with handouts for parents and adolescents. More specific details are available elsewhere in this issue.

Generally, a combination of medication and psychotherapy (ie, IPT or CBT) is recommended for moderate to severe depressions because the acute response, remission, and relapse rates are the best with combined care, especially for the chronic, recurrent, or severely depressed.[14,52,60] However, the use of pharmacotherapy, psychotherapy, or both may vary based on the patient and family's preference

---

Box 7
Reasons for treatment failure

- Lack of adherence to treatment
- Misdiagnosis
- Unrecognized or untreated comorbid psychiatric or medical disorders
- Undetected bipolar disorder
- Inappropriate pharmacotherapy or psychotherapy
- Inadequate length of treatment or dose
- Medication side effects
- Exposure to chronic or severe life events
- Personal identity issues
- Cultural/ethnic factors
- Inadequate fit with, or skill level of, the psychotherapist

Data from Birmaher B, Brent D; AACAP Work Group on Quality Issues, et al. Practice parameters for the assessment and treatment of children and adolescents with depressive disorders. J Am Acad Child Adolesc Psychiatry 2007;46(11):1503–26.

---

along with access to mental health clinicians. Whereas some depressions may be treatment-resistant even with optimal evidence-based treatment, others fail for remediable reasons; a list of which appears in **Box 7**.

Dennis noted that he was suicidal at the time of the appointment with his pediatrician but did not disclose this condition because he was not specifically asked about it. It is crucial that clinicians screen for suicidal ideation along with depression. Whereas prior attempts, self-injurious behaviors, substance abuse, and guns in the home all are known to increase the rates of completed suicide, there is a wider range of other known risk (**Box 8**) and protective factors (**Box 9**) that all clinicians and parents should be familiar with. Inquiry into each area and the careful weighing of the responses are critical for safety assessment. On the most pragmatic level, clinicians and families have to know why a child was suicidal and why they no longer are suicidal to proceed safely. Anything less, including "safety contracts," is not sufficient. Educating families and decreasing risk by removing guns and controlling access to medication (eg, Tylenol ingestion is common for females and families are unaware of its potential lethality) should be part of every treatment plan. Brent and colleagues[14] provide a thorough discussion on assessing suicidal ideation and behavior along with safety planning.

Q&A

Q: Are there additional resources one can provide families or trainees?

A: The usefulness of resources (eg, handouts, books, or Web sites) varies on the educational level, motivation, agenda, and learning style of the individual. Such resources do not serve as alternatives to one-on-one education provided by their clinician. As mentioned earlier, the GLAD-PC toolkit provides helpful educational material for both adolescents and parents. Potentially informative Web sites with resources and recommendations of their own include the following:

Box 8
Risk factors for child and adolescent suicide

Biological

- Mental illness, including mood disorders, psychotic disorders, substance use disorders, and disruptive behavior disorders
- Parental psychopathologic condition
- Chronic medical conditions
- Females (suicide attempts) and males (completed suicide)

Psychological

- Prior suicide attempts
- Childhood adversities/trauma
- Impulsivity
- Self-injurious behaviors (all), particularly ones that warrant medical attention and in locations such as head, neck, and genital areas
- Sexual orientation conflicts
- Impaired thinking or judgment
- Risk-taking behaviors
- Hopelessness
- Negative thinking pattern

Social

- Family or friend who completed suicide
- Contagion behavior (locally or through the media)
- Bullying
- Family distress and dysfunction
- Poor family communication and lower parental monitoring
- Difficulties in school or even just perception that their academic performance is poor, which is independent of intelligence
- Incarceration
- Shameful event
- Access (eg, guns and lethal medication)
- No significant other (ie, no trusted friend or confidante)

Data from Refs.[14,35,38,61–68]

- AACAP – Depression Resource Center (http://www.aacap.org/cs/Depression.ResourceCenter).
- Columbia University's TeenScreen Program (http://www.teenscreen.org/).
- National Institute of Mental Health (http://www.nimh.nih.gov/index.shtml).
- Families for Depression Awareness (http://familyaware.org/).
- National Alliance on Mental Illness Child & Adolescent Action Center (http://www.nami.org/template.cfm?section=child_and_teen_support).
- American Foundation for Suicide Prevention (http://www.afsp.org/).

> **Box 9**
> **Protective factors with regard to child and adolescent stressors and suicide**
>
> - Self-esteem and confidence
> - Self-efficacy
> - Effortful approaches to challenges (eg, taking direction, seeking support) as opposed to automatic approaches to challenges (eg, impulsive, aggressive, or destructive action); similar to engaged and problem-focused coping
> - Family support, adaptability, and communication
> - Future-oriented thinking
> - Sense of family cohesion
> - Positive family relationship
> - School connectedness
> - Hopefulness
> - Religion or spirituality
> - Healthy peer support
>
> *Data from* Refs.[11,66,67]

- Another resource where clinicians can learn about pertinent pediatric topics, including depression, on their own with regard to using case-based modules can be found at http://www.pedicases.org/, which was developed by Bright Futures Center for Pediatric Education at Children's Hospital Boston.

Q: Are there quick suicidal screens one can use in a primary care setting?

A: Columbia Suicidal Severity Rating Scale. The Risk of Suicide Questionnaire is brief and consists of four questions[69]:

- Are you here because you tried to hurt yourself?
- In the past week, have you been having thoughts about killing yourself?
- Have you ever tried to hurt yourself in the past other than this time?
- Has something very stressful happened to you in the past few weeks?

Thought-provoking question: If your patient was actively suicidal and in your office, how would you proceed?

HELEN
Understanding: Biological, Psychological, Social, and Developmental Perspective

Case: Helen is a 10-year-old white female with irritability and has been in and out of foster care placements since she was 4 for severe neglect by her parents and concerns for physical and sexual abuse. She was referred to a child and adolescent psychiatrist because her foster parents are concerned that she has depression and possibly bipolar disorder.

Teaching Points

As children grow they develop fundamental building blocks that will continuously influence their lives across all aspects (ie, personal, social, academic, extracurricular, and occupational). These building blocks develop at different rates and influence one another and include self-regulation, self-identity, self-esteem, and self-efficacy. Their healthy development will promote resiliency against stressors, trauma, and depression. Promoting their development is influenced by relationships from birth on (eg, parental attachment, affective attunement, sensitivity, and responsiveness), environment (eg, secure and stimulating), validation (ie, being able to be who you are and being accepted and loved regardless), and accomplishments.[26,70] Things that interfere with such development (eg, severe adversity, trauma, or parental psychopathology) reduce resiliency and predispose children to developing depression. Schmid and colleagues[71] used longitudinal evidence to show that less maternal stimulation during mother-infant interaction at age 3 months predicted a higher rate of depression and more depressive symptoms in their offspring 19 years later. This study was based on the normal variation of maternal interaction with her child and did not represent extremes such as with Helen.

Many patients who have experienced severe trauma (ie, neglect, sexual, emotional, and physical abuse) get diagnosed with multiple psychiatric diagnoses, including anxiety, mood, or behavioral disorders, and end up being treated with multiple psychopharmacologic agents. A recent metaanalysis suggested that childhood maltreatment was associated with an elevated risk of developing recurrent and persistent depressive episodes in addition to a lack of response or remission during treatment for depression.[72] The complex origins and diverse presentations of the depressive disorders make a thorough understanding of the patient from a biological, psychological, social, and developmental perspective imperative to best guide treatment and prevent unnecessary interventions (eg, a patient is on multiple psychotropic medications because they are available but would likely benefit far more from structure, security, and stability at home along with trauma-informed child-parent psychotherapy—and with fewer side effects).

Helen presented with irritability, and her foster caregivers were concerned with depression and bipolar disorder. As Leibenluft[73] wrote, "Irritability is a common, yet relatively understudied, symptom in pediatric psychopathology." Lack of understanding about irritability has led to controversial diagnosing of bipolar disorder and questionable use of antipsychotic medication. Growing data from longitudinal and pathophysiologic studies indicate that *nonepisodic irritability* is associated with an increased risk for anxiety and unipolar depressive disorders, but not bipolar disorder in adulthood.[73] Those with nonepisodic irritability also differ pathophysiologically from those with bipolar disorder. Understanding the underlying contributory factors and the differential diagnosis of irritability becomes a critical skill and is reviewed in **Box 10**.

Helen's irritability may very well be attributable to both depression and trauma concomitant to the interrupted or altered development of self (-regulation, -identity, -esteem, and -efficacy). Studies are establishing a clearer relationship between trauma, depression, and suicide and are even being described at the neurophysiologic level. Epigenetic studies, including Patrick McGowan's[74] and Michael Meaney's[74,75] work on rats and humans, continue to highlight the important relationship between genes and environment. A more detailed review is discussed elsewhere in this issue.

Although Helen may not currently meet criteria for major depression, she is still at risk particularly because she has not hit puberty. It has become clearer that the onset of puberty and continuation through adolescence raises the risk for the development of depression.[9,76,77] The increased risk of depression associated with puberty is related to biological, psychological, and social factors. Multiple changes are occurring with the brain, entire body, hormones, cognition, emotions, and behaviors.

Box 10
Understanding and diagnosing irritability

- Complete psychiatric review of systems, including evaluation for disruptive behavior disorders (eg, attention-deficit/hyperactivity disorder and oppositional defiant disorder), mood disorders (eg, severe mood dysregulation vs classic symptoms of manic episode), developmental disorders (eg, autism spectrum disorders), and anxiety disorders (eg, generalized anxiety disorder and posttraumatic stress disorder)

- When did it start, and is it getting better, the same, or worse?

- Stress and trauma history

- Parental psychopathology

- Episodic versus nonepisodic irritability

- Triggers, precipitants, and alleviating factors of irritability

- Is the irritability present in all environments?

- Severity of irritability, including duration, influence on function, and damage related to irritability (eg, breaking objects, punching walls, or hurting self or others)

- What are the parenting approach and style and are they consistent?

- What are the home and school environments like (eg, structure)?

- Collateral information representing different domains of patient's life (eg, school and peers) or if possible, observe patient in different environments (eg, in office, waiting room, or even school)

Psychosocially, there may be more difficult transitions (eg, entering high school), more intense stressors (eg, bullying), more complex behaviors (eg, dating and sexual activity), worsened attachments (eg, supports moving from parents to peers, and increasing conflicts with both), greater mismatch between increased emotional reactivity and limited coping skills, and increased self-blame.[9,76] Clearly, Helen is at increased risk for developing depression with her history of trauma, less than optimally developed self, and her potentially altered neurophysiology. Unfortunately, her continued dysregulation will likely lead to social and academic failure, thereby further worsening her self-identity, self-esteem, and self-efficacy, and placing her at further risk for a mental health issue. Negative cognitions, including low self-esteem, self-control, and self-efficacy consistently have been found to be associated with depression.[9]

Fortunately, as for Helen, her pediatrician was aware of a clinic that was devoted to children with traumatic histories and worked with foster care parents using child-parent psychotherapy. Through collaboration between Helen's foster care parents, pediatrician, child-parent psychotherapist, child and adolescent psychiatrist, and school, Helen's irritability slowly improved as she got back on appropriate tracks of development.

Q&A

Q: What are some resources for children or adolescents exposed to adversity, including trauma?

A: Please consider the following:

- The National Child Traumatic Stress Network (NCTSN) is a useful resource, not just for medical trauma but all forms of trauma (http://www.nctsnet.org/).

- The Center on the Developing Child provides useful information on how "toxic stress" can derail healthy development (http://developingchild.harvard.edu/).
- For children who have lost someone in their immediate family there are grief centers throughout the country that help children grieve at their own pace. You may find one closest to you through The Dougy Center, The National Center for Grieving Children and Families (http://www.dougy.org/).

Thought-provoking questions: If the cause of depression is not clearly biological, then why are we so surprised when the efficacy studies of SSRIs are not as impressive as we would like? What are the long-term effects of altering serotonin in a developing brain?

SUMMARY

Depression is a common and highly treatable illness that affects upwards of 20% of the population, with the majority of cases beginning in childhood or adolescence. This incidence makes developing functional competence in the identification, understanding, and intervention strategies with the depressive disorder a vital component for every practitioner working with pediatric populations. Using clinical vignettes, up-to-date research, and expert opinion along with guidelines, resources, and tools, the authors have provided a basic, self-contained toolbox for educators and clinicians alike.

REFERENCES

1. Gardner W, Kelleher KJ, Pajer KA, et al. Primary care clinicians' use of standardized psychiatric diagnoses. Child Care Health Dev 2004;30(5):401–12.
2. Lewy C, Sells W, Gilhooly J, et al. Adolescent depression: evaluating pediatric resident's knowledge, confidence, and interpersonal skills using standardized patients. Acad Psychiatry 2009;33(5):389–93.
3. Sarvet BD, Wegner L. Developing effective child psychiatry collaboration with primary care: leadership and management strategies. Child Adolesc Psychiatric Clin N Am 2010;19:139–48.
4. Stein RK, Zitner LE, Jensen P. Interventions for adolescent depression in primary care. Pediatrics 2006;118(2):669–82.
5. Sudak D, Roy A, Sudak H, et al. Deficiencies in suicide training in primary care specialties: a survey of training directors. Acad Psychiatry 2007;31(5):345–9.
6. Zuckerbrot RA, Cheun AH, Jensen PS, et al. Guidelines for adolescent depression in primary care (GLAD-PC): I. Identification, assessment, and initial management. Pediatrics 2007;120:e1299–312.
7. American Academy of Child and Adolescent Psychiatry Committee on Health Care Access and Economics Task Force on Mental Health. Improving mental health services in primary care: reducing administrative and financial barriers to access and collaboration. Pediatrics 2009;123(4):1248–51.
8. Birmaher B, Brent D, AACAP Work Group on Quality Issues, et al. Practice parameters for the assessment and treatment of children and adolescents with depressive disorders. J Am Acad Child Adolesc Psychiatry 2007;46(11):1503–26.
9. Rao U, Chen LA. Characteristics, correlates, and outcomes of childhood and adolescent depressive disorders. Dialogues Clin Neurosci 2009;11(1):45–62.
10. Shanahan L, Copeland WE, Costello EJ, et al. Child-, adolescent- and young adult-onset depression: differential risk factors in development? Psychol Med 2011; 41(11):2265–74.

11. Shaw RJ, DeMaso DR. Textbook of pediatric psychosomatic medicine. Arlington (VA): American Psychiatric Publishing, Inc; 2010.
12. Cheung AH, Zickerbrot RA, Jensen PS, et al. Guidelines for adolescent depression in primary care (GLAD-PC): II. Treatment and ongoing management. Pediatrics 2007; 120:e1313–26.
13. US Department of Health and Human Services, Agency for Healthcare Research and Quality, US Preventive Services Task Force. Screening and treatment for major depressive disorder in children and adolescents: recommendation statement, March 2009. Available at: http://www.ahrq.gov/clinic/uspstf09/depression/chdeprrs.htm. Accessed October 1, 2011.
14. Brent DA, Poling KD, Goldstein TR. Treating depressed and suicidal adolescents. New York: The Guilford Press; 2010.
15. American Psychiatric Association. Diagnostic and Statistical Manual of Mental Disorders. 4th edition. Washington, DC: American Psychiatric Association; 1994.
16. Pinquart M, Shen Y. Depressive symptoms in children and adolescents with chronic physical illness: an updated meta-analysis. J Pediatr Psychol 2011;36(4):375–84.
17. Manepalli J, Thaipisuttikul P, Yarnal R. Identifying and treating depression across the life span. Current Psychiatry 2011;10(6):20–4.
18. Beardslee WR, Versage EM, Gladston TR. Children of affectively ill parents: a review of the past 10 years. J Am Acad Child Adolesc Psychiatry 1998;37:1134–41.
19. Goodman S, Gotlib I. Risk for psychopathology in the children of depressed mothers: A developmental model for understanding mechanisms of transmission. Psychol Rev 1999;106:458–90.
20. Goodman S, Gotlib I. Children of depressed parents – mechanisms of risk and implications for treatment. Washington, DC: American Psychological Association Press; 2002.
21. Luking KR, Repovs G, Belden AC, et al. Functional connectivity of the amygdala in early-childhood-onset depression. J Am Acad Child Adolesc Psychiatry 2011;50(10): 1027–41.
22. Murray L, Arteche A, Fearon P, et al. Maternal postnatal depression and the development of depression in offspring up to 16 years of age. J Am Acad Child Adolesc Psychiatry 2011;50(5):460–70.
23. Weissman MM, Wickramaratne P, Nomura Y, et al. Offspring of depressed parents: 20 years later. Am J Psychiatry 2006;163:1001–8.
24. Weissman MM, Pilowsky DJ, Wickramaratne PJ, et al. Remissions in maternal depression and child psychopathology: a STAR*D-child report. JAMA 2006;295: 1389–98.
25. Gunlicks ML, Weissman MM. Change in child psychopathology with improvement in parental depression: a systemic review. J Am Acad Child Adolesc Psychiatry 2008; 47(4):379–89.
26. National Research Council and Institute of Medicine. Preventing mental, emotional, and behavioral disorders among young people – progress and possibilities. Washington, DC: National Academy Press; 2009.
27. Beardslee WR, Gladstone TR, Wright EJ, et al. A family-based approach to the prevention of depressive symptoms in children at risk: evidence of parental and child change. Pediatrics 2003;112(2):e119–31.
28. Podorefsky DL, McDonald-Dowdell M, Beardslee W. Adaptation of preventive interventions for a low-income, culturally diverse community. J Am Acad Child Adolesc Psychiatry 2001;40(8):879–86.

29. D'Angelo EJ, Llerena-Quinn R, Shapiro R, et al. Adaptation of the preventive intervention program for depression for use with predominantly low-income Latino families. Fam Process 2009;48:269–91.

30. Solantaus T, Paavonen EJ, Toikka S, et al. Preventive interventions in families with parental depression: children's psychosocial symptoms and prosocial behavior. Eur Child Adolesc Psychiatry 2010;19:883–92.

31. Kearney CA. School absenteeism and school refusal behavior in youth: a contemporary review. Clin Psychol Rev 2008;28:451–71.

32. Trivedi HK, Kershner JD. Practical child and adolescent psychiatry for pediatrics and primary care. Cambridge (MA): Hogrefe & Huber Publishers; 2009.

33. Wang J, Iannotti RJ, Nansel TR. School bullying among adolescents in the United States: Physical, verbal, relational, and cyber. J Adolesc Health 2009;45(4):368–75.

34. Eaton DK, Kann, L, Kinchen S, et al. Youth risk behavior surveillance – United States, 2009. Surveill Summ 2010;59:1–142.

35. Klomek AB, Sourander A, Gould M. The association of suicide and bullying in childhood to young adulthood: a review of cross-sectional and longitudinal research findings. Can J Psychiatry 2010;55(5):282–8.

36. McMahon EM, Reulbacha U, Keeley H, et al. Bullying victimisation, self harm and associated factors in Irish adolescent boys. Soc Sci Med 2010;71(7):1300–7.

37. Frankowski, BL. Sexual orientation and adolescents. Pediatrics 2004;113:1827–32.

38. Kitts RL. Gay adolescents and suicide - understanding the association. Adolescence 2005;40:621–8.

39. Zhao Y, Montoro R, Igartua K, et al. Suicidal ideation and attempt among adolescents reporting "unsure" sexual identity or heterosexual identity plus same-sex attraction or behavior: forgotten groups? J Am Acad Child Adolesc Psychiatry 2010;49(2):104–13.

40. Coker TR, Austin SB, Schuster MA. The health and health care of lesbian, gay, and bisexual adolescents. Annu Rev Public Health 2010;31:457–77.

41. Kitts RL. Barriers to optimal care between physicians and lesbian, gay, bisexual, transgender, and questioning adolescent patients. J Homosex 2010;57(6):730–47.

42. Bowes L, Maughan B, Caspi A, et al. Families promote emotional and behavioural resilience to bullying: evidence of an environmental effect. J Child Psychol Psychiatry 2010;51(7):809–17.

43. Truong J, Jain S, Tan J, et al. Young children's perceptions of physicians wearing standard precautions versus customary attire. Pediatr Emerg Care 2006;22(1):13–7.

44. Drotar D. Physician behavior in the care of pediatric chronic illness: association with health outcomes and treatment adherence. J Dev Behav Pediatr 2009;30:246–54.

45. Stivers T. Physician-child interactions: when children answer physicians' questions in routine medical encounters. Patient Educ Couns 2011. [Epub ahead of print].

46. Fritsch SL, Overton MW, Douglas RR. The interface of child mental health and juvenile diabetes. Child Adolesc Psychiatric Clin N Am 2010;19:335–52.

47. Angell M. Industry-sponsored clinical research: a broken system. JAMA 2008;300(9):1069–71.

48. DeAngelis CD, Fontanarosa PB. Impugning the integrity of medical science – the adverse effects of industry influence. JAMA 2008;299(15):1833–5.

49. Bridge JA, Ivengar S, Salary CB, et al. Clinical response and risk for reported suicidal ideation and suicide attempts in pediatric antidepressant treatment: a meta-analysis of randomized controlled trials. JAMA 2007;297(15):1683–96.

50. Gibbons RD, Hur K, Bhaumik DK, et al. The relationship between antidepressant prescription rates and rate of early adolescent suicide. Am J Psychiatry 2006;163(11):1898–904.

51. Gibbons RD, Brown CH, Hur K, et al. Early evidence on the effects of regulators' suicidality warnings on SSRI prescriptions and suicide in children and adolescents. Am J Psychiatry 2007;164:1356–63.

52. March JS, Vitiello BB. Clinical message from the treatment for adolescents with depression study (TADS). Am J Psychiatry 2009;166(10):1118–23.

53. Meyer RE, Salzman C, Youngstrom EA, et al. Suicidality and risk of suicide—definition, drug safety concerns, and a necessary target for drug development: a brief report. J Clin Psychiatry 2010;71(8):1040–6.

54. Nakagawa A, Grunebaum MF, Ellis SP, et al. Association of suicide and antidepressant prescription rates in Japan, 1999–2003. J Clin Psychiatry 2007;68(6):908–16.

55. David-Ferdon C, Kaslow NJ. Evidence-based psychosocial treatments for child and adolescent depression. J Clin Child Adolesc Psychol 2008;37(1):62–104.

56. Spirito A, Esposito-Smythers C, Wolf J, et al. Cognitive-behavioral therapy for adolescent depression and suicidality. Child Adolesc Psychiatr Clin N Am 2011;20:191–204.

57. Markowitz JC, Weissman MM. Interpersonal psychotherapy: principles and applications. World Psychiatry 2004;3(3):136–9.

58. American Academy of Child and Adolescent Psychiatry's Committee on Collaboration with Medical Professionals. Guide to building collaborative mental health care partnerships in pediatric primary care, June 2010. Available at: http://www.aacap.org/cs/systems_of_care_and_collaborative_models/collaboration_with_primary_care. Accessed October 1, 2011.

59. The United States Department of Health and Human Services. Strategies to support the integration of mental health into pediatric primary care, August 2009. Available at: http://nihcm.org/pdf/PediatricMH-FINAL.pdf. Accessed October 1, 2011.

60. March JS, Silva S, Curry J, et al. The treatment for adolescents with depression study (TADS): outcomes over 1 year of naturalistic follow-up. Am J Psychiatry 2009;166(10):1141–9.

61. Bearman PS, Moody J. Suicide and friendships among American adolescents. Am J Public Health 2004;94:89–95.

62. Bridge JA, Goldstein TR, Brent DA. Adolescent suicide and suicidal behavior. J Child Psychol Psychiatry 2006;47(3–4):372–94.

63. Brodsky BS, Mann JJ, Stanley B, et al. Familial transmission of suicidal behavior: factors mediating the relationship between childhood abuse and offspring suicide attempts. J Clin Psychiatry 2008;69(4):584–96.

64. Burke AK, Galfalvy H, Everett B, et al. Effect of exposure to suicidal behavior in a high risk sample of offspring of depressed parents. J Am Acad Child Adolesc Psychiatry 2010;49(2):114–21.

65. Fleischmann A, Bertolote JM, Belfer M, et al. Completed suicide and psychiatric diagnoses in young people: a critical examination of the evidence. Am J Orthopsychiatry 2005;75(4):676–83.

66. Steele MM, Doey T. Suicidal behavior in children and adolescents. Part I: etiology and risk factors. Can J Psychiatry 2007;52(1):21–33.

67. Walsh E, Eggert LL. Suicide risk and protective factors among youth experiencing school difficulties. Int J Ment Health Nurs 2007;16:349–59.

68. Whitlock J, Knox KL. The relationship between self-injurious behavior and suicide in a young adult population. Arch Pediatr Adolesc Med 2007;161(7):634–40.

69. Horowitz LM, Ballard ED, Pao M. Suicide screening in schools, primary care and emergency departments. Curr Opin Pediatr 2009;21(5):620–7.

70. National Research Council and Institute of Medicine. From neurons to neighborhoods – the science of early childhood development. Washington, DC: National Academy Press; 2000.

71. Schmid BS, Blomeyer D, Buchmann AF, et al. Quality of early mother-child interaction associated with depressive psychopathology in the offspring: a prospective study from infancy to adulthood. J Psychiatr Res 2011;45:1387–94.

72. Nanni V, Uher R, Danese A. Childhood maltreatment predicts unfavorable course of illness and treatment outcome in depression: a meta-analysis. Am J Psychiatry 2011;AiA:1–11.

73. Leibenluft E. Severe mood dysregulation, irritability, and the diagnostic boundaries of bipolar disorder in youths. Am J Psychiatry 2011;168:129–42.

74. McGowan PO, Sasaki A, Alessio AC, et al. Epigenetic regulation of the glucocorticoid receptor in human brain associates with childhood abuse. Nat Neurosci 2009;12(3): 342–8.

75. Meaney MJ. Maternal care, gene expression, and the transmission of individual differences in stress reactivity across generations. Annu Rev Neurosci 2001;24: 1161–92.

76. Patton GC, Olsson C, Bond L, et al. Predicting female depression across puberty: a two-nation longitudinal study. J Am Acad Child Adolesc Psychiatry 2008;47(12): 1424–42.

77. Rao U, Hammen CL, Poland RE. Longitudinal course of adolescent depression: neuroendocrine and psychosocial predictors. J. Am. Acad. Child Adolesc. Psychiatry 2010;49(2):141–51.

Index

Note: Page numbers of article titles are in **boldface** type.

Printed and bound by CPI Group (UK) Ltd, Croydon, CR0 4YY

03/10/2024

01040456-0006